Kinesiology
for the
Occupational Therapy Assistant

Essential Components of Function and Movement

Kinesiology
for the
Occupational Therapy Assistant

Essential Components of Function and Movement

Jeremy L. Keough, MSOT, OTR/L
Life Care Centers of America
Maryville, Tennessee

Susan J. Sain, MS, OTR/L, FAOTA
Academic Fieldwork Coordinator
Roane State Community College
Harriman, Tennessee

Carolyn L. Roller, OTR/L
Supervisor of Occupational Therapy
Tennessee Orthopaedic Clinics
Knoxville, Tennessee

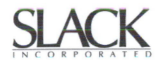

SLACK
INCORPORATED

Kinesiology for the Occupational Assistant: Essential Components of Function and Movement includes ancillary materials available for faculty use. Included are Test Bank Questions and PowerPoint slides. Please visit www.efacultylounge.com to obtain access.

Published by: SLACK Incorporated
                   6900 Grove Road
                   Thorofare, NJ 08086 USA
                   Telephone: 856-848-1000
                   Fax: 856-848-6091
                   www.slackbooks.com

Contact SLACK Incorporated for more information about other books in this field or about the availability of our books from distributors outside the United States.

Library of Congress Cataloging-in-Publication Data

Keough, Jeremy.
  Kinesiology for the occupational therapy assistant : essential components of function and movement / Jeremy Keough, Susan Sain, Carolyn Roller.
      p. ; cm.
  Includes bibliographical references and index.
   ISBN 978-1-55642-967-5 (pbk.)
 1. Occupational therapy. 2. Applied kinesiology. 3. Occupational therapy assistants. I. Sain, Susan. II. Roller, Carolyn. III. Title.
   [DNLM: 1. Occupational Therapy. 2. Kinesiology, Applied--methods. 3. Musculoskeletal Physiological Phenomena. WB 555]
   RM735.K46 2011
   615.8'515--dc23
                          2011012983

Printed in the United States of America.

Last digit is print number: 10 9 8 7 6 5 4 3 2 1

CONTENTS

Kinesiology for the Occupational Assistant: Essential Components of Function and Movement includes ancillary materials available for faculty use. Included are Test Bank Questions and PowerPoint slides. Please visit www.cfacultylounge.com to obtain access.

ACKNOWLEDGMENTS

We would like to thank the following people for their invaluable assistance with preparing this text.

We all wish to express sincere gratitude to the following:

- All of our patients, past and present, for helping us to become better therapists.
- All of our students over the past years, in the clinic and in the classroom, who have taught us so much.
- Our places of employment: Tennessee Orthopaedic Clinics (TOC), Life Care Centers of America, Roane State Community College, and Belmont University for the many opportunities experienced there.
- Jane Harrold Sorensen, mutual friend and mentor, for supporting our efforts and for graciously agreeing to write the foreword to this text.
- Each other; we began this text as coauthors and completed it as friends. We have learned much together!

Jeremy warmly thanks the following:
- Dr. Ruth Huebner for encouraging me to learn the art of writing.
- My wife, Lori, for her support in allowing me to complete this project.

Susan warmly thanks the following:
- My parents, the ultimate role models of all things important in life. My husband, Riley, for his enduring support and belief in me, and for providing balance in my life. My children, Daniel and Ericka, for their patience with me during the process of writing and for the use of their pictures in this text.
- Kathy Payne, Suzanne Peloquin, Jyothi Gupta, and Rene Padilla for their mentorship, including the suggestion and encouragement to write.

Carolyn warmly thanks the following:
- My coworkers for giving me the environment to grow as a therapist, educator, and author. I especially thank Angie Hartman, Robb Seahorn, and Alaina Cope.
- The doctors at TOC for teaching me and sharing their patients with me, especially Brantley Burns and John Harrison.
- Angie Hance, Lauren Foster, Tonya Turner, Jana DuCharme, and Alice Power, who particularly helped me complete this project.
- Lastly, but most importantly, my children, Laura, Sara, and Brad; my amazing grandchildren; my sisters, Margaret and Joy; my mother, Pauline; and my dear friend, Ruby. Thank you all for your love, support, inspiration, and advice.

Teresa warmly thanks the following:
- My students, whose thirst for knowledge compels me to engage in my own pursuit of understanding.
- My partner, whose support and love for learning makes all areas of life more complete.

ABOUT THE AUTHORS

Jeremy L. Keough, MSOT, OTR/L, is currently a staff occupational therapist for Life Care Centers of America. Jeremy earned his undergraduate degree in occupational therapy from Eastern Kentucky University and a post-professional master's degree from Belmont University. His professional experiences include long-term care, inpatient rehabilitation, outpatient rehabilitation, work hardening, acute care, and occupational therapy assistant (OTA) education. Jeremy served as the OTA Program Director at Roane State Community College and instructed the kinesiology course for 3 years. Currently, Jeremy's interests include neurorehabilitation approaches, occupation-based practice, functional movement, and volunteering for the National Board for Certification in Occupational Therapy.

Susan J. Sain, MS, OTR/L, FAOTA, is currently a faculty member and academic fieldwork coordinator at Roane State Community College in Tennessee. Susan earned her undergraduate degree in occupational therapy from the University of Wisconsin at Madison along with a degree in Spanish. She later earned a master's degree in health promotion/health education from the University of Tennessee at Knoxville. Her professional experiences include adult and child psychology, long-term care, pediatrics in a variety of settings, early intervention, and academia. Susan served as the Program Director of the OTA program at Roane State Community College for 11 years and has been the Academic Fieldwork Coordinator for 2 years. Susan has instructed the kinesiology course for more than 12 years. Susan has served in a variety of volunteer positions for state associations, AOTA, and NBCOT. Her current interests include international study opportunities for allied health science students and cultural diversity.

Carolyn L. Roller, OTR/L, is currently Supervisor of Occupational Therapy at Tennessee Orthopedic Clinics, PC, specializing in upper extremity rehabilitation. Carolyn earned her undergraduate degree in occupational therapy from the University of Wisconsin at Milwaukee. Her professional experiences include outpatient rehabilitation, home and job site analysis, ergonomic considerations in the wellness community, and OTA education. Carolyn was an adjunct faculty member at South College in Knoxville, TN, teaching kinesiology in the OTA program. Currently, Carolyn serves as guest lecturer and chairperson of the advisory board for the OTA program at Roane State Community College in Oak Ridge, TN. Her interests include student fieldwork education, hand rehabilitation and prevention of hand injuries in the wellness community.

CONTRIBUTING AUTHOR

Teresa Plummer, PhD, MSOT, OTR/L, ATP, is currently an assistant professor in the School of Occupational Therapy at Belmont University. Dr. Plummer graduated with her Bachelor of Science degree in occupational therapy from the Medical College of Virginia, her Master of Science degree in occupational therapy from Belmont University, and her Doctor of Philosophy degree in occupational therapy from Nova Southeastern University. Dr. Plummer is an assistive technology professional through the Rehabilitation Engineering and Assistive Technology Society of North America (RESNA). She has extensive clinical and teaching experience and is currently an assistant professor and primary professor for assistive technology courses at Belmont University's Entry Level Occupational Therapy Doctorate and Master's Program. Additionally, she is employed by Monroe Carrell Jr. Children's Hospital at Vanderbilt in the seating clinic.

Dr. Plummer's professional experiences include adult rehabilitation, seating, and positioning. Teresa has worked in the field of adult rehabilitation for more than 30 years. She has conducted workshops nationally and internationally in the areas of rehabilitation and assistive technology. Dr. Plummer's research interests include wheelchair assessment, empowerment, and vision and its relationship to posture and mobility.

FOREWORD

This textbook fills a significant gap in educational materials for occupational therapy assistant students. While there are many kinesiology textbooks, most of these have been written by or for physical therapy practitioners or from a strictly body-function point of view. Finally, occupational therapy assistant educators have a textbook that fully embraces occupational therapy tenets. Students can learn the ins and outs of kinesiology while also strengthening their understanding of clients, occupation, and the environment. The authors use the *Occupational Therapy Practice Framework: Domain and Process, 2nd Edition* (OTPF-2) throughout the text to keep students focused on the client and his or her ability to engage in occupations of choice. Movement is an important part of daily function, making knowledge of kinesiology critical to an occupational therapy practitioner's understanding of the client's ability to engage in occupations.

The authors' many years of experience as occupational therapy practitioners and occupational therapy assistant educators come through in every page of this textbook. Each author shares knowledge and insight from his or her own area of expertise and makes the subject of kinesiology understandable and relevant to occupational therapy. Students are given thorough explanations and are provided excellent learning activities to help them put kinesiology into context. The Gold Boxes, pictures, and tables highlight and clarify important concepts and make the study of kinesiology much less daunting for the student. Having a kinesiology book that includes goniometry, muscle testing, and connections to the OTPF-2 is ideal for students, instructors, and practitioners who want a convenient reference book. It provides a seamless integration of theory, fact, and practice. I am delighted to be able to recommend this book and wish it had been available when I was searching for textbooks for occupational therapy assistant students.

Jane Harrold Sorensen, OTR
Former OTA Program Director
South College
Knoxville, Tennessee

INTRODUCTION

The intent of this text is to enable the reader to identify the underlying components that make movement possible and to connect how kinesiology applies to the client. The reader will gain insight into the practice of occupational therapy through solving problems and developing questions needed to assist the client to achieve movement goals. Gross range of motion and manual muscle testing are also introduced to further enable skill development. This text will refer to those who receive occupational therapy services as clients, following the terminology of the *Occupational Therapy Practice Framework: Domain and Process, 2nd Edition*.

This text is divided into nine chapters to encourage learning of the study of movement. Chapter 1, Kinesiology: A Foundation in Occupational Therapy, summarizes kinesiology and how the study of movement applies in occupational therapy. Historical applications are referenced as well as current influences of kinesiology within the profession. The *Occupational Therapy Practice Framework: Domain and Process, 2nd Edition* is also introduced to help unify chapter organization throughout the text. Specifically, client factors and activity demands are discussed to build on the knowledge needed to identify movement in context.

Chapter 2, Human Body Functions and Structures Influencing Movement, identifies anatomical features that impact movement. Such body functions topics include skeletal and neuromuscular. Body structure information includes specific topics on muscles and joints. Body functions are presented prior to body structures in each chapter to build on the top-down approach used in this text. This also helps to maintain the focus on function.

Chapter 3, Factors Influencing Movement, and Chapter 4, Introducing Movement Demands, provide the basis for understanding movement. Information is provided to better understand how and why abnormal and normal movements occur. Factors are also identified that assist the reader in observing movement of interest to the occupational therapy assistant (OTA) during engagement in activity by the client.

Chapters 5 through 9 focus on the essential functions and movement of the trunk and neck, lower extremity, and upper extremity. Information is focused on specific areas relevant to the OTA with an overview of peripheral topics. Chapters 5 and 6 address the trunk and lower extremity first as a basis for support during movement and to allow the student to develop a system for assimilating information prior to progressing to the upper extremity. Chapters 7 through 9 focus on function of the upper extremity including topics on movement. Again, body functions are identified first followed by information related to body structures.

The text is presented in such a way as to encourage the reader to visualize how all the components of movement fit together and affect each other. Information is provided at the OTA level and in a sequence that enhances learning. The authors feel this approach will maximize learning and keep the reader from simply memorizing detailed bits of information that later prove difficult to remember and apply in the practice setting. We hope the reader will gain an understanding that movement is a complex symphony of all body systems working in harmony. More importantly, we hope the reader is able to perceive how movement enables or hinders function and engagement in daily activities and occupations.

UNIQUE FEATURES OF THIS KINESIOLOGY TEXT

Many features strengthen the uniqueness of this kinesiology text to provide an enhanced learning experience for the student and health care professional. Specifically, unique features of this text can be found in the following bullets. Of key interest is that this one comprehensive text should be the only text needed for an OTA kinesiology course. Numerous resources, manual muscle testing and range of muscle norms and procedures, and occupational profiles describing OT interventions are included. The authors believe that these unique features make this kinesiology text superior to other texts available on the market.

- Incorporates the *Occupational Therapy Practice Framework: Domain and Process, 2nd Edition.*
- Occupation/real life-based activities and questions at the end of each chapter.
- "Gold Boxes" with additional key information.
- Occupational profiles to present applications to occupational therapy.
- Implications of function across the lifespan.
- Written for the OTA student at the OTA level.
- Written by occupational therapy practitioners with more than 18 years of combined experience teaching kinesiology to OTA students.
- Answers the charge by the American Occupational Therapy Association (AOTA) Representative Assembly for upper extremity guidelines in education.
- Fills an anticipated need as AOTA moves toward creating a "model curricula" for basic sciences. Kinesiology is a hallmark in occupational therapy and can be traced back as a requirement for graduation from programs over the past century.
- Helps meet Accreditation Council for Occupational Therapy Education (ACOTE) Standards for OTA education.
- Changes and improves sequence of topics to enhance OTA learning.
- Enables range of motion and manual muscle testing to be incorporated in the course with the use of one book.
- Provides a top-down approach to learning with a focus on application of information versus rote memorization.
- Allows for OTA program variability in teaching approach to meet the needs of biomechanical to occupation-based programs and preferences of the instructor.

The text also addresses ease of use for faculty. Instructor's manual materials are provided to include test questions and PowerPoint slides for each chapter. These materials will increase the quality and continuity of learning between reading the text, classroom didactic learning, and the assessment of learning. This also enables the instructor the ability to spend valuable time enhancing his or her course as needed to meet student learning needs as a solid course foundation is provided. Further details about faculty resources can be found at www.efacultylounge.com.

chapter 1

Kinesiology: A Foundation in Occupational Therapy

Jeremy L. Keough, MSOT, OTR/L and
Susan J. Sain, MS, OTR/L, FAOTA

Kinesiology incorporates the study of many areas to provide an understanding of movement. Anatomy, physiology, physics, calculus, and biomechanics all provide information to define or describe how movement occurs. Anatomy provides information on muscles, bones, and joints, which make up the components that produce movement. Physiology describes the body systems and body functions that influence movement. Physics is the study of nature and provides information to understand how force, motion, and energy apply to movement. Calculus can be applied to general physics to explain how change occurs and thus quantify how movement occurs. Lastly, biomechanics refers to the application of mechanical principles to the human being and thus is directly relevant to kinesiology. A formal definition of kinesiology is provided in Gold Box 1-1.

Unfortunately, one area of study cannot fully and adequately describe how or why movement occurs. Occupational therapy (OT) practitioners use information from all of the above-mentioned areas of study and apply this information to individuals and their unique situations to effect change. One consideration is that each treatment session often necessitates a new analysis of movement during the treatment of physical disabilities. Additionally, the therapist may also change the extent of what to consider in the analysis of movement at each treatment session. The multitude of variables to consider is endless; however, the *Occupational Therapy Practice Framework: Domain and Process, 2nd Edition* (OTPF-2) provides a method to identify some of these important variables. The OTPF-2 is presented in greater detail later in this chapter. Another important consideration is whether or not the practitioner is seeking qualitative or quantitative information about the client's movement.

Qualitative information includes information on movement that may come from observation or interview. Examples may include movement analysis through observation, gross range of motion or manual muscle testing, or an interview of a client's perceived performance. Several factors may lead the therapist to choose a qualitative approach. A client may be observed performing activities of daily living (ADL) or may be asked to move a certain way to identify preferred movement patterns and movements available to the client. Formal range-of-motion evaluations may not be indicated, or a lack of time may necessitate a gross range-of-motion or manual muscle testing observation. Another consideration may be impaired cognition that can hamper a client's ability to follow directions and complete a standardized assessment.

On the other hand, **quantitative** information identifies numerical data under standardized situations to gather information. Examples may include obtaining formal range-of-motion measurements with a goniometer, assessing manual muscle testing grade, or using a computer or video

Keough, J. L., Sain, S. J., Roller, C. L.
Kinesiology for the Occupational Therapy Assistant:
Essential Components of Function and Movement (pp. 1-26).
© 2012 SLACK Incorporated.

Gold Box 1-1

Kinesiology: The study of the principles of mechanics and anatomy in relation to human movement.

Merriam-Webster's collegiate dictionary (1991, p. 662)

to analyze movement. Each method requires the practitioner to use a standardized procedure or method to gather data about the client. This provides information that can be assessed at a later date to identify change or progress toward OT goals. The complexity of deciding what is important to include in the analysis of movement and how to attain this information is one reason why kinesiology can be considered one of the hardest courses of study in OT.

As the profession of OT and the use of kinesiology have changed over time, both have become more holistic, returning interest to the qualitative characteristics of movement and occupation. Descriptions on qualitative and quantitative approaches can be expressed in much more detail than this text allows; however, important information will be identified that is needed for entry-level practice as an occupational therapy assistant (OTA). A review of the historical connections of OT and kinesiology will provide a link to understanding current OT practice characteristics.

FOUNDATIONS IN OCCUPATIONAL THERAPY

Educational Requirements Related to Kinesiology

Kinesiology has been a tool OT practitioners have used since the inception of the profession. While the emphasis on kinesiology has changed over the years, the importance of understanding movement and its impact on treatment has remained constant. Kinesiology has always been one of the basic sciences included in OT training programs. One way to examine the emphasis on kinesiology can be found by looking at the training requirements for OT practitioners during the past century.

At the start of the profession during World War I, reconstruction aides were established to meet the rehabilitative needs of returning injured soldiers. Reconstruction aides could specialize in either physical therapy or OT. Kinesiology was one of the lectures provided during the training programs for reconstruction aides specializing in OT (United States Federal Board for Vocational Education, 1918). Following World War I, the American Occupational Therapy Association (AOTA) adopted standards for OT courses in 1923. These standards are reflected in the April 15, 1929 flier describing the Boston School of Occupational Therapy (BSOT, 1929). Figure 1-1 shows students in the classroom at the BSOT in 1925. Courses covering medical, social services, and craft study were provided by the school. In particular, anatomy, kinesiology, hygiene, and physiology were subjects identified under the topic of medical study.

In 1935, the essentials of an accredited school in OT were established by the Council on Medical Education and Hospitals of the American Medical Association in collaboration with AOTA. Again, kinesiology was identified as a required subject listed under the biological sciences (Willard & Spackman, 1947). Kinesiology remained a requirement when the essentials were revised in 1949. Interestingly, kinesiology was viewed as important enough to be included in the first OT master's degree program at the University of Southern California in 1947 (*American Journal of Occupational Therapy*, 1947). A course listed as advanced kinesiology was included for 2 credit hours in the 31 credit hours required to graduate.

The essentials remained in effect until the next major revisions were adopted in 1973. A major change that was incorporated in this revision was that course content and hourly requirements were replaced with terminal behavioral objectives (Huss, 1981). There have been several additional revisions to the essentials or standards since 1973; however, the most recent accreditation

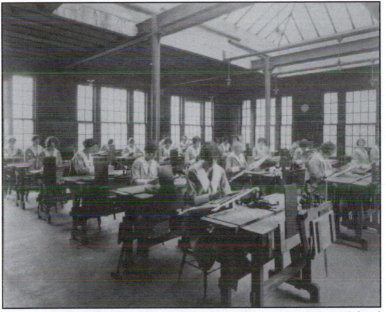

Figure 1-1. Occupational therapists in the making—1925 Boston School of Occupational Therapy. (Reprinted with permission of Tufts University, Digital Collections and Archives, Medford, MA.)

standards for OTA programs continue to present requirements stated through terminal behavioral objectives. The most current revisions were established by the Accreditation Council for Occupational Therapy Education (ACOTE) of AOTA and were adopted in 2006 (ACOTE, 2006). Figure 1-2 presents an image of the OTA program at Roane State Community College and current education in contrast to the 1925 picture of the BSOT.

Terminal behavioral objectives reflect what the OTA student should be able to demonstrate upon completion of an OTA program in preparation for becoming an OTA practitioner. Some terminal behavioral objectives from the 2006 Accreditation Standards for Educational Programs for the OTA are identified in Table 1-1. These terminal behaviors apply to education and learning provided by a course in kinesiology.

While educational standards for OT have changed over time, basic sciences, and specifically kinesiology, remain a constant educational foundation in the educational preparation of the OTA practitioner. Understanding the terminal behavioral objectives that apply to a kinesiology course will enhance learning and aid in comprehending how kinesiology fits within OT. Reviewing entry-level practice as identified by the National Board for the Certification of Occupational Therapy (NBCOT) can also enhance the understanding of how kinesiology fits in OT.

National Board for the Certification of Occupational Therapy

The 2006 ACOTE educational standards can be compared to the picture of entry-level practice identified by the NBCOT. The NBCOT provides the national certification examination that identifies whether minimum standards of knowledge and competency are achieved as an entry-level OTA practitioner. Entry-level practice is described as an OTA practitioner up to the third year of practice. To identify entry-level competencies, NBCOT collects information on current practice through a "Practice Analysis" (NBCOT, 2008a). The most recent analysis and competencies were established in 2008.

Entry-level practice presented by NBCOT is described by four hierarchical components that include domain areas, task statements, knowledge statements, and skill statements (NBCOT, 2008b).

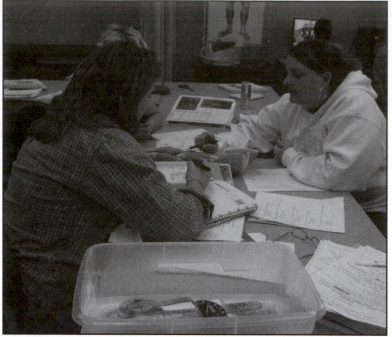

Figure 1-2. Occupational therapy assistants in the making: Roane State Community College, 2010.

Table 1-1	Terminal Behavior Objectives Relevant to Occupational Therapy Assistant Education of Kinesiology
Foundational Content Requirements	
Program content must be based on a foundation of the liberal arts and sciences. A foundation in the biological, physical, social, and behavioral sciences supports an understanding of occupation across the lifespan. Coursework in these areas may be prerequisite to or concurrent with occupational therapy assistant education and must facilitate development of the performance criteria listed below. The student will be able to do the following:	
B.1.4	Demonstrate knowledge and understanding of the structure and function of the human body to include the biological and physical sciences. Course content must include, but is not limited to, anatomy, physiology, and biomechanics.
B.2.7	Exhibit the ability to analyze tasks relative to areas of occupation, performance skills, performance patterns, activity demands, context(s), and client factors to implement the intervention plan.
B.2.10	Explain the need for and use of compensatory strategies when desired life tasks cannot be performed.
B.3.3	Analyze and discuss how history, theory, and the sociopolitical climate influence practice.
B.4.1	Gather and share data for the purpose of screening and evaluation, including, but not limited to, specified screening tools; assessments; skilled observations; checklists; histories; consultations with other professionals; and interviews with the client, family, and significant others.

(continued)

Table 1-1	Terminal Behavior Objectives Relevant to Occupational Therapy Assistant Education of Kinesiology (*continued*)
B.4.2	Administer selected assessments using appropriate procedures and protocols (including standardized formats) and use occupation for the purpose of assessment.
B.4.3	Gather and share data for the purpose of evaluating client(s)' occupational performance in activities of daily living (ADL), instrumental activities of daily living (IADL), education, work, play, leisure, and social participation. Evaluation of occupational performance includes • Client factors, including body functions (e.g., neuromuscular, sensory, visual, perceptual, cognitive, mental) and body structures (e.g., cardiovascular, digestive systems). • Performance skills, including motor (e.g., posture, mobility, coordination, strength, energy).
B.5.1	Assist with the development of occupation-based intervention plans and strategies (including goals and methods to achieve them) based on the stated needs of the client as well as data gathered during the evaluation process in collaboration with the client and others. Intervention plans and strategies must be culturally relevant, reflective of current occupational therapy practice, and based on available evidence. Interventions address the following components: • The occupational profile, including participation in activities that are meaningful and necessary for the client to carry out in home, work, and community environments. • Client factors, including body functions (e.g., neuromuscular, sensory, visual, perceptual, cognitive, mental) and body structures (e.g., cardiovascular, digestive systems). • Performance skills, including motor (e.g., posture, mobility, coordination, strength, energy).
B.5.8	Modify environments (e.g., home, work, school, community) and adapt processes, including the application of ergonomic principles.
B.5.11	Provide training in techniques to enhance mobility, including physical transfers, wheelchair management, and community mobility, and participate in addressing issues related to driving.

Adapted from Accreditation Council for Occupational Therapy Education. (2006). *The 2006 accreditation standards for an educational program for the occupational therapy assistant.* Gaithersburg, MD: Author.

Domain areas identify the major performance components of the profession. Task statements indicate activities performed in the domain area. Knowledge statements describe the minimum knowledge required to perform each task. Lastly, skill statements identify the skill required to perform each task to acceptable standards. The components of entry-level practice that correspond with the ACOTE accreditation standards and are relevant to knowledge of kinesiology are presented in Table 1-2. ACOTE standards that are relevant to kinesiology are identified in the column to the right. Further information of what specific ACOTE standards apply to task, knowledge, and skill statements can be found in the NBCOT document, "Matrix Study: NBCOT 2008 Practice Analysis" (NBCOT, 2008a).

Table 1-2	Similarities of Entry-Level Practice by National Board for the Certification of Occupational Therapy and Accreditation Council for Occupational Therapy Education	
NBCOT Classification Code	**NBCOT Domain Covering Task, Knowledge, and Skill Statements**	**Corresponding ACOTE Accreditation Standard**
Domain 1	Gather information on an ongoing basis using appropriate tools, procedures, and protocols in order to identify factors that impact participation in occupation.	B.1.5, B.2.7, B.2.8, B.4.1, B.4.2, B.4.3, B.5.1
Domain 2	Select and implement evidence-based interventions to support participation in areas of occupation (e.g., ADL, education, work, play, leisure, and social participation) throughout the continuum of care.	B.1.5, B.4.3, B.5.1, B.5.8, B.5.11, B.1.5, B.1.4
Domain 3	Uphold professional standards and responsibilities to promote quality in practice.	B.2.8

Adapted from National Board for the Certification of Occupational Therapy. (2008). Matrix study-NBCOT 2008 practice analysis: Certified occupational therapy assistant COTA. Author.

The ACOTE accreditation standards and the NBCOT practice analysis highlight necessary components of the current practice of OT. The use of kinesiology in the profession of OT can be identified as one of these components. However, this does not provide a more in-depth description of how OTAs apply the knowledge of kinesiology in daily practice. The OTPF-2 does describe in greater detail how kinesiology is applied in OT. First, a look at the history of the profession may help to provide greater insight into current practice trends.

Historical Influences in Occupational Therapy

The current applications of kinesiology in OT can be identified over the past century by looking at prior trends in practice. While the historical practice of OT may not be reflective of present practice settings, core components can be identified that remain true today as well as in the past. The foremost similarity between today and the past is the use of kinesiology as a tool to achieve goals in OT. The multitude of variables affecting the profession of OT allows similar trends to be grouped together. Particular trends in practice (Table 1-3) can be broken down into groups ranging from the 1900s to 1920s, 1930s to 1950s, 1950s to 1970s, and 1970s to present.

The profession of OT emerged at the start of the 19th century during the reconstruction and curative era. The moral treatment movement in the 1800s identified a need to provide a higher quality of life for individuals in institutions. As a result, OT primarily emerged in mental health institutions to enhance individual engagement in craftwork and therapeutic activities. While aspects of kinesiology were not specifically addressed, movement considerations were identified as aspects to consider in craftwork. Specifically, strength was mentioned 10 times, coordination three times, and endurance one time throughout the first textbook in the study of OT, *Studies in Invalid Occupations: A Manual for Nurses and Attendants* written by Susan Tracy (1910).

Table 1-3	Practice Trends in Occupational Therapy
1900s to 1920s	Reconstruction and Curative Era
1930s to 1950s	Reductionistic Era and Orthopedic Model
1950s to 1970s	Medical Era and Kinetic Model
1970s to Present	Occupation Era and Biomechanical Model

With the start of World War I, the professions of OT and physical therapy emerged as reconstruction aides to provide interventions for injured soldiers. Interventions by reconstruction aides in OT not only targeted psychological disorders but also the physical disabilities of returning injured soldiers. General exercise, exercises of certain parts of the body, and kinesiology were identified as techniques of OT in the book *Training for Teachers for Occupational Therapy for the Rehabilitation of Disabled Soldiers and Sailors* (USFBVE, 1918). Reconstruction aides began to consider range of motion for specific limbs. Surgeons prescribing "work" in OT also considered specific joints or muscles (Greene & Roberts, 2005; USFBVE, 1918). OT became more and more accepted as beneficial for individuals with mental and physical disabilities through the provision of curative occupations.

Throughout the 1920s, the emphasis on curative occupations continued to grow in OT. Emphasis was placed on finding specifically chosen purposeful activities for intervention instead of random activities or "busy work." Sands (1928) was able to express this newfound emphasis in her article, "When is Occupation Curative?" She identified that if work was to be called OT, then it should be curative and that the physical objective of curative work was to strengthen weak muscles. She also recommended that joint measurements should be taken, record keeping should be improved, and the use of haphazard occupations should be discouraged. By the end of the 1920s, the art of craftwork and activities most commonly applied at the start of the century were enhanced with the considerations of anatomy and kinesiology. Clearly, a broader influence of the medical field was beginning to take root in OT.

OT gained further acceptance within the medical community over the next several decades from the 1930s to 1950s. OT adopted rational inquiry as did the medical field, which encouraged a reductionistic approach to treatment (Keilhofner & Burke, 1977). This approach encouraged scientific efforts and attempted to identify all therapeutic components that were most beneficial in treatment, even to the smallest element. OT created greater ties within the medical community, and the medical community encouraged OT to further address the motor deficits accompanying physical disabilities (Keilhofner & Burke, 1977). OT responded with the development of the orthopedic model, among other models, to address motor impairments (Greene & Roberts, 2005; Haworth & Macdonald, 1940).

The orthopedic model took into consideration anatomy, physiology, pathology, and kinesiology in addressing client impairments and disabilities. Activities, or occupations, were selected depending on the desired movements. Greater care was also undertaken to record client information, number of treatments, results, and remarks. Haworth and Macdonald (1940) provided information on how to apply the orthopedic model, part of which is displayed in Gold Box 1-2. Few texts and journals were available to further refine this approach, which slowed the development and sharing of professional information.

Following World War II, OT continued its development within the medical era, and the profession further refined an approach to treating physical disabilities with the kinetic model (Greene & Roberts, 2005; Licht, 1950; Willard & Spackman, 1947). This era roughly lasted from 1950 to 1970. The kinetic model provided the basis for future kinesiological approaches to treatment.

Gold Box 1-2

Orthopedic Model

"If the occupational therapist intends to re-educate joints and muscles to perform certain movements it is obvious that she must know something of the structure of joints and the way in which movements are normally produced. A knowledge therefore of anatomy and physiology, of the structure of, and movements performed by, each joint and of the muscles and groups of muscles used in each movement is essential."

Haworth & Macdonald (1940, p. 68)

The first edition of Willard and Spackman's *Principles of Occupational Therapy*, published in 1947, provided three aims of treatment for physical disabilities, which are presented in Gold Box 1-3. Kinesiology is mentioned six times in the text, and significant space is provided to address range-of-motion limitations.

Gold Box 1-3

Kinetic Model

"The aim of Occupational Therapy in the treatment of physical injuries is threefold (1): improve the motion of joints and the strength of muscles, (2): develop coordination, motor skills and work tolerance, (3): prevent building up of unwholesome psychologic reactions."

Willard & Spackman (1947, p. 168)

Increased availability of texts and literature in OT supported the use of kinesiology in treating physical disabilities. The *American Journal of Occupational Therapy* printed several articles on joint measurement in 1947 and 1948. Licht (1950) also provided significant information on how to apply the kinetic model. They identified influential variables of the kinetic model to be cycle of motion, types of muscle contractions, joint range, starting position, realism, and tool variants. Increased scientific efforts and reductionism in the 1950s and 1960s further refined the use of kinesiology in OT. By the third edition of Willard and Spackman's *Occupational Therapy*, 72 pages were provided to describe the restoration of physical function in further depth and clarity (Spackman, 1963).

Renewed interest in occupation re-emerged in the 1970s, and the biomechanical model emerged as a popular model for addressing activity limitations due to impairments in body structure and body functions. The biomechanical model is a restorative approach that attempts to isolate and remediate impairments in body structure and function with the end result of improving occupational performance (James, 2003). Kinesiology is important to help understand and apply this model. This model is commonly used because it fits well in today's medical clinics and medical model to effect quick change in therapy. The biomechanical model is not a holistic approach; however, it can be used effectively and efficiently in conjunction with other treatment approaches. It is accepted that reducing the client's problems to the smallest component does not efficiently or effectively address the complexity of human impairments and disabilities.

Kinesiology is one of the basic medical sciences important to OT practitioners working in the medical model. It is also a common technique or tool used by OT practitioners to address client limitations and disabilities. Kinesiology, through the biomechanical model, provides a structured method of observation to understand human movement. The OTPF-2 can provide a better grasp of how kinesiology and the biomechanical model are used in the current practice of OT.

ENGAGEMENT IN HUMAN OCCUPATION

Describing human nature and behavior can be a daunting task. Perhaps the first thing to reflect on is, "What comprises human occupation?" **Occupation** has individual and unique meanings for each person. In its basic form, occupation can be considered what people do to occupy their time. An occupation can be defined as anything from rest or sleep to work, incorporating everything that occurs throughout the day. Many people define themselves by their occupations or individual daily activities. These chosen pursuits reflect who we are. The anthropologist Bateson (1996, p. 11) wrote, "The capacity to do something useful for yourself or others is key to personhood." Given its importance, occupation cannot simply be reduced to its mechanics or kinesiology alone. Sociological, cultural, emotional, and psychological domains all play important roles in what we engage in and how we perform the occupations of our choosing.

The OTPF-2 gives OT practitioners a structure to identify the mechanics of movement while still considering other aspects of occupation. The OTPF-2 is published by AOTA and provides guidelines for the practice of OT. The most recent revision of the OTPF-2 was adopted in 2008. The format and language of this kinesiology text are based on the 2008 official OTPF-2 document.

World Health Organization: International Classification of Functioning, Disability, and Health

The OTPF-2 is derived from the World Health Organization's (WHO) *International Classification of Functioning, Disability, and Health* (ICF), endorsed May 22, 2001 (WHO, 2009). WHO is a global health organization within the United Nations that promotes the health of all people as a basic and fundamental human right. WHO (2006) adopts a broad definition of health as, "a state of complete physical, mental and social well-being and not merely the absence of disease or infirmity." The practice of OT as reflected in the OTPF-2 embraces this definition of health. The ICF is an international standard used to define and assess health and disability. The most recent revision of this document, accepted in 2001, demonstrates a radically different view of disability that moves focus away from a purely medical or biological perspective. All aspects that may contribute to disability are recognized, such as societal attitudes, context, and environment. This holistic perspective is also a hallmark of OT.

The viewpoint put forth in the ICF implies that having a disease or diagnosis does not necessarily indicate a disability or a decrease in function. A person may have a diagnosis yet function perfectly well. Conversely, a person may not have any diagnosis or medical condition yet not function adequately. Contextual factors such as societal views on illness or disability and environmental factors may impact, positively or negatively, a person's level of functioning. Disability now becomes viewed as a universal human experience affecting all people. This paradigm shift moves the responsibility from the individual alone to society as a whole. The society becomes responsible for allowing an individual condition to become a disabling factor or not. In an article describing the meaning of therapy and the virtues of occupation, Englehardt (1977, p. 672) stated, "people are healthy or diseased in terms of the activities open to them or denied them." In other words, societal attitude, context, and environment can enable or disable a person.

The ICF is divided into three sections: body, activities and participation, and environmental factors. The section on body includes body functions and body structures organized according to major anatomical divisions such as cardiovascular, neuromuscular, skin, sensory, mental, speech, digestive, and genitourinary. Activities and participation includes broader categories that involve actions a person is capable of performing based on body functions and structures. Examples include learning and applying knowledge, communication, mobility, self-care, and community, social, and civic life. Environmental factors span a wide range, from the natural and manmade environment to things such as attitudes of people, services, systems, policies, and technology (WHO, 2002). The OTPF-2 also reflects these categories.

Table 1-4	Comparison of the Medical Model and Social Model	
	Medical Model	**Social Model**
Cause of disability	Diagnosis or disease	Environmental barriers, social stigma, lack of support system
Responsible party	Individual	Society
Treatment, care given to address disability	Surgery, medication, individual therapy	Environmental modifications, policy change, legislation, change of societal perceptions
Disability primarily affects	Individual, family	Community, social system or groups, society as a whole

Body functions and body structures have historically been addressed by medical or rehabilitative models using the principles of kinesiology. The reductionistic approach in the medical model proposes that if the impairments are corrected or improved, function will also improve. This approach, however, does not address the multitude of contextual and environmental factors and furthermore places too much emphasis on the individual.

Contextual and environmental factors are addressed by social models. The social model looks at disability as a socially or environmentally created problem, wherein the physical environment and social or cultural attitudes create the disability by lack of access or acceptance. In the social model, the responsibility for, or cause of, the disability is taken off of the individual and placed on society. This model pays little attention to the disease or disability that may exist. Refer to Table 1-4 for a comparison of these models.

As neither the medical or social model fully captures the nature of disability or functioning, a third model is used in the ICF. This model, known as the biopsychosocial model, attempts to merge the medical and social models, incorporating the strengths of each model. The biopsychosocial model was introduced by George Engel in 1977. His model interconnects biological, psychological, and sociological fields and applies them to health and illness. The shift in focus is toward health and functioning, incorporating all domains, rather than using diagnosis alone as a predictor of success or engagement in occupation. The philosophy reflected in the OTPF-2 is aligned with this holistic approach to health and functioning.

The ICF identifies three levels of human functioning: body or body part, the whole person, and the person in context of the society in which he or she lives. These levels coincide with levels of dysfunction labeled **impairment** (body part), **activity limitation** (individual level or whole person), and **participation restriction** (societal). Refer to the definitions in Gold Box 1-4.

Gold Box 1-4

Activity is defined as "the execution of a task or action by an individual."
Participation is defined as "involvement in a life situation."

WHO (2002)

Table 1-5	Levels of Dysfunction to Body Level Impairments		
Condition	Impairment (Body/Body Part)	Activity Limitation (Individual)	Participation Restriction (Societal)
Severe facial burn	Yes	None	Yes—due to society not accepting how person looks
Lower extremity amputation	Yes	Possibly—gait, sports	No—school, playground, community activities all accessible
HIV-positive	No	Maybe	Yes—denied insurance or services, denied access to certain community activities due to fear and stereotypes

A person may have impairments in a body part, but this may or may not translate into an activity limitation or restriction in social participation. An impairment example at the body part level would be scarring from a severe burn, which may cause limitations in activity or social participation. The person may be physically able to engage in any occupation of choice, therefore demonstrating no activity limitation; however, actual participation may be reduced or denied due to societal stigma and unacceptance of someone who looks different. This would result in participation impairments at the societal level. Conversely, a child with a lower extremity amputation, which is a body part impairment, may be provided with a prosthesis and encouraged to interact as any other child. In this case, there are no activity or participation limitations. Additionally, it is possible to have activity or participation restrictions *without* having an impairment of the body or a body part. A person may be diagnosed with HIV, but currently not have any symptoms or impairments affecting the body level. The person, however, may be limited in activity or denied social participation because of social or cultural stereotyping or stigmatization. This situation creates a restriction at the societal/participation level in the absence of body level impairment. Table 1-5 depicts how activity limitations or participation restrictions relate to body level impairments.

Although the focus of this kinesiology text will be on the categories of body function and body structure as well as the study of movement as it relates to the practice of OT, one cannot ignore the other factors that contribute to health and functioning. As OT practitioners, we are called to use a holistic approach, addressing all domains while treating the total person. The OTPF-2 helps to identify the other factors contributing to health and functioning.

Occupational Therapy Practice Framework: Domain and Process, 2nd Edition

The OTPF-2 serves as a guide to the practice of OT and is designed to help organize and delineate OT services in a uniform manner that is understood by all practitioners. Table 1-6 identifies the aspects of OT's domain. The OTPF-2 does not provide the specific knowledge necessary to practice nor does it espouse a particular theory or model of practice. To adequately address a client's occupational needs, the OTPF-2 was created as a construct from which to manage all of the necessary information related to client interventions. The OTPF-2 is a tool for OT practitioners to use while conducting and planning therapy interventions. OT's focus on function aligns with the

Table 1-6   Aspects of Occupational Therapy's Domain

Areas of Occupation	Client Factors	Performance Skills	Performance Patterns	Context and Environment	Activity Demands
Activities of daily living (ADL)*	Values, beliefs, and spirituality	Sensory perceptual skills	Habits	Cultural	Objects used and their properties
Instrumental activities of daily living (IADL)	Body functions	Motor and praxis skills	Routines	Personal	Space demands
Rest and sleep	Body structures	Emotional regulation	Roles	Physical	Social demands
Education		Skills	Rituals	Social	Sequencing and timing
Work		Cognitive skills		Temporal	Required actions
Play		Communication and social skills		Virtual	Required body functions
Leisure					Required body structures
Social participation					

*Also referred to as basic activities of daily living (BADLs) or personal activities of daily living (PADL)

Reprinted with permission from American Occupational Therapy Association. (2008). Occupational therapy practice framework: Domain and process (2nd ed.). *American Journal of Occupational Therapy, 62,* 628.

Table 1-7	Similarities of the *Occupational Therapy Practice Framework, 2nd Edition* Domains and the *International Classification of Functioning*		
Occupational Therapy Practice Framework, 2nd Edition Domains	*International Classification of Functioning* Body Functions and Structures	*International Classification of Functioning* Activity and Participation	*International Classification of Functioning* Environment
Areas of occupation		x	
Performance skills	x	x	
Performance patterns	x	x	
Context and environment			x
Activity demands	x	x	x
Client factors	x		

WHO's view of health. The classifications and language of the WHO ICF, recognized by health care professionals worldwide, was adopted for use in the OTPF-2.

The OTPF-2 identifies those who receive OT services as *clients*. Clients are categorized into three groups: people, organizations, and populations. The category labeled people refers not only to an individual receiving OT services but to his or her family and caregivers as well. Individuals involved with the client, such as teachers or employers, and any other relevant person are also included at the person level. Organizations, the next level of client group, takes into account groups or associations such as businesses, industries, and clubs. The largest category for clients is populations. Populations include various people in similar situations that can be grouped together (e.g. refugees, people with chronic health conditions, or the elderly) (AOTA, 2008). For the purposes of this kinesiology textbook, focus will be on the personal or individual level. Additionally, this text will refer to anyone receiving OT services as *client* in accordance with the language of the OTPF-2.

The OTPF-2 is further divided into two main sections: domain and process. The OTPF-2 domain section reflects the content of the ICF document reflected in Table 1-7. Section 2, process, relates specifically to the delivery of OT services with clients. The two sections of the OTPF-2, domain and process, are designed to be used together to guide therapy and enhance client engagement in occupation. Expressly, information gathered regarding the client in all components of the domain is used purposely to plan the therapy process, including interventions. This kinesiology text will emphasize aspects of the domain within the larger picture of the OT process.

All aspects of the domain are interrelated and are of equal importance. The areas of the domain encompass building blocks and variables that come together so that a client can engage in an activity of choice. As put forth by the OTPF-2, the domain of OT includes areas of occupation, performance skills, performance patterns, context and environment, activity demands, and client factors.

The domain labeled **areas of occupation** includes a broad spectrum of activities. These range from getting up and performing morning ADL to attending school or contributing at work. Areas of occupation can also include what one chooses to do during free time. General categories in the domain of areas of occupation include ADL, instrumental activities of daily living (IADL), rest and sleep, education, work, play, leisure, and social participation (AOTA, 2008). A specific activity may fit under a variety of occupational areas. How the individual categorizes an activity is based on personal values that may change over time. Not all people will categorize activities similarly. Some people will put an activity in one area of occupation, while others will place the same activity in a different occupational area. This is understandable because different activities mean different things to different people. One person might view cooking as the area of occupation labeled work while another might place cooking in the category of leisure activity or social participation. One individual might see cleaning as an instrumental activity of daily living while another may see it as relaxation or leisure. Gold Box 1-5 lists definitions for some of the areas of occupation.

Gold Box 1-5

Activities of Daily Living (ADL)—Self-care tasks performed to take care of one's body, such as bathing, brushing teeth, dressing, eating, bowel and bladder functions, mobility, etc.

Instrumental Activities of Daily Living (IADL)—More complex tasks than ADL, IADL support daily life and may occur in the community as well as the home. Examples include caring for pets or other people, financial management, meal preparation, shopping, and home management.

AOTA (2008)

Performance skills, another domain, are defined in the OTPF-2 as "the abilities clients demonstrate in the actions they perform" (AOTA, 2008, p. 639). Included in this domain are the interrelated skills of motor and praxis, sensory-perceptual, emotional, cognitive, communication, and social. These skills are learned and developed over time and require that the individual recruit and apply various body functions and structures in specific ways to successfully complete the action. Often, many performance skills are used simultaneously to engage in an occupation. For example, if a person wants to complete a crossword puzzle, he or she must use sensory-perceptual skills and cognitive skills to see and interpret the words and spaces on the paper. This must be accompanied by the fine motor skills and praxis needed to write. Social and communication skills may be required as well if the person seeks assistance from someone else to solve one of the clues.

Performance skills are related to, but distinct from, **performance patterns**. The domain of performance patterns includes habits, routines, rituals, and roles (AOTA, 2008). Performance patterns attempt to describe the manner in which the person uses performance skills. Performance patterns include frequency, consistency, and sequencing and whether the behaviors are automatic, set by culture or personal values, or help to provide structure for daily life. A person may have the ability to perform a skill but, if the skill is not embedded into a pattern, it may not be used enough to be of value. One example is a child who knows how to, and can independently, brush his or her teeth but does not do so unless reminded. The performance of this skill has not developed into a pattern that is used consistently. In another case, the college student who has the performance skills to succeed but has not fully identified with the role of student, has not developed the routine of daily study, and is in the habit of arriving late or missing classes is therefore not utilizing his or her abilities and skills. The result is that the student will most likely do poorly.

All of the domains are affected by the aspects of **context** and **environment**. Human activities do not take place in a vacuum, and all actions are modified and molded by the surroundings in which they occur. Context and environment shape the areas of occupation, performance skills, and patterns. Context is considered in the OTPF-2 to primarily consist of internal conditions, whereas environment is traditionally used to depict the physical or external atmosphere of nonhuman objects as well as the human presence. The attribute of human presence is termed the *social environment*. Specific categories within this domain include cultural, personal, temporal, and virtual contexts as well as the physical and social environment (AOTA, 2008). Performance can be affected either positively or negatively by any of these factors.

The domain of **activity demands** includes all aspects of the actual activity including the objects used. Underlying required actions, body functions, and body structures are taken into consideration when determining whether or not a client can engage in a certain activity. Other things to consider in relation to a specific activity include social components, space or environmental needs, and the timing and sequencing of the activity. The domain of **client factors** includes body structures, body functions, and personal belief systems. Body functions and body structures are based on human anatomy and physiology. Personal belief systems incorporate spirituality, a person's sense of right and wrong, and other thought processes and patterns that influence an individual's life decisions. The domain aspects of activity demands and client factors will be discussed more thoroughly in this chapter.

The focus of this kinesiology textbook will be on the first section of the OTPF-2, which is domain. This textbook will primarily address client factors including body functions, body structures, and values as these relate most directly to kinesiology, biomechanics, and human movement related to function. The additional domains of the OTPF-2 will be attended to, especially within the context of the occupational profiles. Fully presenting the process section of the OTPF-2, which encompasses the delivery of OT services, is not within the intended scope of this kinesiology text.

Client Factors

The domain of client factors is described as things that are mostly internal to the client that may positively or negatively affect performance. Client factors are divided into three sections. The first section includes values, beliefs, and spirituality. This is followed by body functions in the second section, and body structures in the third section. The client factors of values, beliefs, and spirituality are formed over a lifetime of learning and through life experiences. Values, beliefs, and spirituality influence motivation. Body functions and structures relate to the actual anatomic and physiologic make-up of each person. These client factors are for the most part evident at birth. **Body functions** focus on the physiologic functions of body systems such as sensory, neuromuscular, psychological, respiratory, and cardiovascular. Physiologic function can support or hamper engagement in occupations. Anatomy and specific body parts are discussed in the **body structures** section of client factors. Organs, skin, muscles, bones, limbs, and other anatomical features are grouped under body structures. A basic understanding of anatomical features is necessary in order to understand kinesiology, biomechanics, and human movement. The OTPF-2 uses the classifications and definitions found in the ICF to categorize and define body functions and structures. Subsequent chapters in this text will focus in greater detail on body functions and body structures as they relate to kinesiology (AOTA, 2008).

An early kinesiologist and scholar of the symbolic nature of movement, Eleanor Metheny (1954), eloquently incorporated all of the client factors inherent in movement and how they interrelate with one another. Her reflective statement is presented in Gold Box 1-6.

Gold Box 1-6

"The body is the physical manifestation of the person, his mind, his emotions, his thoughts, his feelings. . . . Through its movements he expresses and externalizes the thinking and feeling which makes him a unique person. And as he moves, the very act of movement modifies and affects his thinking and feeling and being."

Metheny (1954, p. 27)

Values, Beliefs, and Spirituality

A person's belief system influences all that he or she does. Each individual's personal set of values and beliefs gives unique meaning to his or her life and guides the manner in which he or she lives life each day. **Values** may be defined as principles and standards that an individual considers to be essential to follow in order to lead a good life. A person might value honesty, integrity, hard work, or family relationships, to name a few. What the person understands as truth and fact make up his or her beliefs. A person's **beliefs** are true to him or her regardless of what another person might say, think, or believe. Some people might believe that a certain president was the best ever, even though not everyone would agree with this. Personal beliefs may not always be accurate. Consider the past when it was a commonly held belief that the world was flat. **Spirituality** is defined as the search for meaning in all that one does, which includes values and beliefs. It is an overarching principle. As implied with the example on beliefs, any of these client factors (values, beliefs, or spirituality) can change over time as a result of life experiences.

Illness or change in personal health status or that of a significant other can alter the way that values, beliefs, and spirituality are interpreted and used. For example, following a heart attack, a client may not immediately have the abilities he or she had previously; therefore, life activities are impacted. Likewise, even after physical improvement, the person's outlook on life may have changed. What was once important (e.g., climbing the corporate ladder) may be replaced with other beliefs or values, such as spending more time with family. Another consideration is that a client may not engage in an activity because of associations or beliefs formed by previous experiences. In this example, the person who had the heart attack experienced it while golfing and may never want to golf again. In the same example, the client, following his or her personal religion, may choose not to include certain medical options available because of his or her beliefs.

Motivation

Client **motivation** is derived from and affected by individual factors such as personality, values, beliefs, and spirituality; however, motivation may also be affected by external factors. A literature review dealing with physical rehabilitation of individuals who had a recent medical diagnosis identified three major groups or theories addressing motivation (Maclean & Pound, 2000). These groups included internal or personality-based theories, external or social theories, and a combination of internal and social factors. One assertion found in the literature review is that the combination of internal and social factors enhances motivation more than using only one or the other. The review also acknowledged the difficulty of studying motivation as there is no consensus on the definition of motivation per se (Maclean & Pound, 2000). An internal factor for the kinesiology student might be feeling good about oneself for reaching a goal. External or social motivators might include a high grade, parental approval, or retention of scholarship monies. As seen, motivation can be intrinsic, coming from internal sources, or extrinsic, reinforced by external factors.

As stated, some experts propose a combination of internal and external motivators. One such model is termed *self-determined extrinsic motivation*. This is defined as when the person will attempt an activity for external reasons, but these external reasons hold value for the person; they have been chosen by the individual because they are important to that person (Dacey, Baltzell, & Zaichkowsky, 2008). External factors need to have significance to the person or have some type of internalized personal value or they will not be motivating. An example of a personally valued or endorsed extrinsic motivator may be appearance.

Self-determined extrinsic motivation grew out of the self-determination theory, which recognizes the importance of autonomy and competence on motivation. Both intrinsic and extrinsic motivators are viewed as important (Dacey et al., 2008). This is a dynamic theory acknowledging that levels of motivation as well as what actually motivates a person are individual and can change throughout the lifespan. For example, exercise may be important to a young individual because it enhances appearance. As this person ages, exercise may become important for health reasons. The person's motivation for exercise has changed. Related to the importance of autonomy and competence on motivation, research by Laliberte-Rudman (2002) has shown that when goals are selected by the client, performance increases.

Another theory describing motivation is named locus of control (Rotter, 1966). Locus of control theory has similarities to self-determination theory, as it also addresses internal and external beliefs. Rotter's theory further postulates that control and motivation are based on personal experience and can be modified by learning, culture, and family. The term **locus of control** refers to who, or what, has impact over outcomes. An internal locus of control indicates that a person believes he or she has control over what will happen to him- or herself. The person believes that his or her actions will make a difference. On the other hand, someone with an external locus of control believes that what happens to him or her is a result of outside influences and that the outcome is not under personal control. The person believes that his or her efforts will not make a difference in the situation. Locus of control theory also acknowledges that an individual's perspective can change over time. Other research has found that the desire to control one's environment is fundamental to motivation (Heckhausen, 2000). This research states that behavior directed at controlling one's environment is broad reaching and can impact any number of functional domains and activities.

Research indicates that several factors impact client motivation to engage in occupation. These factors include internal characteristics inherent in personality, personal values and beliefs, external factors that the client views as important, locus of control or the belief that one's actions have an impact on the outcome, autonomy in decision making, and the desire to control one's environment. Additionally, research indicates that motivational factors are dynamic and can change over the lifespan, as depicted in the following paragraph.

All people begin life with an innate drive for movement and mastery over their environment. In infancy, children have the intrinsic desire to explore and learn about their environment through reaching, grabbing, and mouthing items. This desire to explore continues as the infant's world expands with crawling and later walking. As the child masters basic motor skills with physical maturation, motivation becomes somewhat more extrinsic. Factors such as competition and a desire to prove oneself emerge. In adulthood, motivators commonly include health, appearance, being fit, stress reduction, emotional benefits, and weight reduction. As people age, intrinsic and extrinsic motivation toward physical activity decreases, and motivators such as appearance and weight management are no longer as important. The motivator found to have the greatest positive impact on older individuals remaining physically active is an internal motivator called enjoyment (Dacey et al., 2008).

As OT practitioners, we need to remain mindful of our client's motivational level. We need to pay attention to what is specifically motivating for the client at any given point in time. It is important to remember that motivation can and does change and that motivation may come from internal or external sources.

Activity Demands

Activity demands describe the unique qualities of an activity. These qualities determine the type and amount of effort needed to engage in the activity (AOTA, 2008). OT practitioners can manipulate various activity demands in order to enhance or further challenge a client's engagement in the activity, depending on client need. To enable participation by the client, OT practitioners analyze activities to determine which demands are essential, which can be modified, and how to modify them. Activity demands are broken down into the categories of objects used and their properties, space demands, social demands, sequencing and timing, required actions, required body functions, and required body structures. Changing any one of these areas will impact the other areas as well as the overall activity.

Space demands relate to the physical environment. This can include the room or outdoor space used as well as any physical characteristics of the environment. Characteristics take into account lighting, sound, temperature, humidity, furniture or equipment, and its placement. The structure itself is part of the physical environment. Component parts of the structure, such as the threshold of a door, are also considered. Any or all of these structures and component parts can be altered to enhance functioning and performance. Space demands often need to be modified to accommodate for mobility or movement issues such as the use of a wheelchair. One such example is to use space-saving hinges or remove a door to add width to the opening so that a wheelchair can pass through.

Social demands have to do with the social and cultural aspects of an activity. Social demands may include other people and the need to share, communicate, respect other's viewpoints, or take turns. Social demands also include things like the rules of a game. Cultural aspects may relate to the activity itself or to the participants. Cultural demands can vary greatly. Cultural and social demands may even have an impact on when or how a person gains a skill. For example, many children adopted from other countries are asked to play pat-a-cake when initially assessed by the pediatrician in the United States. This is not a universally practiced activity with children, so the child is unable to do it. After exposure to the activity, the child who is functioning normally quickly learns the game. Social demands, such as rules to a game, can be easily modified. A one-on-one game could become a team effort with one team playing against another. Cultural aspects are usually more difficult to modify as they reflect underlying beliefs and practices of the individual and his or her society. Sequencing and timing of activities are as crucial to successful performance as the physical ability to carry out the activity. A client might have the physical ability to perform an ADL such as bathing; however, the client may not be able to complete this activity independently if unable to plan and sequence each step. When bathing, for example, the water must be turned to the correct temperature to avoid scalding. The person must remember to undress prior to entering the tub or shower. The person must allocate enough time to complete the bathing activity before he or she needs to leave the home. If even one of these activity demands is not met, the task may not be completed successfully. Often, the OT practitioner initially needs to assist the client in breaking the activity down into manageable steps, then direct the client to perform the steps in the correct sequence. Required actions, performance skills, and body functions and structures will be covered throughout this text. These activity demands incorporate the anatomy and physiology required to carry out an activity as well as the skill sets that need to be learned in order to perform the activity. These include not only physical abilities but cognitive, sensory, perceptual, and communication skills to name a few.

Summary

Kinesiology is a specific topic that can be traced back through the history of OT and certainly can be noted in the current practice trends of the profession. Knowledge of kinesiology is an expectation of entry-level practitioners and is often used to assist clients in participating or engaging in areas of occupation or purposeful activities of interest. The role of kinesiology in OT cannot be fully appreciated by using a minimal, reductionistic approach to understanding how or why movement occurs. As a result, the OTPF-2 provides the most comprehensive approach to understanding how and why movement occurs within the practice of OT. Incorporation of the OTPF-2 supports a focus on occupation and the top-down approach to addressing client problems.

APPLICATIONS

The following activities will help you identify domains of the OTPF-2, which will be highlighted in this text. Activities can be completed individually or in a small group to enhance learning.

1. **Qualitative Versus Quantitative Information:** The purpose of this activity is to help identify what is qualitative information versus quantitative information. Qualitative information includes information that may come from observation or interview. This may include information that can be different depending on the situation. Quantitative information identifies numerical data under standardized situations to gather information. As long as the information follows the standardized format, it should yield

similar comparable information. Through observation of the classroom, identify examples of information that might be qualitative or quantitative. A qualitative example might include the comfort of the seat for students. A quantitative example that is measurable might be the temperature of the room. Individually or within groups, see how many other examples you can find.

2. **Variation of Health Condition Related to Levels of Dysfunction: T**he purpose of this activity is to help the student to see how the impact of health conditions may vary depending on the client. This activity supports the view of health and disability put forth in the ICF and OTPF-2 that a diagnosis does not always imply a disability. It is possible that the client may have impairments, activity limitations, and/or participation restrictions. Individually or in groups, identify the possible results of the health condition related to the problem identified in Table 1-8.

   Questions:
   A. What category was most difficult to identify for the result of the problem?
   B. Were all levels of dysfunction impacted?
   C. Can you provide solutions to each level of dysfunction to alleviate each concern?

3. **OTPF-2 Areas of Occupation:** The purpose of this activity is to help identify the areas of occupation, which are of key interest to the OT practitioner. Areas of occupation include ADL, IADL, rest and sleep, education, work, play, leisure, and social participation (AOTA, 2008). Areas of occupation include those individual daily activities that have meaning and purpose in our lives. Identify those daily activities in Table 1-9 that apply to you at this time in your life. Try to only place the activity in the most applicable column, realizing that an activity can apply to more than one area of occupation.

   Questions:
   A. At other times in your life, would you have checked different domain categories? Can you identify current or past activities for each category of areas of occupation that applied to you?
   B. Compare your perspective to that of family or friends for this same activity. How do your friends and family compare to your selections? Were there specific similarities or differences?
   C. If you could, what area of occupation would you engage in more to make your life more balanced? Your perspective can have an impact on how you view and categorize

Table 1-8	Variation of Health Condition Related to Levels of Dysfunction	
Health Condition	**Levels of Dysfunction**	**Result of Health Condition Related to the Problem**
Broken humeral bone following a car accident	Impairment (body part)	Decreased mobility . . .
	Activity limitation (individual or whole person)	School, playground . . .
	Participation restrictions (societal)	Stereotypes about people with disabilities . . .
Diagnosed with the flu	Impairment (body part)	
	Activity limitation (individual or whole person)	
	Participation restrictions (societal)	

Table 1-9	*Occupational Therapy Practice Framework, 2nd Edition* **Domain Aspect: Areas of Occupation**						
Areas of Occupation							
ADL	IADL	Rest and Sleep	Education	Work	Play	Leisure	Social Participation
Brushed teeth	*Swept floor*	*Slept 4 hours*	*Kinesiology OTA class*	*Sandwich artist*	*Tennis, video game*	*Titans football*	*Student OTA association*

your activities or occupations. If you are stressed and categorize everything as work, then you will have little time for play or leisure in your life. You may also procrastinate and put off doing things, resulting in even less time available for required tasks. If you can alter your perspective and consider, for example, the time spent preparing a meal as a relaxing, leisure/hobby time (either solitary or social depending on your preference) and enjoy the process rather than dreading it, you will be more satisfied and use your time more efficiently.

4. **OTPF-2 Activity Demands:** Activity demands include all aspects of the actual activity, which also include the objects being used. Underlying required actions, body functions, and body structures are all considered. The purpose of this activity is to be more mindful of the life demands that impact what appears to be a simple activity. This activity should raise your awareness of what is really involved in completing an activity. It is important to realize that you have control over many of these demands and can modify or change them to enhance your overall success in performing the activity. Identify an activity and area of occupation in Table 1-10 that is relevant in your life and its associated activity demands.
    Questions:
    A. Are there activity demands that interfere with the completion of an activity? Identify them with a negative sign (−), and identify activity demands that promote an activity with a positive sign (+).
    B. Is there an example where one student identified a negative activity demand and another student identified that same activity demand as a positive?
    C. What activity demands do you feel are out of your ability to control? How can you change any of the activity demands with a negative sign to enable your engagement in the activity?

5. **OTPF-2 Consideration of Health Condition:** The purpose of this activity is to help the student "bring the OTPF-2 all together" in considering health conditions. Again, the OTPF-2 was created as a construct to manage all of the necessary information related to client interventions. Having a disease or diagnosis does not necessarily indicate a disability or a decrease in function. Levels of dysfunction identified by the ICF include impairment, which occurs at the body part, activity limitation, which occurs at the individual level, and participation restriction, which occurs at the societal level. Health conditions are identified in Table 1-11. For each health condition, identify which domain aspects

Table 1-10	**Occupational Therapy Practice Framework, 2nd Edition Activity Demands**							
Activity and Areas of Occupation	Objects Used	Space Demands	Time Demands	Sequencing and Timing	Required Actions	Required Body Functions	Required Body Structures
Studying: *Area of occupation is education*	*Books, notes, paper, pencils, computer, friends*	*Minimal desk, seating, good lighting*	*At least 2 hours per week per credit hour*	*Work, child care, no big blocks of time, what to do first—prioritizing*	*Create schedule, consider lowering work hours, find child care*	*Cognitive, motor, sensory*	*Nerves, muscles, eyes, ears*

Table 1-11   *Occupational Therapy Practice Framework, 2nd Edition* Consideration of Health Condition

Health Condition	Domains	Domain Aspects	Broken Nose		Sprained Ankle	
			Level of Human Functioning	Level of Dysfunction	Level of Human Functioning	Level of Dysfunction
Impact of health condition on OTPF-2 domains	Areas of occupation	Activities of daily living				
		Instrumental ADL				
		Rest and sleep				
		Education				
		Work				
		Play				
		Leisure				
		Social participation				
	Client factors	Values, beliefs, and spirituality				
		Body functions				
		Body structures				
	Performance skills	Sensory perceptual				
		Motor and praxis				
		Emotional regulation				
		Cognitive				
		Communication and social				

(continued)

Table 1-11	Occupational Therapy Practice Framework, 2nd Edition Consideration of Health Condition (continued)					
Health Condition	Domains	Domain Aspects	Broken Nose		Sprained Ankle	
			Level of Human Functioning	Level of Dysfunction	Level of Human Functioning	Level of Dysfunction
Impact of health condition on OTPF-2 domains	Performance patterns	Habits				
		Routines				
		Roles				
		Rituals				
	Context and environment	Cultural				
		Personal				
		Physical				
		Social				
		Temporal				
		Virtual				
	Activity demands	Objects used				
		Space demands				
		Social demands				
		Sequencing and timing				
		Required actions				
		Required body functions				
		Required body structures				

are affected and their associated level of dysfunction. Additionally, identify the level of human functioning that is being affected. This would either be the body part level, individual level, or societal level.

Questions:

A. For each health condition, what OTPF-2 domain appears to be the most affected?

B. Were there any domain aspects that could have been answered either yes or no? Why do you think there is this variability?

C. Is it possible to make changes to that domain aspect to eliminate the level of dysfunction? Provide some examples.

D. Was it difficult to identify the level of human functioning and its corresponding level of disability? Explain your reasoning.

REFERENCES

Accreditation Council for Occupational Therapy Education. (2006). *The 2006 accreditation standards for an educational program for the occupational therapy assistant.* Gaithersburg, MD: Author.

American Journal of Occupational Therapy. (1947). Special notices: Master's Curriculum at USC. *American Journal of Occupational Therapy, 1,* 57.

American Occupational Therapy Association. (2008). Occupational therapy practice framework: Domain and process (2nd ed.). *American Journal of Occupational Therapy, 62,* 625–683.

Bateson, M. C. (1996). Enfolded activity and the concept of occupation. In R. Zemke & F. Clark (Eds.), *Occupational science: The evolving discipline* (pp. 5–12). Philadelphia, PA: F. A. Davis.

Boston School of Occupational Therapy. (1929). *Training young women for a new profession* [Brochure]. Boston, MA: Author.

Dacey, M., Baltzell, A., & Zaichkowsky, L. (2008). Older adults' intrinsic and extrinsic motivation toward physical activity. *American Journal of Health Behavior, 32*(6), 570–582.

Englehardt, T. (1977). Defining occupational therapy: The meaning of therapy and the virtues of occupation. *American Journal of Occupational Therapy, 31,* 666–672.

Greene, D. P., & Roberts, S. L. (2005). Kinesiology: Movement in the context of activity (2nd ed.). St. Louis, MO: Elsevier-Mosby.

Haworth, N. A., & Macdonald, E. M. (1940). *The theory of occupational therapy.* London, UK: Bailliere, Tindall, & Cox.

Heckhausen, J. (2000). Evolutionary perspectives on human motivation. *American Behavioral Scientist, 43*(6), 1015–1029.

Huss, A. J. (1981). From kinesiology to adaptation. *American Journal of Occupational Therapy, 35*(9), 574–580.

James, A. B. (2003). Biomechanical frame of reference. In E. B. Crepeau, E. S. Cohn, & B. A. Boyt-Schell (Eds.), *Willard & Spackman's occupational therapy* (10th ed., pp. 240–242). New York, NY: Lippincott Williams & Wilkins.

Keilhofner, G., & Burke, J. P. (1977). Occupational therapy after 60 years: An account of changing identity and knowledge. *American Journal of Occupational Therapy, 31*(10), 675–689.

Laliberte-Rudman, D. (2002). Linking occupation and identity: Lessons learned through qualitative exploration. *Journal of Occupational Science, 9*(1), 12-19.

Licht, S. (1950). Kinetic occupational therapy. In W. R. Dunton & S. Licht (Eds.), *Occupational therapy principles and practice* (pp. 63–69). Springfield, IL: Charles C. Thomas Publisher.

Maclean, N., & Pound, P. (2000). A critical review of the concept of patient motivation in the literature on physical rehabilitation. *Social Science and Medicine, 50,* 495-506.

Metheny, E. (1954). The third dimension in physical education. *Journal of Health, Physical Education, and Recreation, 25,* 27–28.

Merriam-Webster's collegiate dictionary (9th ed.). (1991). Springfield, MA: Merriam-Webster.

National Board for the Certification of Occupational Therapy. (2008a). Matrix study-NBCOT 2008 practice analysis: Certified occupational therapy assistant COTA. Gaithersburg, MD: Author.

National Board for the Certification of Occupational Therapy. (2008b). Validated domains, tasks, knowledge and skill statements for the certified occupational therapy assistant COTA. Gaithersburg, MD: Author.

Rotter, J. B. (1966). Generalized expectancies for internal versus external control of reinforcement. *Psychological Monographs, 80*(1), Whole No. 609.

Sands, I. F. (1928). When is occupation curative? *Journal of Occupational Therapy and Rehabilitation, 7,* 115–121.

Spackman, C. S. (1963). Occupational therapy for the restoration of physical function in occupational therapy. In H. Willard and C. Spackman (Eds.), *Willard and Spackman's occupational therapy* (pp. 167–239). Philadelphia, PA: J. B. Lippincott Co.

Tracy, S. E. (1910). *Studies in invalid occupations: A manual for nurses and attendants.* Boston, MA: Thomas Todd Co.

United States Federal Board for Vocational Education. (1918). T*raining for teachers for occupational therapy for the rehabilitation of disabled soldiers and sailors.* Washington: GPO.

Willard, H. S., & Spackman, C. S. (1947). *Principles of occupational therapy.* Philadelphia, PA: J. B. Lippincott Company.

World Health Organization. (2002). *Towards a common language for functioning, disability and health, ICF.* Retrieved from WIIO/EIP/GPE/CAS/01.

World Health Organization. (2006). *Basic documents* (45th ed.), Supplement. Retrieved from http://www.who.int/governance/eb/who_constitution_en.pdf.

World Health Organization. (2009). *International classification of functioning, disability and health.* Retrieved from http://www.who.int/classifications/icf/en/.

chapter 2

Human Body Functions and Structures Influencing Movement

Susan J. Sain, MS, OTR/L, FAOTA

The *Occupational Therapy Practice Framework, 2nd Edition* (OTPF-2) considers body functions and structures as inter-related parts under client factors. Body functions focus on the physiological functions of body systems, whereas body structures focus on the underlying anatomy. Both areas reflect capacities residing within the body. For functional use, or engagement in occupation, these innate capacities need to be converted into performance skills by the client. Many, if not most, of these skills rely on movement to complete the action.

BODY FUNCTIONS

Movement constitutes a basic drive for all people. Even before birth, the fetus has the potential and need to move. Indeed, movement is what enables people to survive, gather or hunt for food, communicate, and, among multiple other things, engage in daily activities or occupations. "Movement is a fundamental behavior essential for life itself. Life processes such as blood circulation, respiration, and muscle contraction require motion, as do activities such as walking, bending, and lifting" (Whiting & Rugg, 2006, p. 6). More energy is used for locomotion and movement than for any other purpose of the body (Alexander, 1992). Consequently, it is important to move in an efficient manner. Fortunately, the body on its own strives to move efficiently. Research by Alexander (1992) indicates that animals, including humans, automatically adjust gait patterns to use the most efficient pattern available for the speed that they are traveling. The most efficient use of energy is near the middle of the speed range for whatever type of gait that is used. More energy is consumed at the beginning or end of the speed range for gait. For example, when hiking, it is much easier and less tiring to hike at your own pace, or in your stride, than to speed up or slow down in order to stay in pace with a partner. Additionally, a slower speed of travel requires increased control. This phenomenon is well known by the fly-fisherman, who slips and falls less when "rock hopping" versus trying to carefully put each foot on the next rock.

One might ask what causes us to move and what allows us to move efficiently without apparent thought? Many inter-related systems interact to enable our ability to move. Some of these systems include neuromuscular, muscular, and skeletal structures. Without the muscular system and muscle contractions creating force, we could not move. Perhaps due to this fact, more muscle tissue exists in the body compared to any other kind of tissue (Alexander, 1992). On average, muscle tissue makes up 40% to 50% of the body weight in humans (Thompson & Floyd, 2004). There are

Keough, J. L., Sain, S. J., Roller, C. L.
Kinesiology for the Occupational Therapy Assistant:
Essential Components of Function and Movement (pp. 27-54).

three primary types of muscle: skeletal, smooth, and cardiac. This chapter will focus on skeletal muscle and its relationship to movement. Smooth and cardiac muscle allow all other body and organ systems to function.

For muscle tissue to contract, the muscle must be connected to a nervous system. Additionally, if skeletal muscle is going to be able to move the body, it also needs to be attached to a bony system. The human bony system, the skeleton, provides support as well as allows movement at the joints.

Some of these body systems, such as the respiratory and cardiovascular, both rely on and contribute to the functioning of the skeletal muscular system. Additionally, adequate sensory systems and mental functions, such as cognition, motivation, and perception, are necessary for functional movement. Again, this chapter will identify how these inter-related systems work together to provide us with desired movement.

Neuromuscular and Movement-Related Functions

Muscles cannot be active without nerve innervations; therefore, we will begin our discussion by looking at the nervous system. The nervous system can be broken down into two major parts: the **central nervous system** (CNS) and the **peripheral nervous system** (PNS). The entire nervous system is made up of sensory and motor neurons. **Motor neurons** are generally regarded as **efferent**, or exiting the CNS, and terminate on muscle fibers, causing a contraction. **Sensory neurons** are **afferent**, or ascending to the CNS, and send sensory information to the cortex for interpretation (Solomon, 2009). Sensory input can be received from any stimulation, internal or external, to the body. Touch is an example of external stimulation, whereas a muscle ache is a source of internal stimulation. Table 2-1 contains definitions of important terms in this chapter.

Table 2-1	**Nervous System Definitions**
Autonomic nervous system (ANS)	Part of the peripheral nervous system; efferent or motor innervation controlling the viscera; innervates smooth and cardiac muscle as well as glands; supplies information from the *internal* environment.
Central nervous system (CNS)	The division of the nervous system that includes the brain and spinal cord.
Motor neuron	Also called efferent; relays information from the CNS to structures that need to react or respond; carries information away from the CNS.
Peripheral nervous system (PNS)	The division of nervous system that links the CNS with the muscles and glands; provides sensory information to the CNS; further subdivided into autonomic and somatic divisions.
Sensory neuron	Also called afferent; transmits signals from receptors to the CNS; carries information toward the CNS.
Somatic division	Subdivision of the PNS; sensory receptors and nerves related to the *external* environment; nerves linking these to the CNS, and efferent nerves returning to the skeletal muscle.
Viscera	Organs located within body cavities.

Adapted from Kiernan, J. A. (2009). *Barr's the human nervous system: An anatomical viewpoint* (9th ed.). Baltimore, MD: Lippincott, Williams, and Wilkins.; Solomon, E. P. (2009). *Introduction to human anatomy and physiology.* St. Louis, MO: Saunders Elsevier.

The CNS is commonly defined as the brain and spinal cord and ends at the point where nerve fibers exit the spinal cord. Motor neurons in the CNS are referred to as upper motor neurons (UMNs). UMNs provide the connection of neurons that target particular muscles via their connection to the PNS (Kiernan, 2009). The remainder of the nervous system components or all nervous tissue that is not part of the CNS is called the PNS. The motor neurons found in the PNS are called lower motor neurons (LMNs). Cell bodies of the LMNs are located in the anterior horn of the spinal cord and are sometimes referred to as anterior horn cells. The anterior horn cells mark the last synapse of the CNS and the beginning of the PNS for motor neurons. The axons of LMNs are found outside of the spinal cord. LMNs innervate skeletal muscle.

The PNS is further divided into the somatic nervous system and the autonomic nervous system (ANS). The **somatic** division is primarily responsible for responding to the external environment, or things happening outside of the body. The **autonomic** division helps maintain an internal balance as it responds to internal stimuli, providing functions such as maintaining body temperature, regulating heart rate, and regulating blood pressure (Solomon, 2009). Interestingly, the ANS has cell bodies in both the CNS and PNS. The ANS regulates the function of our vital organs (Farber, 1982). The ANS is split into the sympathetic and parasympathetic divisions. The sympathetic system is responsible for the fight or flight reaction experienced during stressful or emergency situations. In contrast, the parasympathetic system maintains and restores energy. Further review of the ANS can be found in anatomy and physiology texts.

Functionally, there is a significant difference in outcome if the CNS system, or UMN, is injured as compared to an injury to the PNS, or LMN. An UMN lesion, such as seen in a cerebrovascular accident (CVA), usually causes *spastic* **paralysis**, increased muscle tone (**hypertonia**), exaggerated **stretch reflexes**, and little to no **atrophy** except with prolonged disuse. In contrast, a LMN injury, either at the anterior horn cell or a peripheral nerve axon, results in *flaccid* **paralysis,** decreased muscle tone (**hypotonia),** loss of the stretch reflex, and significant atrophy. Examples of LMN injuries may include poliomyelitis or a deep cut on a limb that severs a peripheral nerve (Kiernan, 2009). Gold Box 2-1 includes an interesting fact related to an LMN injury.

Gold Box 2-1

Peripheral nerves have the capacity, to a certain degree, for regeneration and repair if the cell body remains intact. In general, peripheral nerves regenerate at about 2 to 4 mm per day.

Kiernan (2009)

The CNS is often divided into five levels of control, each with its own responsibilities. These divisions of control anatomically include the cerebral cortex, basal ganglia, cerebellum, brainstem, and spinal cord. Basically, the cerebral or motor cortex is concerned with voluntary movement. The basal ganglia regulates posture, equilibrium, and learned movements. The responsibilities of the cerebellum include timing, intensity, and refinement of smooth, coordinated movements. Integration of all CNS activity occurs in the brainstem, which allows it to regulate things such as muscle tone and respiratory rhythm. Finally, the spinal cord integrates various reflexes and higher-level activities in order to send neural messages to most of the body (Thompson & Floyd, 2004).

As each CNS division has its own specific roles, it makes sense that damage to each area will result in different functional outcomes. Injury to the motor cortex, such as in a CVA, will affect voluntary movement, which often leads to paralysis. Damage to the basal ganglia will cause dyskinesias, or movement disorders, including chorea. Cerebellar injury will cause errors in rate, range, direction, and force of movements, resulting in ataxia. Injury to the brainstem can cause a great variety of outcomes, depending on the location of the lesion. Effects of injury to the brainstem may include vertigo, facial paralysis, and tremor. Injury or disease of the spinal cord can also produce a wide variety of symptoms depending on the level and specific location of the injury (Angevine & Cotman, 1981; Kiernan, 2009).

Sensory systems that provide afferent information to higher levels of the CNS profoundly affect movement. Some sensory input elicits immediate reflex activity, such as in flexor withdrawal, which is an automatic reaction that acts to protect a limb or body part from injury. Other sensory input is relayed to the cerebral or motor cortex for interpretation and may be determined irrelevant so the body ignores it. An example of this might be the buzzing of the overhead lights in your classroom. The majority of sensory input is analyzed by the cortex and then used or discarded to direct movement. Various sensory systems provide us with the ability to use pain, sight, hearing, taste, smell, touch, temperature, and **vestibular** and **proprioceptive** feedback to modify movement. Sensory receptors are defined as exteroceptors or interoceptors. Table 2-2 highlights definitions of key terminology.

In summary, the neuromuscular system describes the interdependency of the nervous system's innervations and its communication with the muscular system to enable movement. These two systems relay information back and forth between each other in order to coordinate movement and respond to stimuli. If there is a malfunction in either system, movement will be affected.

Cardiovascular and Respiratory System Functions

On a basic anatomical level, muscles need oxygenation and nutrition via the lungs and blood to thrive. The cardiopulmonary system delivers, among other things, oxygenated blood to all organs, allowing each organ to survive. Adequate cardiopulmonary function also supports endurance. Muscles metabolically generate the energy they need to execute movement via nutrients obtained in vascular and interstitial tissues. Additionally, the cardiovascular and respiratory systems remove carbon dioxide and other waste products to keep the muscles and organs functioning at optimum levels. In other words, the muscular component of movement relies on the cardiovascular and respiratory systems in order to function. Likewise, the cardiovascular and respiratory systems rely on the skeletal muscular system to operate properly. An example occurs when there is a contraction of muscles in a limb that aids the return of blood to the heart and decreases the occurrence of **edema** in the extremities. Regarding the respiratory system, certain skeletal muscles also aid in both the inspiration and expiration phases of respiration.

Disease or limitations in the cardiovascular or respiratory systems can have a negative impact on skeletal muscular function and therefore on movement (Cronin & Mandich, 2005). One example of a respiratory system disease that affects skeletal muscle function and movement is chronic obstructive pulmonary disease (COPD). COPD is characterized by degenerative changes of the alveoli, resulting in breathlessness on exertion, even if the exertion is minimal. The oxygen-carbon dioxide gas exchange is lessened, causing less oxygen to travel to other tissues, fatigue, less energy production, and decreased functioning overall (Steadman, 1982). A person with COPD may have a difficult time breathing and often will prop him- or herself on the elbows in a standing position. This position allows the recruitment of additional skeletal muscles to aid the breathing process. Because breathing is more difficult during movement, the person becomes more sedentary.

Other body functions, such as mental functions, are also involved in the choice to become more sedentary in a person with COPD. In the OTPF-2, mental functions include cognitive areas, such as memory and judgment, as well as affective and perceptual functions that may include temperament and attention span. In the case of the client with COPD, anxiety is associated with the fear that breathing will be further diminished. Increased anxiety puts further strain on breathing and oxygen uptake. In addition, leaving the home often causes increased anxiety and requires more energy expenditure. The person may then decide to remain at home, at rest, to decrease anxiety

Table 2-2	Definitions of Common Terms
Ataxia	Incoordination; inability to execute coordinated voluntary movement; loss of smooth execution of movement; ataxic gait often described as "drunken."
Atrophy	Wasting of tissue, especially in muscle due to lack of use.
Chorea	Irregular, involuntary movements of the limbs or facial muscles, often described as dance-like motions.
Dyskinesia	Difficulty in performing voluntary movements; *dys* meaning bad or difficult, *kinesia* referring to movement.
Edema	Accumulation of excessive amounts of watery fluid in cells, tissue, or serous cavities.
Exteroceptors	"External receivers," afferent nerve endings that respond to stimulation by external agents, specialized in receiving information from the external environment, such as the eyes.
Flexor withdrawal	Sometimes referred to as flexor reflex, protective; the withdrawal of a limb in response to painful stimulation.
Flaccid	Relaxed, without tone.
Hypertonia	"Above or over tone"; extreme tension of the muscles.
Hypotonia	"Under tone"; having a lesser degree of tension; diminished muscular tone.
Interoceptors	"Internal receivers," afferent nerve endings or receptors that respond to stimulation from within the body, primarily from visceral organs.
Tone	Also called muscle tone—the normal state of tension of muscles caused by partial contraction of some of the muscle fibers.
Paralysis	Loss of power of voluntary movement in a muscle through injury or disease to its nerve supply.
Proprioceptor	A sensory end-organ in muscles, tendons, joint capsules, and inner ear allowing us to know the location of one body part in relation to another; activated by movement or action of the organism itself.
Spasticity	A state of increased muscular tone.
Stretch reflex	Slight stretching of a muscle lengthens fibers, causing stimulation of sensory endings, which leads to contraction of the muscle. This is a protective reflex to avoid overstretching. One role of the muscle spindle is to detect stretch and respond to it via the stretch reflex; this phenomenon is in constant use and provides adjustment to muscle tone.
Vestibular	Related to the vestibule of the ear; a vestibule is a small space or region at the entrance of a canal; vestibular organ—the organ of equilibrium.

Adapted from Angevine, J. B., & Cotman, C. W. (1981). *Principles of neuroanatomy.* New York, NY: Oxford University Press, Inc.; Kiernan, J. A. (2009). *Barr's the human nervous system: An anatomical viewpoint* (9th ed.). Baltimore, MD: Lippincott, Williams, and Wilkins.; Solomon, E. P. (2009). *Introduction to human anatomy and physiology.* St. Louis, MO: Saunders Elsevier.; Steadman, T. (1982). *Steadman's medical dictionary* (24th ed.). Baltimore, MD: Williams and Wilkins.

and enhance breathing. Thus, a negative cycle begins. The decreased ability for efficient breathing leads to decreased movement, decreased movement leads to an even further decrease in capacity for the lungs to perform their job, and so on. Many such examples of decreased functional performance in respiratory or cardiovascular systems exist, which in turn will affect movement. Other texts are dedicated to describing the disease process and can be referred to for detailed information on a specific diagnosis. The goal of this text is that the reader will gain an appreciation of how all body systems are inter-related and affect movement abilities and choices.

Muscular Functions

As your study of human movement progresses, you will find that no two people perform the same movements in the same way. Indeed, one person might perform the same movement in different ways at different times, depending on the level of fatigue, pain, motivation, or other factors. Keep in mind that although people often do not use ideal movement patterns in daily activities, they are still able to function at required levels, usually without undue stress on body systems (Fisher & Yakura, 1993). Occupational therapy (OT) may become involved when a client's movement patterns stray far enough from ideal that they do cause the client excessive stress. The inefficient movement patterns may increase energy consumption or become ineffective for daily occupations; thus, the client seeks intervention. To move efficiently, people incorporate the laws of physics, biomechanics, and physiology. These concepts and how they affect movement will be discussed in depth in subsequent chapters of this text.

One focus of this chapter is skeletal muscle. Skeletal muscles are a primary feature influencing movement. Skeletal muscles are not only responsible for movement but also provide a degree of protection, especially for internal organs. In addition, skeletal muscles support posture and produce body heat.

Muscles are able to perform a variety of roles that allow for both mobility and stability against gravity. Muscles must act in cooperation with one another to produce either movement or stability. Muscles are capable of maintaining or switching these roles instantaneously to meet the demands of the movement required. The various roles a muscle can perform are defined in greater detail in Table 2-3.

When a muscle is activated, it can only develop tension. Muscles produce force or tension by contracting. There are two main types of contractions, isometric and isotonic. Both types of contractions have roles in most movements. Isotonic contractions can be further divided into concentric and eccentric contractions.

The word **isometric** literally means *same measure*. The Greek origins of this word tell us its meaning. *Isos* translates as equal, and metric is derived from *metron*, meaning measure (Steadman, 1982). During an isometric contraction, muscle tension develops, but the muscle length does not change. This means that the joint angle or measurement does not change either. Isometric contractions may be thought of as static as they maintain the joint angle in a relatively stationary, nonmoving position. An example of an isometric contraction is when a person is holding the rail on a moving bus or tram while standing. The person's arm muscles produce tension to maintain posture against the forces of acceleration and deceleration, but there is little or no change in joint positions of the arm.

The term **isotonic** is derived from the Greek words *isos* (equal) and *tonos*, translated as tension (Steadman, 1982). Isotonic contractions maintain the muscle at equal tension. This means that the length of the muscle changes, causing joint movement. Isotonic contractions may be thought of as dynamic because the tension produced by the contraction causes movement.

An isotonic contraction is considered **concentric** when the muscle shortens and the joint angle is decreased. This occurs at the elbow when you bring a glass to your mouth. If the muscle contracts with less force than needed to overcome the resistance, an **eccentric** contraction occurs (Solomon, 2009). Resistance may include gravity, an object, or other muscles. In the case of an eccentric contraction, the muscle is actually *lengthening* under stress. Eccentric contractions work to *decelerate* the movement, as a brake would do for a car. Consider the movement of placing your glass back on the table. Eccentric contractions keep the glass from crashing into the table in an

Table 2-3	**Muscle Roles**
Agonists	Sometimes referred to as *movers*, a muscle that *concentrically* contracts causing movement at a joint; at most joints, several muscles act together, each as an agonist, causing the movement. In this situation, some texts refer to primary agonists and assistant agonists; agonists are usually active during acceleration of a body segment.
Antagonists	Muscles with actions opposite those of the agonist, muscles acting against a position or movement, often located on the opposite side of the joint as the agonist; during many movements, the antagonists are passive or perform an *eccentric* contraction slowing the movement; antagonists are usually active during deceleration.
Coactivation	Sometimes referred to as co-contraction; limited to simultaneous action of agonist and antagonist to provide stability, to increase *torque* at a joint, when learning a new movement.
Neutralizers	Muscles that prevent unwanted accessory actions or substitutions or cancel out multiple actions by the same muscle. When a muscle with multiple actions contracts, it attempts to perform all of its actions, unable to determine which one is necessary for the movement. For example, the biceps brachii both flexes the elbow joint and supinates the forearm. If elbow flexion is the desired goal, neutralizers will cancel out the supination action of the biceps muscle.
Stabilizers	Sometimes referred to as *fixators*; muscles that surround a joint or body part to stabilize the joint against unwanted movement. When muscles contract, the insertion can move toward the origin, or vice versa. Stabilizers prevent motion at one of these locations in order to allow controlled movement at the other location; during normal muscle use, these muscles stabilize the origin of the agonist; muscles that stabilize a portion of the body against a particular force, which may be internal from other muscles or external such as gravity or a weight being lifted.
Synergists	Muscles that are not prime movers but assist the agonist in the motion and also help to cancel out undesired motions.

Adapted from Hall, S. (1999). *Basic biomechanics* (3rd ed.). Boston, MA: WCB/McGraw-Hill.; Solomon, E. P. (2009). *Introduction to human anatomy and physiology*. St. Louis, MO: Saunders Elsevier.; Thompson, C. W., & Floyd, R. T. (2004). *Manual of structural kinesiology* (15th ed.). Boston, MA: McGraw Hill.; Whiting, W. C., & Rugg, S. (2006). *Dynatomy: Dynamic human anatomy*. Champaign, IL: Human Kinetics..

uncontrolled manner. If eccentric contractions of the elbow flexor muscles were not occurring in response to the resistance provided by gravity and the weight of the glass, the glass would crash into the table. Eccentric contractions allow for slow, smooth, and controlled movements. Lieber and Bodine-Fowler (1993) believed that muscle injury and soreness are more often associated with eccentric, or lengthening, contractions. The specific structures used by the muscle to contract will be discussed later in this chapter.

Various muscle properties determine how much a certain muscle can shorten or lengthen. Four properties defined in the literature include contractility, extensibility, elasticity, and irritability. **Contractility** has been defined as a muscle's ability to shorten in length; however, as discussed previously, not all contractions result in muscle shortening. Perhaps a more accurate description of contractility refers to a muscle's ability to develop tension against resistance. The **extensibility** of a muscle depicts its capacity to be stretched or lengthened. Conversely, **elasticity** describes the muscle's ability to return to its original length after it has been stretched. **Irritability** is the term used to describe the capacity of the muscle to receive and respond to a stimulus, whether the stimulus is chemical, electrical, or mechanical (Hall, 1999; Thompson & Floyd, 2004). The term **excursion ratio** refers to the difference between how long the muscle is when stretched as compared to its length when contracted. For most muscles, this ratio is 2:1, indicating that most muscles are capable of stretching twice as long as they can shorten (Gench, Hionson, & Harvey, 1999).

Sequencing and timing of muscle contractions also influence the type and quality of movement. Some movements require sudden bursts of speed, such as swinging a bat or throwing a ball. Other motions, such as kneading bread, should be performed more slowly. Certain movements require precise control, as in writing, while other movements only need gross coordination, such as walking. The speed and precision of a muscle contraction is dependent on many variables. Variations can occur in the speed of a muscle contraction, the frequency of contractions, and the strength of the contraction. Often, one of these variables is gained at the loss of another. For example, the faster a group of muscle fibers shorten, the less force they can exert (Alexander, 1992).

The speed of muscle contractions can be affected by the diameter of the axon, the thickness of the myelin sheath, or the properties of the muscle fibers themselves. In general, as the speed of a muscle contraction increases, the potential for fatigue also increases. Conversely, muscles that are slower to contract are better suited for activities that require endurance. To help combat fatigue, different motor units are activated in sequence, rather than all units being activated at the same time. In this manner, a certain number of motor units are relaxing at all times. Some muscle fibers have a longer refractory period than others, meaning that more time passes before they can be activated and are able to produce tension again.

The strength of a muscle contraction is dependent on the number of muscle fibers recruited, the size of the muscle fibers, and the size of the axon. The larger that each of these is, the stronger the contraction will be (Gench et al., 1999). Amazingly, the CNS automatically matches the speed and strength of muscle contractions to the requirements of each and every individual movement to produce efficient, smoothly executed motions. The CNS can spontaneously increase or decrease the number of motor units activated, select between types of motor units, or make numerous other adjustments. These adjustments allow us to perform the activities of our choosing without need for any conscious input on our part.

Skeletal Functions

The skeletal system provides the framework for the body. It also gives support and protection to other systems of the body. The bones of the thorax, or trunk, protect vital organs such as the heart and lungs, while the skull protects the brain. The skeleton consists of a series of bones connected to each other at joints. The joints allow movement to occur. In addition, the skeleton provides attachments for muscles, which enable movement at the joints. The bones of the skeleton also perform other important functions, such as blood cell formation in the bone marrow and storage of certain minerals (Thompson & Floyd, 2004).

Articulations of bones, more commonly known as joints, are of immense functional importance. All skeletal movement in the body occurs at joints. When there is disease or injury at a joint, movement will be negatively impacted. Several factors influence the amount of stability provided, or movement allowed, at each joint. Some of these factors include the type and shape of the joint, the structures surrounding the joint, and the number of degrees of freedom available at the joint.

A joint system based on movement includes three classifications of joints, which are labeled synarthrodial, amphiarthrodial, and diarthrodial. **Synarthrodial** joints are immovable, such as the suture joints of the skull. **Amphiarthrodial** joints, sometimes called cartilaginous joints, allow for limited movement as in the pubic symphysis. The joint classification allowing for the most movement is the **diarthrodial** joint, which is considered freely movable. Its movement is limited primarily by muscle, tendon, and ligaments rather than by the joint structure itself. Diarthrodial joints are enclosed within a joint capsule that secretes synovial fluid to lubricate the joint; thus, these joints are also referred to as **synovial** joints. The majority of the joints in the body are diarthrodial joints (Solomon, 2009; Thompson & Floyd, 2004).

Although diarthrodial joints allow for the most movement, there are still significant variations in movement ability from one diarthrodial joint to another. These differences are based on the number of axes a joint can rotate around and the number of planes the joint can move in. This is also referred to as degrees of freedom. If a joint only has one axis and can move in only one plane, it is said to have one degree of freedom. An example of this would be a hinge joint, such as that found at the elbow joint. Similarly, if the joint has two axes and can move in two planes, it is said to have two degrees of freedom. The metacarpophalangeal (MCP) joints in the hand represent joints with two degrees of freedom. The most freely moving joint can have a maximum of three degrees of freedom. An example of this joint type is the ball and socket joint of the hip. This joint can move in all three planes around three different axes. Joints with one degree of freedom provide more stability but less mobility, while joints with three degrees of freedom allow for more mobility but less stability. As noted, the trade-off for increased mobility is a loss in stability (Hall, 1999). Specific voluntary joint motions and the planes they occur in will be discussed later in this chapter.

In addition to voluntary motions, **accessory motions** increase the pain-free movement available at a given joint. Accessory movements cannot be performed voluntarily. They occur between the articular surfaces of a joint in conjunction with voluntary movement. There are three types of accessory motions, which are called roll, spin, and glide. Roll is sometimes referred to as rocking, and glide is often called slide or translation. Spin is similar to the motion of the tiny point on a toy top spinning in one location on the larger surface of the table or floor (Thompson & Floyd, 2004). Although accessory motions are available at most joints, they are readily apparent in the knee and glenohumeral joint, where one joint surface is significantly different in size than the companion joint surface. Accessory motions at these joints allow for the larger surface of one bone to remain in contact with the smaller surface of the adjoining bone, thus allowing greater range of motion.

As previously noted, in order for muscles to act at joints, they must attach to the bones. These areas of attachment are generally referred to as bony landmarks. Interestingly, fields such as anthropology or forensic medicine use bones and bone markings to determine many things about a person, such as age, gender, race, occupation, health, or even whether or not a person had certain diseases when he or she died (Moore, 1985). Bony landmarks tend to be more prominent in people who performed more physical labor or were more athletic than others. Certain bony landmarks, particularly those that protrude, will be discussed further in this text. Functionally, these bony landmarks are important for two key reasons. The first reason is that they are often used as the axis for goniometric joint measurements, discussed further in subsequent chapters. The second reason relates to clients who are less mobile. For these clients, certain bony landmarks need to be observed or examined periodically to inspect for **decubiti.** Decubiti are more commonly referred to as bed sores and will often form when pressure is maintained over a bony protuberance.

BODY STRUCTURES

A brief overview of anatomical structures, including their impact on movement, will be presented in this section. As outlined in the OTPF-2, body structures are listed under client factors. Client factors include specific characteristics that may affect performance; however, despite their importance, these characteristics do not guarantee successful movement. Conversely, impairments in, or lack of, these structures does not necessarily indicate difficulty carrying out individual occupations of interest to the client (AOTA, 2008). Body structures are just one part of the complex picture that OT practitioners must observe in order to guide the client toward increased functional performance. The World Health Organization (WHO, 2001) defines *body structures* as the anatomical parts that support body functions. Structures include everything from the microscopic cell to the organ or limb.

Nervous System

A summary of the basic functions of the nervous system was presented in the first part of this chapter. The specific structures that permit these basic functions will be further defined and illustrated in this section. There are 12 pairs of cranial nerves and 31 pairs of spinal nerves. Cranial nerves transmit information directly to the brain. Spinal nerves link the spinal cord with sensory receptors and with other parts of the body. The spinal nerves are all mixed nerves, transmitting sensory information to the spinal cord through afferent neurons and also relaying motor information from the spinal cord to the various parts of the body using efferent neurons. Spinal nerves have two points of attachment with the spinal cord. The dorsal root contains afferent neurons or sensory fibers. The ventral root consists of motor neurons or efferent fibers (Solomon, 2009).

This division into sensory or motor distribution is observed in the PNS (Thompson & Floyd, 2004). Dorsal, afferent sensory receptors may be located in any organ system, including skin and muscle. Sensory receptors located in the skin are responsible for sensations such as pain, light touch, and temperature. Each dorsal nerve root receives feedback from a specific area of skin on the body. This specific area is labeled a **dermatome**. When injury occurs to even a single nerve root, sensation in the dermatome supplied by that nerve root will be diminished or altered (Moore, 1985). Refer to Figure 2-1 to see a representation of sensory dermatomes.

Efferent or motor innervations can be segmental or provided by a plexus. Segmental innervations refer to innervations supplied directly by a single nerve root to a nearby region. In contrast, a plexus represents a network, or interconnection of nerves, that then separates into various nerves named for the region of the body they innervate. One example is the brachial plexus

Figure 2-1. Distribution of sensory dermatomes. (Angevine, J., & Cotman, C., *Principles of Neuroanatomy*, 1981, p. 122; By permission of Oxford University Press, Inc.)

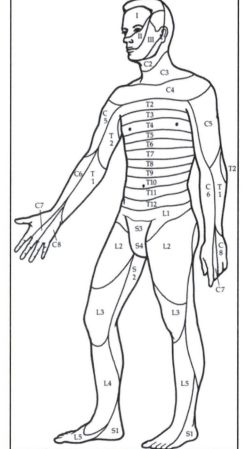

(Steadman, 1982). Table 2-4 gives examples of nerves originating from the brachial and lumbosacral plexuses.

Most innervations of skeletal muscles in the trunk are segmental. Motor innervations to the extremities tend to be via a plexus. Plexuses are thought to provide neuromuscular protection in that if a single nerve root is damaged, muscles innervated by a plexus will continue to have some ability to function. The two plexuses this text is most interested in are the **brachial plexus** and the **lumbosacral plexus**.

The brachial plexus is composed of spinal nerve roots from the fifth cervical nerve (C5) through the first thoracic nerve (T1) and supplies the upper extremities. A representation of the brachial plexus can be seen in Figure 2-2. The lumbar plexus is formed by spinal nerve roots

Table 2-4	Plexus and Nerves		
Plexus	**Nerve Roots**	**Name of Nerve**	**Area of Body Innervated**
Brachial	C5 through T1	Ulnar	Medial forearm, 4th and 5th digits
		Radial	Dorsal aspect of arm, forearm, and hand
Lumbosacral	L1 through L4 L5 through S3	Femoral	Anterior thigh
		Sciatic	Posterior leg

Adapted from Kiernan, J. A. (2009). *Barr's the human nervous system: An anatomical viewpoint* (9th ed.). Baltimore, MD: Lippincott, Williams, and Wilkins.; Solomon, E. P. (2009). *Introduction to human anatomy and physiology.* St. Louis, MO: Saunders Elsevier..

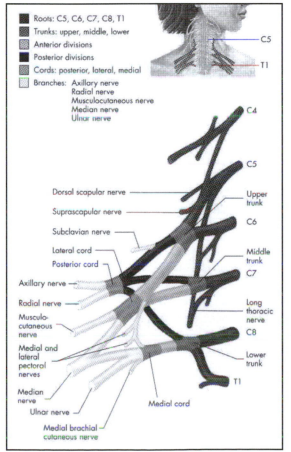

Figure 2-2. The brachial plexus, anterior view, nerve roots C5 through T1. (Seely, R. R., Stephens, T. D., & Tate, P., *Anatomy and Physiology*, 6th ed., 2003; Reprinted with permission from The McGraw-Hill Companies.)

Figure 2-3. The lumbar plexus, anterior view, nerve roots L1 through L5. (Thompson, C., & Floyd, R. T., *Manual of Structural Kinesiology*, 15th ed., 2004; Reprinted with permission from The McGraw-Hill Companies.)

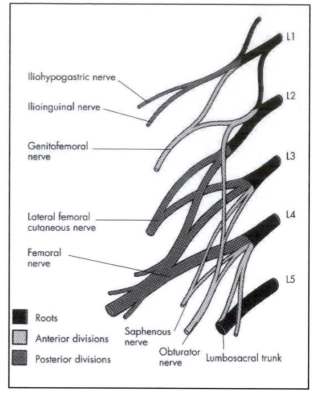

beginning with the first through fourth lumbar nerves (L1 through L4) as shown in Figure 2-3. The sacral plexus, depicted in Figure 2-4, is made up of the fourth and fifth lumbar nerve roots (L4, L5) in addition to the first, second, and third sacral nerve roots (S1 through S3). The lumbar and sacral plexuses are often considered together as the lumbosacral plexus. The combined lumbosacral plexus, consisting of nerve roots L1 through S3, innervates the lower extremities (Moore, 1985; Steadman, 1982).

Muscles

According to Thompson and Floyd (2004), there are more than 600 muscles in the body, including 215 pairs of skeletal muscles. Other sources indicate a lesser number of muscles. What is important to note is that there are a lot of muscles in the body that influence multiple types of movement. Muscles can be described in many ways, such as by shape, location, fiber orientation, size, origin, insertion, or function. Regardless of how skeletal muscles are described, they all react in a similar way.

A brief review of the muscle is presented here. A muscle is composed of several motor units. A motor unit is defined as one motor neuron and all the muscle fibers it innervates (Thompson & Floyd, 2004). Motor units are the building blocks of muscle tone and allow us to perform graded muscular contractions (Hall, 1999). Although the response of a motor unit is all or none, the strength of the response of the entire muscle is determined by the number of motor units activated. A motor unit is made up of fasciculi that are organized into functional groups of varying sizes. A fasciculus is several muscle fibers bundled together.

Each fasciculus or motor unit is made up of the same type of muscle fibers, although the entire muscle itself is usually made up of a combination of fiber types. Most muscle fibers are of the twitch type, meaning that they produce tension in response to a single stimulus. Twitch-type fibers are further divided into fast twitch and slow twitch. Fast twitch fibers are those that reach

Figure 2-4. The sacral plexus, anterior view, nerve roots L5 through S3. (Thompson, C., & Floyd, R. T., *Manual of Structural Kinesiology*, 15th ed., 2004; Reprinted with permission from The McGraw-Hill Companies.)

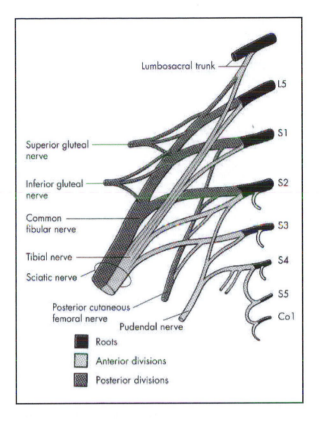

maximum tension very quickly. Conversely, slow twitch fibers take up to seven times longer to reach their peak tension. A single motor unit may contain anywhere from 100 to 2,000 muscle fibers. Fine motor and precise movement are coordinated by motor units containing relatively few muscle fibers. On the other hand, movements requiring gross motor skills and increased force utilize motor units containing a maximum number of muscle fibers (Hall, 1999).

A muscle fiber is the muscle cell. Fiber is the name given to a muscle cell because of its narrow, elongated shape. The sarcomere is the contractile unit in the muscle cell. This is where the actin and myosin are located. Neither actin nor myosin can change in length. Rather, the length of the muscle shortens as the overlapping of the actin and myosin fibers becomes greater (Solomon, 2009).

The structural arrangement of fibers within muscle helps to determine the muscle's function. Shorter fibers, such as those in a pennate arrangement, are specialized to produce more force. Longer fibers, such as those in a parallel arrangement, seem to favor larger excursion or movement and less force (Lieber & Bodine-Fowler, 1993). The two major types of skeletal fiber arrangement are those listed above, pennate and parallel. The term *pennate* is derived from the Latin word for feather. The muscle fibers in a pennate arrangement are oblique or at an angle to the tendon, similar to a feather. Examples of pennate muscles include the peroneus longus and peroneus brevis, as well as the deltoid. On the other hand, fibers in a parallel arrangement run the length of the muscle. The sartorius and biceps brachii muscles are examples of muscles with a parallel fiber arrangement. These two structural arrangements of muscle are further subdivided according primarily to the shape of the muscle. Pennate fibers can be classified as unipennate, bipennate, or multipennate depending on the number of branches. Figure 2-5 depicts the rectus femoris, a muscle with bipennate fibers, which is a subclassification of the pennate arrangement. Parallel fibers may be categorized as flat, fusiform, strap, radiate, or sphincter. Figures 2-6 through 2-8 are all examples of the parallel fiber arrangement; however, each one is slightly different, relating

Figure 2-5. Bipennate muscle fibers can be seen in this picture of the rectus femoris muscle. The bipennate classification is a subclassification of the pennate arrangement. (Reprinted with permission from Carolyn Roller.)

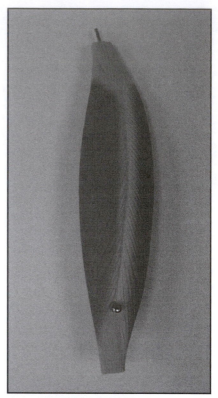

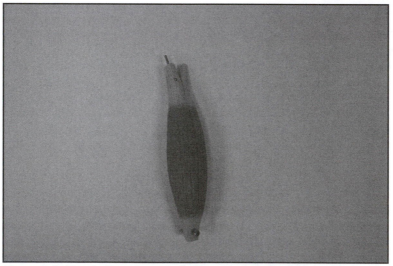

Figure 2-6. Muscle fibers in a parallel arrangement, further classified as the fusiform shape, are seen here in the biceps brachii muscle. (Reprinted with permission from Carolyn Roller.)

to the categorization of the muscle. Flat muscles are usually thin and broad. Fusiform muscles are spindle shaped with a wider belly in the middle and thin ends. An example of this is in Figure 2-6, which depicts the biceps brachii muscle, a muscle with parallel fiber arrangement further categorized as fusiform. Strap muscles are usually uniform in diameter and longer than other muscles. The sartorius muscle is an example of a strap muscle and is depicted in Figure 2-7. Radiate muscles are sometimes described as fan shaped or triangular. Two examples of radiate muscles, the deltoid

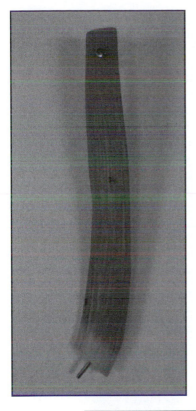

Figure 2-7. The sartorius muscle as an example of a strap-shaped muscle of the parallel fiber arrangement. (Reprinted with permission from Carolyn Roller.)

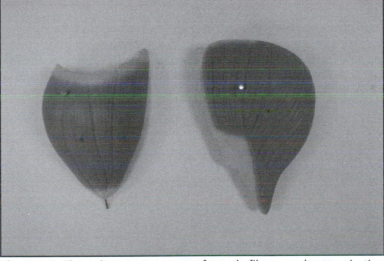

Figure 2-8. The radiate arrangement of muscle fibers, a subcategorization of the parallel fiber arrangement, is depicted here in the deltoid and gluteus maximus muscles. (Reprinted with permission from Carolyn Roller.)

muscle and gluteus maximus muscle, are observed in Figure 2-8. Sphincter muscles are circular and are basically neverending strap muscles that surround openings. Their function is to close an opening when they contract, as in the mouth (Thompson & Floyd, 2004).

Many other terms are also used to describe muscles. Fortunately, most of these are used in the muscle's name and will give clues as to the function, location, size, or other characteristics of the muscle. When identifying a muscle, think about each component of its name. The name itself may indicate the location, action, or other characteristic of the muscle. One such example is the extensor carpi radialis longus. One action of this muscle described in its name is extension. It further designates the location, the wrist (carpi), on the radial side (radialis). Finally, it indicates that more than one muscle exists for this purpose. Because this muscle is the longus, it must have a shorter counterpart, the brevis. If there was not a shorter counterpart, longus would not be part of its name. Nomenclature used to characterize muscle includes descriptions of size, shape, location, action, direction of fibers, number of divisions, points of attachment, or a combination of these. Examples of nomenclature for certain muscles can be found in Table 2-5. Word origins for certain muscle names are listed in Gold Box 2-2.

In order to locate a muscle and know its action, one must know the origin and insertion. The **origin** describes where a muscle begins, or originates. This point is usually proximal, or closer to the trunk or middle of the body, and is often considered to be more stable. The end point for the muscle is termed the **insertion**. The insertion is usually distal or farther away from the trunk and

Table 2-5	Muscle Categorizations
Shape	Rhomboid, trapezius
Size	Teres major, teres minor
Location	Tibialis anterior, latissimus dorsi
Action	Extensor digitorum, supinator
Direction of fibers	Internal oblique, transverse abdominus
Number of divisions	Biceps brachii
Points of attachment	Sternocleidomastoid, coracobrachialis
Action and shape	Pronator quadratus
Action and size	Adductor magnus, extensor carpi radialis longus
Size and location	Vastus lateralis
Shape and location	Serratus anterior, tibialis posterior
Location and attachment	Brachioradialis
Location and number of divisions	Triceps brachii, biceps femoris

Adapted from Thompson, C. W., & Floyd, R. T. (2004). *Manual of structural kinesiology* (15th ed.). Boston, MA: McGraw Hill.

Gold Box 2-2

Word Origins from Latin

Carpus: Or carpi, wrist or pertaining to the wrist.
Magnus: Large, great, denoting a structure of large size.
Teres: Round, smooth, cordlike; as in teres major or pronator teres muscles.
Pollicis: Thumb or first digit of hand.
Quadratus: Square, having four equal sides, denoting the number four.
Rectus: Straight; as in rectus femoris or rectus abdominus.
Sartor: A tailor; as used in the muscle sartorius, which allows us to sit, crossing our legs, in the tailor position.
Serratus: A saw; notched, toothed.

Steadman (1982)

midline of the body and is considered the most movable part. Usually, during muscle activation, the insertion moves toward the origin; however, at times, the origin can move toward the insertion. **Reversal of muscle function** is the terminology used when the insertion is stable and the origin moves toward the insertion (Thompson & Floyd, 2004). Examples include stabilizing the hands during a push-up or elevating and propelling the trunk forward during crutch walking.

Still other terminology describes the general location and function of certain muscle groups. Both the lower and upper extremities have intrinsic and extrinsic muscles. These terms are relative to the ankle or wrist joints. **Intrinsic** muscles originate distal to the joint while **extrinsic** muscles originate proximal to the joint. Some sources define intrinsic muscles as muscles within or acting solely on a specific body part, such as in the hand, and extrinsic muscles as those that originate outside of the body part on which they cause action (Thompson & Floyd, 2004). Intrinsic muscles allow for dexterity, fine movements, and coordination, whereas extrinsic muscles provide for more gross motor skills and strength.

Skeleton

The skeleton is divided into two parts, the axial skeleton and the appendicular skeleton. The skull and trunk comprise the **axial skeleton**. The trunk consists of the vertebral column, ribs, and sternum. The **appendicular skeleton** is composed of the shoulder and pelvic girdles, the upper extremities, and the lower extremities. Most of the long bones of the body are in the appendicular skeleton. Long bones allow for greater range of motion for movement. The surface of bones is not smooth; rather, bones have bumps, depressions, and holes. The bony markings appear wherever tendons, ligaments, and fascia are attached (Moore, 1985). The long bones of the body have many such markings, as several muscles attach to long bones. Table 2-6 identifies a partial listing of bony projections, examples, and their relevance to movement or the formation of decubiti. Openings in bone, such as the obturator foramen, transverse foramen of the cervical vertebrae, or the greater sciatic notch, provide protection to vital structures such as blood vessels and nerves.

Most voluntary movement occurs in the joints of the appendicular skeleton. Joints allow for different amounts of movement depending on the shape of the joint and the number of axes it

Table 2-6	**Examples of Bony Projections**			
	Marking	**Description**	**Example**	**Consideration**
Processes: attachments for tendon, ligament, or fascia; axis for movement or risk for decubiti	Crest	Linear elevation, ridge, narrow	Iliac crest, crest of tibia	Decubitus
	Epicondyle	Rounded projection proximal to condyle	Lateral epicondyle of humerus	Axis for elbow flexion and extension, decubitus
	Process	Any notable projection	Olecranon process	Decubitus
	Spine	Sharp elevation or projection, slender	Anterior superior iliac spine	Axis for hip abduction and adduction; decubitus
	Trochanter	Very large projection, rounded or blunt	Greater trochanter of femur; malleolus	Axis for hip flexion and extension; axis for ankle plantar and dorsi flexion; both—decubitus

Compiled from Moore, K. L. (1985). *Clinically oriented anatomy* (2nd ed.). Baltimore, MD: Williams and Wilkins.; Thompson, C. W., & Floyd, R. T. (2004). *Manual of structural kinesiology* (15th ed.). Boston, MA: McGraw Hill..

rotates around. Joint axes and motions are determined by the planes in which the joint can move. The body is divided into three imaginary planes: the frontal plane, the sagittal plane, and the transverse plane. Each plane has an axis that corresponds to it. The axis is always perpendicular, or at a right angle, to the plane it is associated with. Movement occurs around the axis and is parallel to the plane. Gold Box 2-3 identifies each plane with its alternate name.

Gold Box 2-3

Alternate Names for Planes and Axes

- **Frontal** can be referred to as **coronal**.
- **Transverse** can be referred to as **horizontal**.
- **Sagittal** can be referred to as **anteroposterior**.
- **Vertical** can be referred to as **longitudinal**.

Compiled from Solomon (2009); Thompson & Floyd (2004).

The three planes of the body are depicted in Figures 2-9 and 2-10. Figure 2-9 is an anterior view of the body, while Figure 2-10 is a lateral view. The frontal plane (A) divides the body into anterior and posterior, or front and back sections. The sagittal plane (B) divides the body into left and right sides. The horizontal plane (C) divides the body into upper and lower portions. Movements available in each plane will now be described.

The frontal plane divides the body into anterior and posterior sections. The axis for movement in the frontal plane is called the sagittal axis. Rotation around the sagittal axis, and parallel to the frontal plane, allows for the movements of abduction, adduction, radial deviation, ulnar deviation, and lateral bending. The position of the lower extremities in abduction and the upper extremities in adduction during the beginning stance of a golf swing can be seen in Figure 2-11. The sagittal plane divides the body into left and right sides. The axis for the sagittal plane is termed the frontal axis. Rotation around the frontal axis, and parallel to the sagittal plane, consists of flexion

Figure 2-9. Anterior view of the planes of the body: (A) frontal, (B) sagittal, and (C) horizontal. In this view, the frontal plane appears as the background. (©2003 Jennifer Bridges, PhD. All Rights Reserved. Denoyer.com.)

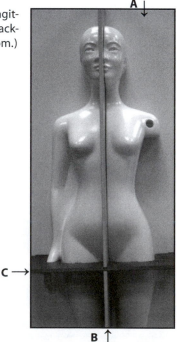

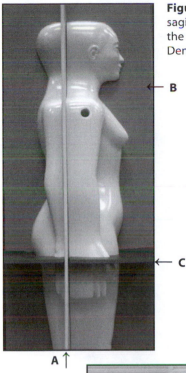

Figure 2-10. Lateral view of the planes of the body: (A) frontal, (B) sagittal, and (C) horizontal. In this view, the sagittal plane appears as the background. (©2003 Jennifer Bridges, PhD. All Rights Reserved. Denoyer.com.)

← B

← C

A ↑

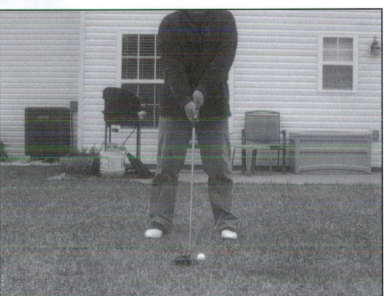

Figure 2-11. Abduction observed in lower extremities; adduction demonstrated in upper extremities during golf stance. (Reprinted with permission of Jeremy Keough.)

and extension. Some sources identify hyperextension in addition to extension, which would also occur in the sagittal plane. Gold Box 2-4 discusses hyperextension. A functional example of flexion, a child exiting a toy car, can be seen in Figure 2-12, whereas extension is seen in Figure 2-13. Extension is observed in the neck, trunk, hips, knees, and elbows of the girl in Figure 2-13.

Gold Box 2-4

Extension or Hyperextension?

Roughly half of the available sources use the term *hyperextension* to describe a posterior movement from the anatomical position. The other half of the available sources use the term *hyperextension* to denote movement in the direction of extension that is beyond normal limits. While a joint may normally be able to move through its available range of motion past the starting position in extension, such as the shoulder joint, this movement may be abnormal for other joints. MCP hyperextension may be an example when the MCP joint is hyperextended past the starting position due to a stretch of the involved body structures.

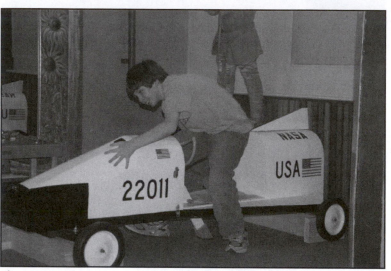

Figure 2-12. Flexion observed in the neck, trunk, hips, knees, ankles, and left elbow of this boy. (Reprinted with permission from Angela Grussing.)

Figure 2-13. Extension observed in the neck, trunk, hips, knees, and elbows of this girl. (Reprinted with permission from Angela Grussing.)

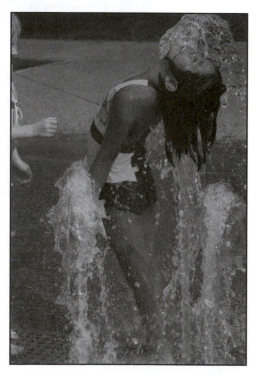

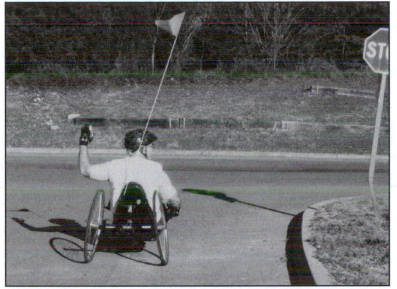

Figure 2-14. External rotation observed in the left arm, which is demonstrating the traditional hand signal for a right turn.

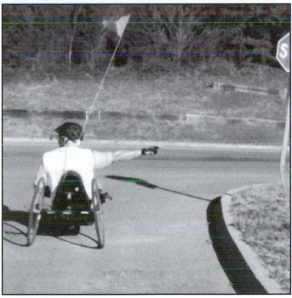

Figure 2-15. Abduction of the right arm, as seen in the more commonly used right hand turn signal.

The horizontal plane divides the body into upper and lower portions. The axis for movement in the horizontal plane is the vertical axis. The movements about this axis are termed *internal* or *medial rotation, external* or *lateral rotation, rotation to the right or left, horizontal abduction* and *adduction, supination,* and *pronation.* Internal rotation and external rotation are depicted in the hand signals used by the competitive hand cyclist in the above pictures. The traditional signal for a right hand turn, in Figure 2-14, incorporates external rotation. This movement or signal originated for vehicle drivers who could not reach across the car to point out of the passenger window toward the right. The cyclist felt it important for the reader to know that simply pointing to the right with the right hand, as seen in Figure 2-15, is the signal more commonly used by cyclists today. The signal to slow down or stop uses internal rotation as in Figure 2-16. Figure 2-17 portrays the motion of horizontal abduction with the right arm as the arm pulls the arrow back on a bow. The left arm remains in a neutral position between horizontal abduction and horizontal adduction. Supination is observed in the left hand in Figure 2-18, while pronation is observed in the right hand during the functional activity of removing cookies from a pan. Descriptions and examples of movement can be found in Table 2-7.

Figure 2-16. Internal rotation observed in the left arm, which is demonstrating the hand signal for stop or slow down.

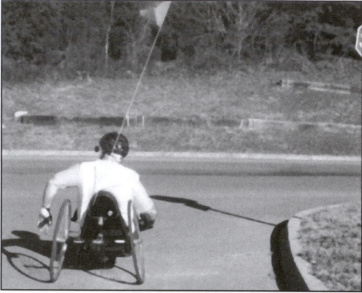

Figure 2-17. Horizontal abduction of the right arm is demonstrated in the picture. As the girl pulls the arrow backwards, her arm moves in the direction of horizontal abduction. The legs are in abduction. (Reprinted with permission from Riley Sain.)

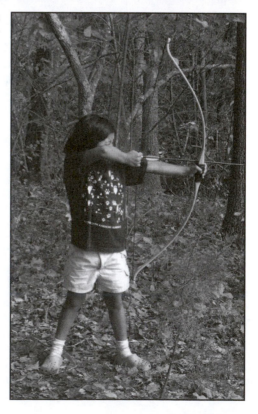

In addition to the degrees of freedom, the shape or type of the joint also helps to determine the movements available. Joint types include **ball and socket**, **hinge**, **saddle**, **pivot**, **gliding**, and **condyloid**. These are descriptive terms for synovial joints. Table 2-8 gives examples of each joint type in addition to the degrees of freedom available, planes, axes, and typical movements.

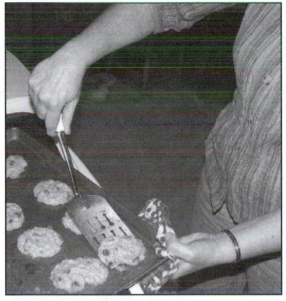

Figure 2-18. The left hand is held in supination as it stabilizes the cookie tray while the right hand is postured in pronation as it holds the spatula to remove the cookies.

Table 2-7	Movement Definitions and Examples	
Movement	**Definition**	**Example**
Abduction	Lateral movement away from midline or center of body	Arm and leg position in upward stroke of jumping jack exercise
Adduction	Medial movement toward midline or center of body; opposite of abduction	Normal resting position while seated or standing of arms at side of body
Flexion	Bending of joint; usually reduces joint angle; two bones moving closer together	Occurs at elbow when bringing fork to mouth
Extension	Joint angle increases, straightening; opposite of flexion	Knee position in standing
Circumduction	Combination of flexion, extension, abduction, and adduction leading to circular motion	Stirring or churning a large vat of apple butter or molasses
Lateral (external) rotation	Rotary movement around vertical axis of bone away from midline of body	Combing back of head, fastening necklace behind neck
Medial (internal) rotation	Rotary movement around vertical axis of bone toward midline of body; opposite of lateral rotation	Reaching into pants pocket
Pronation	Position of forearm when palm is facing down	Position of hands on computer keyboard when typing

(continued)

Table 2-7	Terms Describing General Movement (*continued*)	
Supination	Position of forearm when palm is facing up; opposite of pronation	Position of hand when holding a handful of small candies and fingers are open, not fisted
Horizontal abduction	Humerus positioned in horizontal plane, arm raised to 90 degrees, with movement away from midline and toward back of body	Movement of arm while pulling the string back on a bow to shoot the arrow
Horizontal adduction	Humerus positioned in horizontal plane, arm raised to 90 degrees, with movement toward midline and front of body; opposite of horizontal abduction	When in driver's seat, reaching across chest with right arm to reach shoulder belt
Lateral flexion (side bending)	Movement of head, neck, or trunk laterally away from midline or center of body; abduction of the spine	Leaning over sideways while seated to pick something up off of the floor

Adapted from Solomon, E. P. (2009). *Introduction to human anatomy and physiology.* St. Louis, MO: Saunders Elsevier.; Thompson, C. W., & Floyd, R. T. (2004). *Manual of structural kinesiology* (15th ed.). Boston, MA: McGraw Hill.

Table 2-8	Characteristics of Synovial Joint Types				
Type of Joint	Joint Example	Degrees of Freedom	Plane(s)	Axis and Axes	Movement Examples
Ball and socket	Shoulder and hip joints	3 Triaxial	Frontal	Sagittal	Hip abduction, adduction
			Sagittal	Frontal	Hip flexion, extension
			Horizontal	Vertical	Hip internal and external rotation
Hinge	Elbow and knee joint	1 Uniaxial	Sagittal	Frontal	Elbow flexion, extension
Saddle	Thumb carpometacarpal joint	2+ Bi- or multiaxial	Sagittal	Frontal	Flexion, extension
			Frontal	Sagittal	Abduction, adduction
			Multi	Multi	Opposition
Pivot	Radioulnar joint; atlantoaxial	1 Uniaxial	Horizontal	Vertical	Supination, pronation neck rotation
Gliding	Carpal bones	Variable	Variable	Variable	Accessory motions
Condyloid	Metacarpophalangeal joints 2 through 5	2 Biaxial	Frontal	Sagittal	Abduction, adduction
			Sagittal	Frontal	Flexion, extension of the lesser digits

Adapted from Gench, B. E., Hionson, M. M., & Harvey, P. T. (1999). *Anatomical kinesiology.* Dubuque, IA: Eddie Bowers Publishing, Inc.; Thompson, C. W., & Floyd, R. T. (2004). *Manual of structural kinesiology* (15th ed.). Boston, MA: McGraw Hill.

Table 2-9	**Anatomical Directional Terminology**
Term (alternate name in parenthesis)	**Orientation or Description**
Anterior (ventral)	Toward the front of the body, toward the belly
Posterior (dorsal)	Toward the back of the body or buttocks, relating to the back
Superior (cephalic)	Toward the head, upward, higher than another structure
Inferior (caudal)	Toward the feet, downward from another body part, below in relationship to another structure
Medial (internal)	Toward the middle of the body or midline
Lateral (external)	Toward the sides of the body, away from the midline, on or to the side
Proximal	Toward or closer to the attachment to the trunk or origin, nearer to the center of the body
Distal	Away from or further from the midline of the body or attachment to the trunk, farther from the point of reference or origin
Superficial	Toward the surface of the body, used to describe relative depth of muscles or other tissue
Deep	Toward the inside of or within the body, below the surface
Contralateral	Opposite sides of body, right versus left
Ipsilateral	On the same side of the body; right arm and right leg are ipsilateral to each other
Prone	Lying on stomach in a face-down position
Supine	Lying on back in a face-up position

Adapted from Solomon, E. P. (2009). *Introduction to human anatomy and physiology.* St. Louis, MO: Saunders Elsevier.; Thompson, C. W., & Floyd, R. T. (2004). *Manual of structural kinesiology* (15th ed.). Boston, MA: McGraw Hill.

When describing movement, it is important to be able to give an accurate description of what actions are observed. Reference positions and anatomical directional terms are used in order to do this effectively and in a manner that others will understand. Two reference positions that may be used to describe movement and illustrate planes are the anatomical position and fundamental position. The **anatomical position** is the reference position most widely used and is also the reference position for the definitions used in this text. For both reference positions, the subject is standing in an upright posture, eyes looking forward, feet parallel with toes pointed forward, and the arms slightly abducted at the side of the body. In the anatomical position, the palms are facing forward. If the palms face the side of the body, the person is in the **fundamental position** (Solomon, 2009). Commonly used anatomical directional terminology can be found in Table 2-9.

It should now be evident that functional movement requires complex interactions of multiple body systems, including the nervous, skeletal, and muscular systems as well as major organ systems. Every component or system has an effect on one another and contributes to the overall function of the body or lack thereof (Lieber & Bodine-Fowler, 1993). Only through the synchronization of the body's anatomical systems and structures can we use functional movement patterns in our daily lives (Whiting & Rugg, 2006).

APPLICATIONS

The following activities will help you apply knowledge of the functions and structures of body systems to real-life situations. Activities can be completed individually or in a small group to enhance learning.

1. **Muscle Contractions:** The purpose of this task is to help you better understand the need for both types of contractions, concentric and eccentric, and how they work together. The area of the body where the muscles contract is listed for you. The contraction for each muscle group might be a different type. First, determine the type of contraction used while performing the activity listed. Next, hypothesize as to what would happen if the muscle was not contracting in the manner identified. Complete the grid in Table 2-10. In all of the examples using eccentric contractions, what is the one common force or resistance acting on the muscle?

2. **Determining Joint Types:** The purpose of this application is to help the reader identify types of joints in common objects to better understand how similar joints in the body function. The type of joint will determine, to some extent, the amount and type of movement allowed. Recall that the types of joints include ball and socket, hinge, saddle, pivot, gliding, and condyloid. Not all types are easily found in the environment. Complete Table 2-11.

3. **Planes and Axes:** The purpose of this application is to enable the reader to better understand the planes of motion and the axes associated with them. Fill in the grid in Table 2-12 according to the example given.

4. **Bony Landmarks:** Certain bony landmarks are identified in therapy for measuring range of motion. Other bony landmarks are areas of concern because decubiti can form over them. For these reasons, it is important for the practitioner to be able to find these landmarks. Use an anatomy book for reference, if needed. Working with a partner, find the following bony landmarks by palpating gently:
   4.1. Lateral malleolus
   4.2. Head of the fibula
   4.3. Lateral epicondyle of humerus

Table 2-10	Muscle Contractions: Concentric or Eccentric		
Movement	Muscle Group Used	Type of Contraction	Why Is This Contraction Needed?
Putting book on table	Elbow flexors	Eccentric concentric	Book would smash through table
	Finger flexors		You would lose grasp and drop book
Lowering buttocks to sit on chair	Quadriceps		
Raising hand in class	Shoulder flexors		
Stepping down to the next stair with right leg	Left quadriceps		
While seated, raising leg to tie shoe	Quadriceps		
Your example here			

Table 2-11	Types of Joints in Common Objects		
Object	Joint Type	Movements Allowed	Degrees of Freedom
Door	Hinge	Open and close or back and forth	One
Computer mouse—type with ball in base			
Sliding side door on van			
Standard stick shift on car			
Your example here			

Table 2-12	Planes and Axes Application		
Functional Activity	Joint Movements	Plane of Motion	Axes of Motion
Walking up stairs	Hip flexion	Sagittal	Frontal
	Knee flexion	Sagittal	Frontal
Performing jumping jacks	Shoulder _____	_____	_____
	Hip _____	_____	_____
While driving, turning head to look over shoulder before merging	Neck _____	_____	_____
	Trunk _____	_____	_____
Washing hair	Shoulder _____,	_____	_____
	_____,	Frontal	_____
	_____	Horizontal	_____
	Wrist _____,	_____	_____
	Wrist ulnar and radial deviation	_____	Vertical
Sitting cross legged on the floor	Hip _____,	_____	_____
	_____,	_____	_____
	_____	_____	
Your example here			

4.4. Greater trochanter

4.5. Anterior superior iliac spine

4.6. Styloid process of ulna

5. **Other Body Systems:** The purpose of the following activities is to allow for a greater understanding of how other body systems affect movement. Although a person may not be able to know what it is like to have a certain disease or disability unless that person truly has it, a better understanding can be developed through simulation. The following activities will try to simulate movement as experienced with a decrease in various body systems. Follow the steps listed next:

5.1.   Select an activity of your choice, such as walking, brushing hair, or eating a snack.

5.2.   Select one of the body system simulations listed below.

5.3.   Equip yourself with the decreased function listed.

5.4.   Perform your selected activity.

5.5.   For each activity/simulation, answer the questions listed at the end.

Potential simulations for body system dysfunction include the following:

- Occlude vision using a blindfold.
- Inhibit proprioceptive and tactile feedback by wearing gloves and donning boots that are several sizes too big. Stuff the boots with newspaper or extra layers of socks.
- Spin in a circle several times to alter your vestibular system.
- Wear earmuffs or sound-eliminating headphones to occlude hearing.

Answer these questions:

A. Could you perform the task? Could you complete your entire day with this "disability"? What overall effect would this have on your day?

B. Was the activity harder to perform? If so, how?

C. Did it take longer to perform? Why?

D. Were you less accurate in your movements? Describe how. Why do you think this happened?

E. Did you move in a different manner than usual? Why? Did you make any accommodations to your usual way of doing this? If so, what were they?

REFERENCES

Alexander, R. M. (1992). *Exploring biomechanics in animals.* New York, NY: Scientific American Library.

American Occupational Therapy Association. (2008). Occupational therapy practice framework: Domain and process (2nd ed.). *American Journal of Occupational Therapy, 62*, 625–683.

Angevine, J. B., & Cotman, C. W. (1981). *Principles of neuroanatomy.* New York, NY: Oxford University Press, Inc.

Cronin, A., & Mandich, M. (2005). *Human development and performance throughout the lifespan.* Clifton Park, NY: Thomson Delmar Learning.

Farber, S. D. (1982). *Neurorehabilitation: A multisensory approach.* Philadelphia, PA: W. B. Saunders.

Fisher, B., & Yakura, J. (1993). Movement analysis: A different perspective. *Orthopaedic Physical Therapy Clinics of North America*, 1-14.

Gench, B. E., Hionson, M. M., & Harvey, P. T. (1999). *Anatomical kinesiology.* Dubuque, IA: Eddie Bowers Publishing, Inc.

Hall, S. (1999). Basic biomechanics (3rd ed.). Boston, MA: WCB/McGraw-Hill.

Kiernan, J. A. (2009). *Barr's the human nervous system: An anatomical viewpoint* (9th ed.). Baltimore, MD: Lippincott, Williams, and Wilkins.

Lieber, R. L., & Bodine-Fowler, S. C. (1993). Skeletal muscle mechanics: Implications for rehabilitation. *Physical Therapy, 73(12).*

Moore, K. L. (1985). *Clinically oriented anatomy* (2nd ed.). Baltimore, MD: Williams and Wilkins.

Solomon, E. P. (2009). *Introduction to human anatomy and physiology.* St. Louis, MO: Saunders Elsevier.

Steadman, T. (1982). *Steadman's Medical Dictionary* (24th ed.). Baltimore, MD: Williams and Wilkins.

Thompson, C. W., & Floyd, R. T. (2004). *Manual of structural kinesiology* (15th ed.). Boston, MA: McGraw Hill.

Whiting, W. C., & Rugg, S. (2006). *Dynatomy: Dynamic human anatomy.* Champaign, IL: Human Kinetics.

World Health Organization. (2001). *International classification of functioning, disability and health* (ICF). Geneva, Switzerland: Author.

chapter 3

Factors Influencing Movement

Susan J. Sain, MS, OTR/L, FAOTA

People live and exist in relation to their environment and within the context of their lives. Thus, it stands to reason that context and environment can have a significant impact on function and functional movement. Modifying or changing the context or environment may enhance a client's ability to participate in occupations of choice. Both the World Health Organization (WHO) *International Classification of Functioning and Disability* (ICF) and the *Occupational Therapy Practice Framework, 2nd Edition* (OTPF-2) discuss the impact of contextual and environmental factors on function and disability. The WHO (2001) essentially states that a client's disability resides within the society, and not within the individual. In other words, a client with a disabling condition or diagnosis is hindered by societal norms, expectations, environmental accessibility, and other factors. The client with a diagnosis is not disabled by the actual medical condition. In this sense, if no stereotypes or stigmas existed and universal design was widely accepted, then an individual with a medical disability should be able to function independently in all aspects of society.

The ICF lists two groups of contextual factors: personal and environmental. Within the ICF, personal factors are considered intrinsic, or internal to the person, while environmental factors are considered extrinsic, or external to the individual. The key is how these factors impact the person's ability to function by either facilitating or hindering performance. The OTPF-2 lists cultural, personal, physical, social, temporal, and virtual aspects as factors of the context and environment. As in the ICF, environment refers to external situations. However, environment includes both physical and social aspects in the OTPF-2. Gold Box 3-1 defines context and environment as presented in the OTPF-2. This chapter will follow the definitions of the OTPF-2 as they relate to context and environment.

CONTEXTUAL AND ENVIRONMENTAL FACTORS

Contextual Factors

The domain of context and environment in the OTPF-2 is divided into six areas. Context includes a cluster of four inter-related variables that may exist both within the individual or external to the individual. This cluster of interconnected perspectives includes all of the cultural, personal, temporal, and virtual aspects of a person's life (American Occupational Therapy Association, 2008). The domain subsection of environment, as stated earlier, includes both social and physical aspects pertaining to the overall environment of the individual.

Keough, J. L., Sain, S. J., Roller, C. L.
Kinesiology for the Occupational Therapy Assistant:
Essential Components of Function and Movement (pp. 55-84).

Gold Box 3-1

Context: "…a variety of interrelated conditions that are within and surrounding the client. Contexts as described in the OTPF are cultural, personal, temporal, and virtual."

Environment: "…external physical and social environments that surround the client and in which the client's daily life occupations occur."

Physical environment: "…natural and built nonhuman environment and all objects in them."

Social environment: "…the presence, relationships, and expectations of persons, groups, and organizations with whom the client has contact."

AOTA (2008, p. 642)

The context of culture incorporates values, ideas, behaviors, language, traditions, daily practices, expectations, and attitudes adhered to by a certain group of people. These tend to be passed down from one generation to the next. Culture defines what is acceptable to a certain society. Culture shapes how many things are done. It must be noted that not all members of a certain culture will adhere to the expectations of their culture in the same manner. A person must refrain from stereotyping people based on cultural norms; however, knowledge of generalizations regarding certain cultural norms may help practitioners to provide care that is more meaningful to the client. A stereotype is to "repeat without variation" (*Merriam-Webster Online Dictionary*, 2010). As such, a stereotype is limiting, often derogatory, and usually ends any type of meaningful communication. On the other hand, a generalization serves as a place to begin discussion with a client. A generalization may include common assumptions related to a particular culture, but the person holding the assumption does not force this trait or attribute on all people within that cultural group.

For example, your client is an elderly Hispanic woman receiving inpatient occupational therapy (OT). A generalization about Latin American families is that the extended family, including elders, is very important. Knowing this generalization about family values can guide discussion related to discharge planning for your elderly client. If, on the other hand, based on the generalization, you automatically assume the client will return home and be cared for by family members, that is a stereotype. The generalization leads to discussion sensitive to perceived cultural standards while the stereotype assumes that all people of a given culture will act the same way all the time. The practitioner should not simply assume that he or she knows the cultural norms for a certain group of people, nor assume that these norms have value for a particular client. Behaving in this way would be stereotyping. Additionally, cultural norms may differ from one socioeconomic group to another, even within the same cultural group. Knowledge of cultural norms can lead to dialogue and greater understanding of the individual and how the person internalizes that cultural norm. This information can then be used to aid communication, select therapeutic activities, and tailor an intervention program best suited for the particular client. In this way, incorporating the cultural context makes the intervention more meaningful to the client.

One example of a functional activity affected by cultural standards is mealtime. Many countries in Europe and North, Central, and South America use silverware to eat. Most Asian countries, however, use chopsticks. In Morocco and India, the first three fingers on the right hand are used for eating. All of these forms of eating require different use of the fingers and associated joints and muscles. The time of the meal also varies greatly. In Spain and several Latin American countries, the main meal is eaten at about 2 p.m. In many of these countries, businesses and schools close for 2 to 4 hours during the middle of the day to allow time to eat a large meal and rest afterwards. The evening meal is often eaten at about 10 or 11 p.m., much later than bedtime for most children from the United States! In Japan, it is customary to sit on cushions on the floor while eating at a low table. Imagine how differently this custom may impact the elderly population with limited mobility or a person in a wheelchair as compared to another custom. For these populations, the standard in the United States of sitting on a chair at a higher table might prove easier. This one activity of daily living, eating, and the skills and movements necessary to accomplish this task vary greatly from one cultural group to another.

Cultural standards can also impact child development. For example, in Guatemala, it is not uncommon for women who sell at market to carry infants and young children in a sling near their body or contain them in a box that they cannot climb out of while the women work. These practices keep the child safe and from wandering away. Sometimes, these children are referred to as "box babies." These children often exhibit delays in walking and crawling, primarily due to lack of experience. When given the opportunity, they usually master these gross motor skills quickly. In this situation, it is both the culture and the environment that are influencing movement. Many developmental markers that are used in the United States are not commonly used elsewhere. Examples include the pediatrician encouraging a child to play pat-a-cake or asking an older child to draw a house. Many times, it is the foreign infant's first exposure to the game of pat-a-cake; therefore, the game is not repeated or imitated. This should not be recorded as a lack of learning, knowledge, or ability on the child's part. Rather, it may simply be a lack of experience or exposure. Similarly, during the draw-a-house activity, children who have been living in refugee camps will draw a tent, not a house. These children may have never lived in a house before coming to this country. Depending on the assessment instrument used, a tent drawing might not be scored as passing or age appropriate. These examples of cultural norms indicate how culture may influence behavior, affect movement, guide communication, and have an impact on what is acceptable to an individual. OT goals and intervention must reflect the cultural context of the client in order to be of most benefit and interest to the client.

Personal context includes primarily internal factors such as age, gender, intelligence, temperament, learning style, and personality. Most of the internal personal factors cannot be modified or changed. Other factors that are less intrinsic to the individual may include, but are not limited to, socioeconomic status and educational level. These factors may be modified during one's lifetime. Personal contextual factors can affect a person's motivation to move or determine the selection of movement activities. Activity patterns may change over the lifespan, with younger people tending to choose activities that require more energy expenditure, such as soccer. An older individual may select a less aggressive sport, perhaps golf. However, golf is a relatively expensive sport, so the person in a lower socioeconomic group may not be able to participate, even if interested. Thus, one can see that the personal context does indeed impact a person's ability and opportunity to function.

The third contextual variable listed is the temporal context. According to the OTPF-2, the "temporal context includes stages of life, time of day or year, duration, rhythm of activity, or history" (AOTA, 2008, p. 642). Rhythmicity can also refer to the rhythm or routine timing of basic physiologic functions such as eating, sleeping, and voiding (Cronin & Mandich, 2005). Circadian rhythm, or a person's sleep-wake cycle, may also be included here. Some other factors that may be included are sequence of activity, synchronization of movements for an activity, or synchronization of the activity itself. Also, normative life experiences are included, such as beginning kindergarten or getting married. The activity and movement requirements for each of these temporal situations are different. How each person interprets and responds to a temporal contextual factor is unique to that individual. Consider the life stage referred to as the "empty nest." Some people celebrate this return to prior activities and patterns and enjoy the newly found freedom. For other people, this stage in life can initiate a loss of role identity, a loss of feelings of worth, too much free time, and a feeling of general sadness. Another example relates to sequencing of activities. The sequence you use to brush your teeth may be different from your classmate's. One person might wet the toothbrush and then apply toothpaste, whereas the other person may put the toothpaste on first, then wet the toothbrush and toothpaste. Neither sequence is better than the other; they both work equally well. Although temporal context may affect involvement in movement and activity, it does not dictate any specific way of accomplishing these tasks.

The final contextual variable listed is the virtual environment. The virtual environment can be described as one that occurs in the absence of physical contact. In most situations, the virtual environment refers to some type of communication or interaction between two or more individuals; however, the interaction could be solely between an individual and an electronic system. There are many forms of virtual environment which include, but are not limited to, computers; airway transmissions for hand-held electronic devices; television, radio, and satellite transmissions; home environmental control systems; and video courses or conferencing.

The use of the virtual context is almost limitless and can be incorporated in many areas of occupation, such as play, work, leisure, education, and health care (Cronin & Mandich, 2005). Telemedicine, or the more recent development of telehealth, represents one way that health care is becoming more virtual. Telemedicine focuses more on treatment, whereas telehealth focuses on prevention as well. These systems can monitor the status of the client in his or her own home. So, whether our clients are interested in the virtual world or not, it is encroaching on their lives! The virtual context requires different skills and knowledge than the real environment. For some individuals, the virtual environment has greatly expanded the ability to interact with others in society.

The four contextual factors, which are cultural, personal, temporal, and virtual, are inter-related with one another. Accordingly, each area impacts another. For example, within the *virtual* environment of text messaging, the *temporal* concept changes from that used with other forms of communication. People tend to reply immediately to a text message whereas they may return a phone call, e-mail, or letter hours or even days later. Considering the *personal* context, younger people tend to text more than those in retirement years. Additionally, *cultural* standards are different in the virtual realm. Behavior standards related to what is acceptable are often altered. Different behaviors are considered appropriate or acceptable in the virtual context, such as texting using abbreviations and acronyms, whereas these would not be acceptable in a real environment, such as an English composition class. A person's engagement in any occupation is affected by these factors. Each factor has the potential to aid or hinder movement and involvement in occupation. Therefore, modifying or changing one factor may enhance or interfere with occupational performance overall. Not only are the four factors of context inter-related with each other, they are also intertwined with environmental factors.

Environmental Factors

According to the OTPF-2, engagement in an occupation occurs in an environment. That environment is embedded in, and thus affected by, the four contexts discussed above. The environment is divided into the categories of social environment and physical environment (AOTA, 2008). This division is consistent with the philosophy of the WHO, which states that health, function, and participation are also based on external factors and are not solely based on factors within the individual. The ICF definition of environment includes the physical, social, and attitudinal surroundings in which people carry out their lives. Items or categories included in the classification of environmental factors within the ICF are products, technology, natural and human-made features of the environment, attitudes of people, services, systems, and policies (WHO, 2001). Focus will be on the social and physical environment classifications put forth in the OTPF-2. While studying these environmental variables, keep in mind that many of them can be modified by the OT practitioner to enhance functional movement. Additionally, a client's needs and movement demands will change depending on the environment and the context in which the client is performing the task. In other words, one functional movement pattern or option is not sufficient; clients will need a range of movement options to meet the ever changing conditions encountered daily.

The social environment consists of things like relationships, expectations, fads, and organized sports. The social aspect may include other people as well as animals. The expectations of other people with whom the client interacts comprise yet another aspect of the social environment. As indicated in the ICF, attitude as an environmental factor incorporates consequences of social interactions that affect the person individually and on the societal level (WHO, 2001). Societal level consequences may include limiting factors, such as stereotypes, or supportive factors, such as legislation mandating that people with differing abilities are treated equally. Fads related to dress can impact what a person wears. Different sport groups may imply different behavioral norms. For example, those playing rugby are often considered rough and crude as compared to other athletes. Real or perceived expectations of other people greatly impact a person's choice of, and engagement in, an occupation. This is often seen in parents' desires regarding their children's employment or educational occupations. For example, children may be expected to work in the family business, regardless of what the child wants. Some occupations are chosen because they encourage interaction with the social environment, such as being in a choir. Other occupations are chosen because they limit the social interactions required, e.g. reading. As with the contextual factors, the social environment may enhance or impede engagement in occupation. When considering involvement in occupation, the social environment must be taken into account.

The physical environment can include the built or man made environment and natural phenomena. Humans can impact the environment in many ways. One of these is the *built or man-made physical environment,* which includes buildings, roads, bridges, communication towers, flood walls, and numerous other structures. In addition, human impact can cause widespread changes in the environment that affect daily lives. Some examples include pollution, environmental disasters, and war. The *natural physical environment* includes things such as terrain, bodies of water, sensory aspects including climate, scents, plants and animals, and forces, such as gravity and friction. Some of these forces and their relationship to motion have been described by Sir Isaac Newton. Newton's three laws of motion will be described as they impact functional movement, including how these concepts can be applied to OT. Other factors related to gravity, the center of gravity in the body or in an object, and stability against competing forces will also be discussed in this chapter. Other natural phenomena can also alter the environment, often in negative ways, causing significant and lasting change that affects human performance and engagement in occupation. Some examples include hurricanes, earthquakes, mudslides, and excessive or insufficient rainfall. The impacts of these natural occurrences are beyond the scope of this text.

The *built or man-made environment* can have a significant impact on an individual's ability for independent engagement in occupation. Structures, including buildings and roads, that are properly designed and adhere to the laws related to accessibility can enable engagement in occupation and increase functional mobility. On the other hand, structures that are not adequately constructed can have a huge negative impact on function. Accessibility is regarded as a beginning point when considering impact on function. A building or bathroom can be accessible but not functional. Consider the bathroom that is large enough for a wheelchair, has grab bars for transfers, and has a door that is easy to maneuver.

What could hinder independent functioning? Perhaps the toilet paper dispenser is out of reach once the person has transferred to the commode. This is a common occurrence impairing the individual's use of the bathroom. The ability of the person to interact with the environment and independently use common features, such as a toilet paper dispenser, is part of a more comprehensive approach named **negotiability**. Negotiability implies that the built environment is also designed so that features such as doors, household appliances, light switches, and sinks are usable by everyone. Negotiability is related to the concept of universal design. The intent of universal design is to simplify life for all people, regardless of age or ability, by making all environments (built, social, print, and virtual) usable by as many people as possible (Center for Universal Design, 2008). Universal design is more valuable and cost effective if items are initially designed and constructed in a way that is usable for the most people without later having to make adaptations. The concept of universal design has been applied to many areas in addition to the construction of buildings. One such example is a professor providing handouts electronically. In this way, a student with visual deficits can independently and privately enlarge the print for enhanced personal use. Computerized lecture handouts could also benefit the student who has problems with handwriting, spelling, or grammar. If keyboarding is more efficient for this student, notes can be taken electronically with the automatic spell and grammar check activated. It may also benefit the student who has no particular physical deficits but would prefer to access notes from a home computer late at night. When working with clients who have movement impairments or who are not engaging in their occupations of choice, the OT practitioner needs to assess the man-made environmental features to determine what, if anything, is impeding function. Often, modifying the built physical environment will increase engagement and enhance functional movement. Accessibility, negotiability, and universal design are defined in Gold Box 3-2, and examples of each, related to a specific condition, are given in Table 3-1.

The *natural physical environment* can also affect function in many ways. Geographic terrain can impair or enhance movement. It is easier to walk, ride a bike, propel a wheelchair, or rollerblade on a hard, smooth, flat, even surface than on an uneven, rough, steep terrain strewn with rocks. Climate, especially heat and humidity levels, can decrease function in people of all abilities. For a person with cardiovascular and respiratory problems, increases in temperature and humidity can constitute a significant health risk. For the generally healthy individual, these same excesses can decrease endurance and enjoyment of an activity. Sensory aspects including aromas, plants, and animals may pose a problem for people with allergies or asthma while for other individuals these sensory qualities may enhance the experience. Perhaps of more importance to the study of

---

Gold Box 3-2

Accessibility: ". . .removing barriers that prevent people with activity limitations from the use of services, products, and information. . ." (Cronin & Mandich, 2005, p. 351).

Negotiability: ". . .the ability to access a feature of the environment and use it for its intended purpose in a manner acceptable to the person" (Cronin & Mandich, 2005, p. 351).

Universal Design: "Universal design is the design of products and environments to be usable by all people, to the greatest extent possible, without the need for adaptation or specialized design" (Mace, 2008).

Table 3-1	Definitions and Examples of Accessibility, Negotiability, and Universal Design		
	Accessibility	Negotiability	Universal Design
Wheelchair use in home	Ramps, elevators, grab bars	Automatic doors, lower light switches	Original construction with 17" high toilet (customary is 14" to 15"), curbless showers, stepless entrances; *flexibility, ease of use*
Severe visual impairments in academics	Braille, white cane, seeing eye dog	No clutter in hallways, sound notification crosswalks	*Varied and flexible* means of attending, teaching, engaging students, testing
Weak grasp, mealtime	Adapted utensils, containers opened by others, pre-cut food	Lightweight utensils with easy-grip handles, lightweight glasses or use of straw to drink	In this situation, universal design principles are similar to examples in negotiability

kinesiology and movement is an examination of the various forces in the natural environment that impact movement. Forces in nature can produce motion, stop motion, or modify motion. Additionally, once something is in motion, force can increase or decrease the speed of the motion or change the direction of the motion (Luttgens & Hamilton, 1997). A force can either produce a push, also termed *compression*, or a pull, also called *tension*, on an object. When both of these force types are balanced, the object is said to be in equilibrium. Movement occurs when the forces are not balanced or are not in equilibrium (Smith, Weiss, & Lehmkuhl, 1996). Newton developed his laws of motion while studying various natural forces.

In order to fully appreciate Newton's laws of motion, it is helpful to first have a basic understanding of some of the forces at work in nature that affect one's ability to move. Force can be generated from internal or external sources. The most common internal force is the force produced by muscles. Muscular force is discussed in other chapters of this text. External forces include fluid forces such as wind or water resistance, contact forces including friction and normal reaction, and gravity. These primary forces can in turn lead to three secondary forces acting on the body. The first secondary force is joint compression, while the second is joint distraction. The third secondary force is pressure on body surfaces (Luttgens & Hamilton, 1997; Smith et al.,1996). Primary forces will be presented first.

The first external force listed, fluid resistance, includes air and liquids, such as water. The dynamic forces of water and air are both subject to the same laws and principles. These are all forms of resistance and include buoyancy, drag, and lift. **Buoyancy** is commonly considered a phenomenon of water and is defined as an upward force equal to the weight of the displaced liquid. A body displaces air. Therefore, this principle is also applicable, albeit the buoyancy of air has a much smaller impact on movement. Due to the increased buoyancy in water relative to air, water can support a body more easily than air. For example, a client whose muscles are not strong enough to overcome the effects of gravity may be able to perform graded underwater exercises to increase strength. OT practitioners may also use the medium of water to unload weight from painful joints, such as occurs with arthritis, in order to allow the client to experience pain-free range of motion or other exercises. However, due to the increased **drag**, or resistance to forward motion, of water over air, water exercise can also be used to increase resistance. Water is considered to provide more drag or resistance than air, so increasing the speed of a movement in water will make the movement more difficult to complete, and it will require more energy expenditure. Additionally, adding an object with a large surface area, such as a paddle, will cause increased drag or resistance as it moves through the water. The final principle, **lift**, refers to a change in fluid pressure as a result of differences in air or liquid flow velocities around an object. Lift is produced when flow over one side of the object is faster than the flow over the opposite side of the same object. Lift acts perpendicular to the direction of fluid flow and is best exemplified in the ability of heavy planes to remain in the air, as described in the Bernoulli Principle (Luttgens & Hamilton, 1997). Drag and lift can only occur if there is velocity occurring either in the object or in the fluid. The greater the velocity, the greater the effects of drag and lift.

These various effects—buoyancy, drag, and lift—can be felt if you place your hand out of a car window while the car is in motion. If your hand is perpendicular to the ground, you experience drag; pressure is felt on the surface of the hand facing the front of the car, and turbulence is felt on the opposite side. Streamlining reduces drag, allowing for easier and faster movement through the fluid. If you gradually lower your hand toward a position parallel to the ground, the drag decreases as the contact surface area lessens, and less pressure is felt on the hand. When the hand is parallel to the ground, you experience much less drag or resistance because the surface area of your fingertips is much less than that of the palm of your hand. However, before your hand reaches the parallel-to-the-ground position and is tilted with the fingers slightly upward, you will feel lift—the air flow is faster under your fingers and thus tends to push them upward, the effect of lift. Because fluid forces have a greater impact on movement as velocity increases, or when the body is in water, they present less of an impact on daily occupations than do the other forms of force. Contact forces, such as normal reaction and friction, have a greater impact on functional movement and are easier to manipulate in daily life activities.

The second external force listed is contact force and occurs when one object comes in contact with another object, creating force between the objects. Categories of contact force include normal reaction and friction. In normal reaction, each object must contact the other with the same magnitude or amount of force. Normal reaction is related to the idea that forces must be paired and opposite to each other. The two opposing forces are sometimes called interaction pairs or action-reaction forces. Without these interaction pairs, there would be no motion. A child hanging from a jungle gym pulls down on the equipment at the same time and with the same force as the equipment pushes back up on the child. This concept is exemplified in Newton's third law of motion: for every action, there is an equal and opposite reaction. This law and its applications to functional movement will be discussed later in the chapter.

Another type of contact force, **friction,** is described as force acting in the *opposite* direction to the desired movement and occurring at the area of contact between the two surfaces. Friction can also be described as a force that opposes the efforts of one object to slide or roll over another object. Friction can be considered a special type of shear force. A shear force is a force that attempts to move one object against another; however, in this case, the force acts *in the same* direction as the desired or attempted movement (Hall, 1999; Levangie & Norkin, 2005). A shear force might be described as a sliding or rubbing in the same direction as the movement. Shear forces are important to consider in therapy as they can cause skin damage or breakdown. One example of shear force is if a client is not properly seated in the wheelchair and the buttocks are sliding forward toward the front of the chair. There is force, or rubbing, between the person's skin, clothing, and seat of the chair. Both the skin and clothing are moving forward, but perhaps not at the same speed. Additionally, there is pressure between the surfaces due to body weight. This sliding or shear force can damage the skin. Considering movement or resistance in opposite directions, friction can either enable the activity or make it more difficult to complete depending on the desired outcome. Friction is preferred during the push-off phase of walking so the foot does not slip across the floor, causing a fall. Friction in this case can be increased by wearing rubber-soled shoes. On the other hand, too much friction is undesirable for the dancer trying to glide across the floor. In this example, friction is decreased by the smooth leather sole of the ballet shoe moving against the polished surface of the hardwood dance floor. Yet another example is observed when using the hands to grasp an object. Friction is desired on the tennis racquet so that the racquet does not fly out of the hand. The gymnast decreases friction with the use of chalk so both hands will rotate easily around the uneven bars. The amount of friction is often manipulated in therapy to enable functional movement. As friction has an impact on every motion, the applications in therapy are endless. Refer to Gold Box 3-3 for examples of how to modify friction to enable participation.

Gold Box 3-3

Examples of ways to *increase* friction to enable client participation and independence include using gloves for wheelchair propulsion, placing gripper pads under throw rugs, using dycem or gripper pads under dishes while eating or cooking, and using sticky or tacky finger cream to count or separate money or turn pages in a book.

Examples of ways to *decrease* friction to enable client participation and independence include placing a plastic bag in the seat of a chair to help the client slide forward or pivot in the chair; placing tennis balls over the feet of a walker or on chair legs to make them easier to slide across the floor; and placing heavier items (such as a pan of water) on a smooth cloth or pillow case before sliding them over the counter, floor, or other surface.

The final external force mentioned is a force that affects absolutely every movement and occupation in which we engage. It is known as gravity. The direction of the force of gravity is always toward the center of the earth. Gravity is measured as the weight of the body through its **center of gravity** (**COG**). The COG of an object is the point around which the body's mass is evenly distributed. Mass and weight are not the same thing. Mass is defined as the quantity of matter contained in an object, whereas weight is the amount of gravitational force exerted on a body or object (Hall, 1999). It is true that weight is proportional to mass, or stated another way, the greater the mass, usually the greater the weight, especially on the earth. However, if a person were to travel to the moon, the body mass would remain the same while the body weight would decrease as a result of the decreased effects of gravity at that distance from the center of the earth. Even though gravity exerts a constant, unchanging force on our bodies, one can modify its effects. For example, an OT practitioner may have an extremely weak client begin exercises in a gravity-reduced position. If the movement is elbow flexion, gravity-reduced options may include having the client place the upper extremity on a table and positioning the arm horizontal to the floor or using a mobile arm support. Figure 3-1 shows a client working in a gravity-reduced plane. In addition, a cloth is placed under the client's arm to reduce friction, thus making the activity even easier to complete.

All of the external forces discussed, as well as the internal force provided by muscles, share some common features. Force is a vector quantity, which means that it has qualities of both magnitude and direction. Force is also considered to have a specific point of application or area where the force contacts the object. The magnitude of a force refers to its size or the amount of force exerted. The direction of a force is the path the force follows. The path of movement can be either linear or rotary motion. Linear movement may be categorized either as moving along a straight line or curvilinear, moving along a curved line. Rotary motion occurs around an axis. Combinations of linear and rotary movements occur together for most functional human movements. This is called general motion. In many situations, the direction of movement is a downward direction following the pull of gravity. Forces other than gravity often have a different direction vector; for example, a toy car pushed across the floor would follow a perpendicular path to, or move horizontal to, the direction vector for gravity. For muscles, the direction of force is the line of pull of the muscle. The point of application of a force in the body is at the point of insertion of the muscle tendon. For objects, the point of application is through the center of gravity for linear movements. If the point of

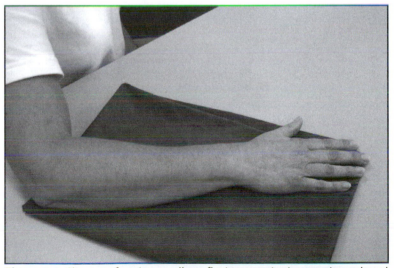

Figure 3-1. Client performing an elbow flexion exercise in a gravity-reduced plane. A cloth is placed under the client's arm to reduce the effects of friction, further grading the exercise to meet the client's weakened state. (Reprinted with permission of Carolyn Roller.)

application is not through the center of gravity, a rotary movement will occur (Luttgens & Hamilton, 1997). An example of both linear and rotary movement can be observed during the activity of pushing a heavy box. If the box is pushed in the middle, through its COG, the box will slide across the floor in a straight line, or in a linear fashion. If the box is pushed at a point toward one of the ends and not through its COG, the box will rotate. Rotary movement also occurs under the conditions of a force couple. A **force couple** is defined as two or more forces with similar magnitude but opposite or significantly different **direction** vectors. These forces must be applied to the same object at the same time and always produce rotation. The forces act on opposite sides of the axis of the object. The **axis** is the center, or point, around which the object rotates. A force couple allows for greater strength in movement. A common example in daily life of a force couple is a steering wheel. While one hand pulls in a downward direction, the other hand is pulling in an upward direction. These opposite, but combined, movements cause the wheel to turn with more power than if only one hand is used. This is especially evident when the power steering mechanism is not working. In the case of the steering wheel, the axis is the steering column. The forces are provided in opposite directions on each side of the steering wheel by the upper extremities. The rotary force generated is called torque (Levangie & Norkin, 2005). Greater torque is created when turning the wheel without power steering than when the power steering is functioning. Definitions of terms in bold are located in Gold Box 3-4.

Gold Box 3-4

Axis: The point or line passing through the two poles of a spherical body, about which the body may rotate.

Force couple: Always produces rotary motion; two or more forces of equal magnitude, but opposite direction, applied to the same object but at different points of application, working together to cause movement.

Linear motion: Movement along a path pertaining to or representing a line that may be straight or curved; all parts of the object move in the same direction at the same speed.

Magnitude: Size, amount; the basic unit of measurement in the United States for the magnitude of force is the pound.

Point of application: The point on the object where the force is applied; for a muscular force, this is commonly considered to be at the insertion of the muscle to the bone.

Rotary motion: Turning or movement about an axis; parts of the object further from the axis move at a greater speed than those close to the axis.

Torque: The turning or rotary effect of a force.

Vector: A physical quantity or force possessing both magnitude or size and direction; can be represented by a straight line.

From Steadman (1982); Hall (1999).

The primary forces discussed above include fluid force, contact force, gravity, and objects acting on the body. These forces in turn lead to three secondary forces that act on the body, including joint compression, joint distraction, and pressure on body surfaces (Luttgens & Hamilton, 1997; Smith et al., 1996). Joint **compression** is the pushing together of both sides of the joint toward the center of the joint. Joint compression occurs naturally in the ankles, knees, and hips during walking or jumping and in the joints of the upper extremity when doing a push-up. Joint **distraction,** a pulling apart of the two joint surfaces, is also sometimes referred to as traction. Joint distraction is often produced by external forces, such as in the use of an external fixator, to help a broken bone realign for proper healing. Joint distraction occurs naturally in the shoulder, elbow, and wrist

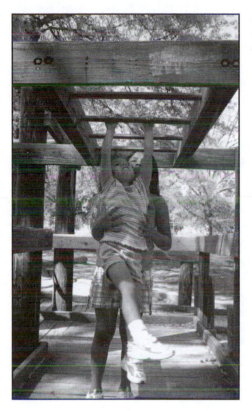

Figure 3-2. Naturally occurring joint distraction (mild separation of the bony ends of the joint) of the upper extremities as a child plays on the monkey bars.

joints as a child swings across the monkey bars, as seen in Figure 3-2. Lower extremity knee and hip joint distraction can be observed in the child hanging upside down with legs wrapped around a jungle gym.

Pressures on body surfaces pose a potentially serious problem in OT. Repeated pressure over a small surface area, such as the back of the heel for a bed-ridden client, can easily lead to decubiti, more commonly known as bed sores. In the fabrication of splints, the therapist needs to be exceedingly careful to avoid areas of pressure, as this can also cause pain, discomfort, and skin breakdown. In general, if the pressure can be distributed over a larger surface area, the likelihood of skin breakdown, tissue death, or bruising is lessened. The concept of diffusing pressure over a larger surface area is evident when comparing high-heeled shoes that have a very small heel size to tennis shoes. If someone steps on your toe with a spiked heel, it will hurt much more than if someone steps on your toe while wearing tennis shoes. This is because the pressure exerted by the weight of the person wearing tennis shoes is distributed through the much larger surface area of the entire bottom of the shoe.

When considering a client's functional movement, the practitioner must always consider the forces at work that impact movement. Just as primary forces can be manipulated during OT treatment, secondary forces are also important to consider in therapy. Two examples of manipulation of primary forces discussed include increasing or decreasing friction and reducing the effects of gravity to aid movement. Secondary forces such as joint manipulation, including compression or traction, may also be used or modified by the practitioner to enhance range of motion. Additionally, the effects of pressure need to be continually monitored to avoid skin breakdown and tissue damage.

Newton's laws of motion stem from his observations of the forces at work in nature, especially the primary forces. His laws describe the forces that produce, modify, or stop motion. Newton's laws, as he originally penned them, are printed here. "Newton published his findings in 1687 in a book called *Philosophiae Naturalis Principia Mathematica (Mathematical Principles of Natural Philosophy)* commonly known as the *Principia*.

- Newton's Law of Inertia: Every object persists in its state of rest or uniform motion in a straight line unless it is compelled to change that state by forces impressed upon it.
- Newton's Law of Acceleration: Force is equal to the change in momentum (mV) per change in time. For a constant mass, force equals mass times acceleration [expressed in the famous equation $F = ma$].
- Newton's Law of Action and Reaction: For every action, there is an equal and opposite reaction (Ravilious, 2010).

To better understand Newton's first law of motion, the concept of inertia needs to be addressed. **Inertia** is defined as "the state of a physical body in which it resists any force acting to move it from a position of rest or to change its uniform motion" (Steadman, 1982). If an object is at rest, a force must act on the object to initiate movement. If, however, an object is already in motion, it will remain in motion, moving at the same speed and progressing in the same direction unless a force modifies or stops its motion. Considering this concept, it stands to reason that it takes more effort or energy for a person to begin moving than it takes to remain in motion. This is why many long-distance hikers prefer not to stop to take breaks; getting started again uses more energy than continuing on does. A skateboarder demonstrates the impact of this law as it acts on the skateboard as well as on the skateboarder. The skateboard will stop abruptly when it hits the curb; however, the skateboarder will not stop because his or her body did not have a force act on it. The skateboarder will continue moving forward, through the air, at the same speed and in the same direction until the force of gravity pulls the direction of his or her movement downward and ultimately contact with the ground stops his or her motion. The use of seat belts in cars, lap belts on wheelchairs, and straps in baby strollers help provide the force needed to stop the body's motion when the moving object the body is riding in stops abruptly.

The law of acceleration, commonly referred to as Newton's second law, describes why an object with less mass will move faster than an object with greater mass, given the same push or force. Inversely, this law states that a greater force or push is required to move (or stop) an object of larger mass than what is required to move (or stop) an object of smaller mass. **Acceleration** may be defined as "the rate in change of velocity with respect to time" (*Merriam-Webster Online Dictionary*, 2010). This law can be observed easily in the health care setting. One example is that it takes less force, or simply stated, is easier, to propel a small, lightweight person in a wheelchair than it does to propel a heavier person. The practitioner needs to keep this law in mind when working with clients who have general weakness. If a greater force is required to move something that is heavier, the practitioner needs to exhibit caution when using assistive devices, adaptive equipment, or splints. These devices increase the weight of the extremity being moved, thus requiring more force to produce and maintain movement for a functional activity such as eating. If, however, for safety reasons, a client's speed in propelling his or her own wheelchair or walker needs to be decreased, adding weight would help.

Newton's third law, the law of action and reaction, implies that there must be two forces present. Each force acts on the other, with the direction of the forces being opposite and the magnitude of the forces being equal. This concept is observed when a person leans against the wall. The wall supports the person by "pushing" back with equal force to the weight and pressure of the person pushing against the wall. Otherwise, the wall would cave in. In relation to functional movement, this concept can enable or hinder client independence. For example, it is much harder for a person to walk on a sandy beach, in which some sand is displaced prior to the equal and opposite reaction taking effect, than when the person walks on a paved sidewalk. Similarly, it is more difficult for the weak client to stand from a soft chair or sofa than it is to rise from a hard-surfaced chair.

When considering functional movement, it is essential for the OT practitioner to consider Newton's laws of motion in relation to client performance. Understanding these laws allows the practitioner to assess movement and make adjustments to the environment, objects in the environment, or the activity itself in order to increase independence or to create the right challenge for the client. Additionally, recognizing the ever-present consequences of these laws will enhance safety awareness and compliance.

RELATED FACTORS

Further factors that can influence functional movement and the practice of OT are included here. Simple machines, created to lessen the amount of effort required to perform a task or movement, will be discussed. Aspects of joint and muscle properties not discussed elsewhere in the text will also be addressed. These include insufficiency, kinematic chains, and open- or close-pack joint positions.

Simple Machines

There are six simple machines consisting of the inclined plane, wheel and axle, pulley, screw, wedge, and lever. These machines cannot reduce the amount of work required, but they do lessen the effort needed to perform the task. Work consists of both the amount of force needed and the distance over which the force is applied. Work is defined by *Merriam-Webster Online Dictionary* (2010) as "the transference of energy that is produced by the motion of the point of application of a force and is measured by multiplying the force and the displacement of its point of application in the line of action." There is a trade-off when using simple machines; although the effort or force required is lessened, the distance over which a person must apply the force is increased. Machines can also allow us to change the direction of the force applied, such as in the use of a pulley. Gold Box 3-5 describes the six simple machines.

Gold Box 3-5

Inclined plane: Used for elevating objects; a flat surface or plane that is at an angle to the horizontal surface it is placed upon.

Wheel and axle: Used to move things over a greater distance; a circular object that rotates around a shaft.

Pulley: Used to change the direction of force or the point of application of force; consists of a rope around a small wheel that has a grooved rim to keep the rope in place.

Screw: Technically, a type of inclined plane, converts rotary motion into linear motion, either forward or backward.

Wedge: Converts downward force into perpendicular force, separating or splitting the object; a tool that is wide at one end and narrow at the other.

Lever: A rigid bar that rotates about an axis or fulcrum; downward motion at one end causes upward motion at the opposite end.

Adapted from *Free Dictionary On-line* (2010) and *Merriam-Webster Online Dictionary* (2010)

An example of the use of an inclined plane in therapy or functional movement for the person in a wheelchair is the ramp. The ramp requires the wheelchair to move over a greater distance but requires less effort than moving in a vertical direction, such as that of a step. Inclined planes are sometimes presented as slant boards in OT and can be used to grade activities. If a client is unable to lift an object straight up from its resting surface, the activity can be made easier by sliding the object up the slant board. The wheel and axle and the pulley may be used in therapy with exercise equipment, scooter boards, arm boards, mobile arm supports, and other devices to aid movement. The screw and wedge are tools used more often in construction-type activities to either hold things together or to separate them. The simple machine that is of most significance related to the practice of OT is the lever.

A lever functions on the basis of using torque or rotation. All levers consist of a rigid bar rotating about an axis. The lever has three main components. These include the axis, the point at which force or effort is applied, and the point at which resistance is encountered. Also of importance is the length of the bar, or arm, from the axis to either the force or resistance. These are labeled force arm and resistance arm. The length of these arms can be altered, which, in turn, will make a task either easier or harder to complete. In general, lengthening the force arm makes the task easier; conversely, shortening the force arm would render the task more difficult. Similarly, shortening the resistance arm makes the task easier, whereas lengthening the resistance arm causes the task to be more difficult to complete. Refer to Gold Box 3-6 for further description of these parts. In the body, the axis is generally considered be the joint, the force or effort is produced by muscles, and the resistance is the weight of the limb or body in addition to any external load, such as a bag of groceries or a textbook.

Gold Box 3-6

Axis: Also called fulcrum or pivot, the point about which the rigid bar turns; in diagrams, often referred to as "A."

Force: The effort or energy used to move or hold the object; in diagrams, often referred to as "F."

Force arm: Also called effort arm or moment arm; distance from the axis to the point of application of the force; in diagrams often referred to as "FA."

Resistance: The object one is trying to move, sometimes referred to as weight or load; in diagrams, often referred to as "R."

Resistance arm: Distance from the axis to the point of application of the resistance or load; in diagrams, often referred to as "RA."

Dail, Agnew, & Floyd (2011)

Levers can serve various functions. They can overcome a large resistance with less effort, provide balance, increase the speed of the motion, or increase the distance the resistance is moved. There are three types or classes of levers, and each class is designed to serve one of these functions. The difference in the classes of levers is dependent on the relationship of the three components to each other.

1.   In a first-class lever, the axis is between the force and the resistance. A common example of this is a seesaw. The first-class lever is designed for balance. In the seesaw, the axis is in the middle and is the point of rotation for the board resting on it. The force and resistance are the children at either end of the seesaw. In the case of the first-class lever, the direction of the force and direction of the resistance are the same, downward toward the pull of gravity. The force arm and resistance arm, however, move in opposite directions; as one goes up, the other goes down. In this type of lever, it does not matter which arm is longer; either the force arm or the resistance arm can be longer than the other. Examples of first-class levers in the body are limited. Dail et al. (2011) refer to the head balancing on the vertebral column as a first-class lever. The axis is the vertebra, the resistance is the weight of the head, pulled forward by gravity, and the force is supplied by the posterior muscles contracting to keep the head erect. First-class levers are used in OT with devices such as the mobile arm support balancing the forearm for functional use and in splinting a finger to decrease deformity. The axis or balance point for the splint is over the joint, while effort and resistance are applied equally on either side of the joint axis. Refer to Figures 3-3 through 3-5 for pictures of first-class levers.

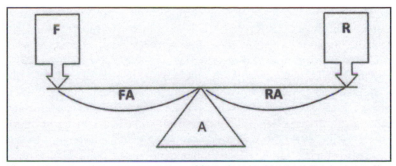

Figure 3-3. Graphic representation of first-class lever where the axis is in the middle. **A** represents axis, **F** represents force, and **R** represents resistance. The arrows depict the direction of the force and resistance. **RA** indicates the length of the resistance arm, and **FA** indicates the length of the force arm. First-class levers are designed for balance.

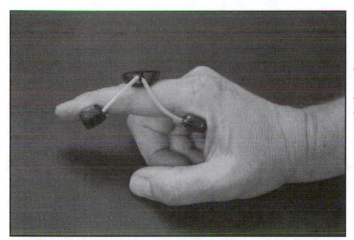

Figure 3-4. A finger splint designed using the principles of a first-class lever. The axis in this situation is the joint. Pressure (force and resistance) is balanced on both sides of the joint to encourage extension at the joint. (Reprinted with permission of Carolyn Roller.)

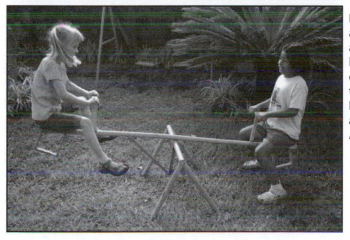

Figure 3-5. A seesaw is an example of a first-class lever. When both children are approximately the same weight, balance occurs. If the children are of different weights, the length of the force arm, the resistance arm, or both can be changed to facilitate balance. (Reprinted with permission of Angela Grussing.)

2. Second-class levers give the mechanical advantage of force. With a second-class lever, a person can move a large resistance with a relatively small amount of force. In the second-class lever, the axis is at one end, the resistance is in the middle, and the force is at the end opposite the axis. In this type of lever, the force arm must always be longer than the resistance arm. As stated earlier, a longer force arm makes the task easier to perform.

Unlike in the first-class lever, the direction of force and the direction of resistance are opposite. Additionally, the force arm and resistance arm in the second-class lever move in the same direction. A common example of this type of lever is the wheelbarrow. The force exerted is in an upward direction moving the force arm upward while at the same time lifting the resistance or load, thus moving the resistance arm upward also. Whether or not second-class levers exist within the body is debatable. Some sources say that there is an example of this; others insist it is not so. This debate will be left to the researchers. Second-class levers are often used in therapy to make a task easier. If the OT practitioner lengthens the force arm on various devices, less energy is needed for the client to use the device. This principle can be observed in extending the handles on a nutcracker, a lever faucet, or a three-ring hole punch. Examples of second-class levers can be seen in Figures 3-6 through 3-9.

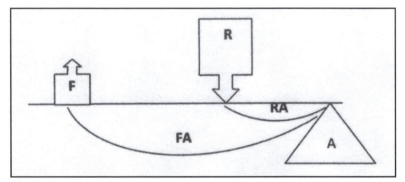

Figure 3-6. Graphic representation of a second-class lever where the resistance is in the middle. **A** represents axis, **F** represents force, and **R** represents resistance. The arrows depict the direction of the force and resistance. **RA** indicates the length of the resistance arm, and **FA** indicates the length of the force arm. A second-class lever is designed so that less force or strength is required to move a heavy item.

Figure 3-7. A wheelbarrow is an example of a second-class lever. The weight or resistance is between the axis and force, in this case inside the bucket. A heavy load is easier for a person to move due to the longer force arm (handles) in comparison to the short resistance arm (distance from weight in bucket to wheel axle).

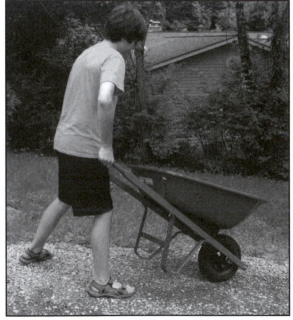

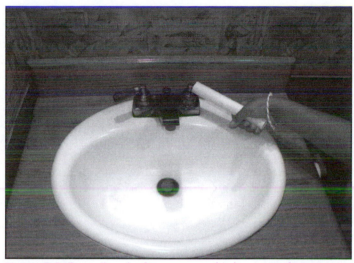

Figure 3-8. Extending the force arm on this lever-type faucet makes it easier to move the handle to turn the water on. This faucet is also a second-class lever.

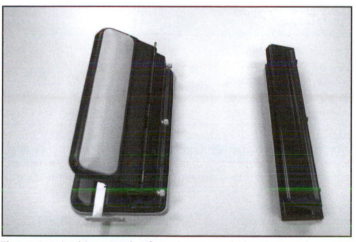

Figure 3-9. In this example of another second-class lever, a three-hole punch, the example on the left has a longer resistance arm, making it easier to punch holes in a large stack of paper. (Reprinted with permission of Carolyn Roller.)

3. Effort is between the axis and the resistance in the third-class lever. As such, the resistance arm always needs to be longer than the force arm. A longer resistance arm requires more effort or force to use; however, the pay-off is increased speed and range of motion. Similar to the second-class lever, the directions of the force and the resistance are opposite, but both arms move in the same direction in the third-class lever. Unlike second-class levers, there are few external examples and more examples within the human body. In fact, most of the levers at work in the human body are third-class levers. External examples of third-class levers include a golf club and a baseball bat: the athlete's body is the axis, the force is applied through muscular action where the hands grasp and swing the club or bat, and the resistance is the ball. An internal example, or one within the body, occurs when a person uses the biceps brachii and other elbow flexors to overcome the resistance of a full glass of water as it is lifted to the mouth. In this case, the elbow is the axis, the point of insertion of the muscles is the force, and the resistance is the pull of

gravity or the weight of the forearm plus the weight of the glass and water. This class of levers does require a fair amount of force or effort, but in turn it allows a person to move the distal segment of a limb across a wide range of motion, to do so with speed, or both. These factors are necessary in order to carry out most functional activities. An example of a third-class lever commonly used in OT is the reacher. A reacher may be used by clients when they have decreased range of motion and cannot reach items (e.g., items dropped on the floor). Basically, the reacher extends the resistance arm. This makes the item feel heavier or harder to pick up; however, the greater range of motion granted does allow the client to retrieve the dropped item. A word of caution should be expressed here. Because extending the resistance arm makes the object seem heavier, only relatively light-weight items should be picked up with a reacher. Once again, the axis is the elbow, the force is the point of muscle insertion, and the resistance is the weight of the reacher plus the sock or other item being picked up. Examples of third-class levers can be found in Figures 3-10 through 3-12.

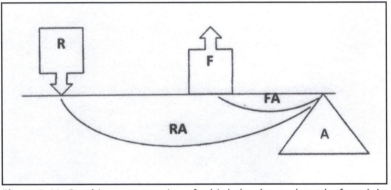

Figure 3-10. Graphic representation of a third-class lever where the force is in the middle. **A** represents axis, **F** represents force, and **R** represents resistance. The arrows depict the direction of the force and resistance. **RA** indicates the length of the resistance arm, and **FA** indicates the length of the force arm.

Figure 3-11. In this example of a third-class lever, the batter's torso is the axis, the point of application of force is the hands on the bat, and the force is the batter's muscle strength. The resistance is the ball. The third-class lever gives advantage to range of motion and speed, as observed in the trajectory of a well-hit ball.

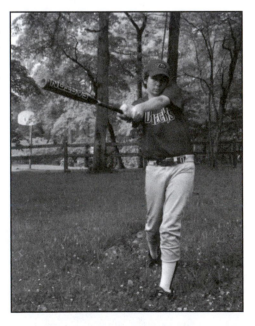

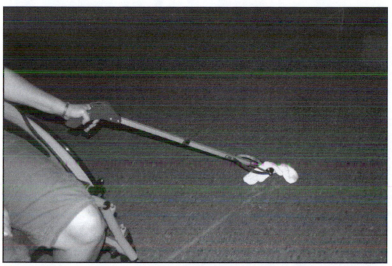

Figure 3-12. The reacher is also an example of a third-class lever. In this situation, the axis is the elbow joint; the force is composed of the action of the elbow flexor muscles; and the resistance is the sock, the weight of the limb, and the weight of the reacher combined. In this case, the resistance arm is lengthened by the distance from the hand to the end of the reacher. The advantage gained is range of motion; the cost is increased effort or energy and strength required to pick up the sock. (Reprinted with permission of Carolyn Roller.)

While working with clients, remember to use the lever class that matches the desired outcome. If balance and stability are desired, the first-class lever is appropriate. If the goal is to make a task easier to do, requiring less force or effort to complete the task, then the second-class lever is the better choice. If increasing speed or range of motion in an activity is necessary, the third-class lever is helpful. It is also important to understand the principles behind the lever system, for example, knowing that extending the resistance arm will make the resistance seem greater is applicable in the use of a reacher, carrying an item close to the body, or when using weights on an extremity for strengthening purposes.

Active and Passive Insufficiency

Certain aspects of joints and muscles that affect movement will be included here. One such aspect is that of insufficiency. Many muscles in the human body cross or act at two or more joints simultaneously. These muscles can affect motion at all the joints they cross. The amount and type of motion occurring at each joint crossed is dependent on several factors such as location of attachment or other muscles acting on the same joint. At times, the fact that a muscle may span two or more joints is advantageous; at other times, this is a disadvantage. The disadvantage occurs with a phenomenon called insufficiency. *Insufficiency* indicates that the muscle is not able to work to its full potential at all joints at the same time. Insufficiency is often defined as "lack of completeness of function" (Steadman, 1982). Insufficiency can occur in two different ways. **Active insufficiency** occurs when a muscle cannot shorten or contract any further and fails to shorten to the extent required for simultaneous full range of motion at all joints crossed. Conversely, **passive insufficiency** occurs when a muscle cannot be stretched any further, yet it has not stretched the amount required for full range of motion at all joints crossed at the same time. Active insufficiency occurs when the client is actively contracting muscle to cause movement. The muscle cannot actively contract enough to cause full range of motion at all joints. Often, the client feels a cramp in the muscle when nearing active insufficiency. Passive insufficiency occurs without

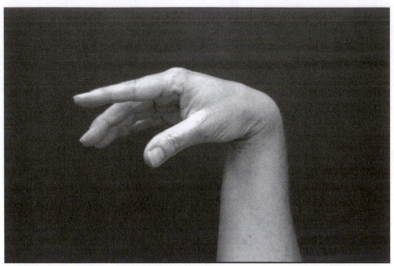

Figure 3-13. Passive insufficiency of the long finger extensor muscles observed in lack of complete finger flexion while the wrist is positioned in full flexion. (Reprinted with permission of Carolyn Roller.)

active muscular contraction by the client. Passive insufficiency occurs in response to a stretch. The muscle cannot be stretched enough to allow full range of motion at all joints crossed. In this case, the client often feels more of a burn or heat in the muscle, not a cramp. Consider the wrist and fingers as an example. If you actively and fully flex your wrist, it will be difficult to close your fingers into a fist. This is due to active insufficiency of the long finger flexors, which cross several joints, including the wrist. If you fully extend your wrist, your fingers tend to flex on their own and it is difficult to straighten or extend them with the wrist in full extension. This is an example of passive insufficiency of the long finger flexors. The second example, passive insufficiency of the long finger flexors, can be used to the advantage of a client with a weak or insufficient grasp. This is referred to as a tenodesis grasp. Tenodesis literally means to "stabilize a joint by anchoring the tendons which move that joint" (Steadman, 1982). In some clients, shortening of the long finger flexors is actually encouraged to enhance the effects of passive insufficiency. In a tenodesis grasp, grip is possible, and strength is increased by placing the wrist in extension, causing the fingers to flex. Tenodesis splints have been designed to take greater advantage of this effect of passive insufficiency. Refer to Figures 3-13 and 3-14 to note the positioning of the fingers related to passive insufficiency of the long finger extensors and long finger flexors, respectively.

Kinematic Chains

Functional movement occurs in a sequence influenced by a concept referred to as a kinematic chain. Some sources refer to this as a kinetic chain. This text will use Levangie and Norkin's (2005) terminology of a kinematic chain. The term *kinematics* is derived from the Greek word for things that move. The common term for movies, *cinema*, is derived from this same word. In relation to the human body, kinematics refers to movements of each part of the body, body movements in relation to one another, and the form or pattern of movement in relation to time. A chain is generally a linear structure composed of rigid segments interconnected with moveable joints or parts. In a chain, motion in one area leads to motion in subsequent areas, causing a type of ripple effect along the entire chain. A **kinematic chain** therefore depicts a combination of these two concepts. The human kinematic chain may be defined as the bones and joints moving in sequence following a specified pattern depending on whether the chain is open or closed. In an **open kinematic chain**, the distal segment is freely moving, and, therefore, one joint can move without impacting

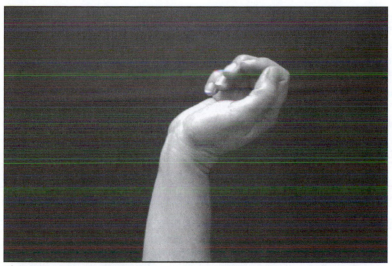

Figure 3-14. Passive insufficiency of the long finger flexor muscles observed in lack of complete finger extension while the wrist is positioned in full extension. (Reprinted with permission of Carolyn Roller.)

movement of the other joints. Using the upper extremity as an example, holding the hand in the air would position the distal segment, the hand, to be freely moveable. In this case, the person can greet a friend by making waving motions at the wrist without having to also move the elbow or shoulder. Similarly, the person could move at the elbow, such as in chopping, and not move the wrist or shoulder joints. The idea is that one joint can move in isolation, or independently, from other joints. In contrast, in a **closed kinematic chain,** the distal segment is fixed or stabilized so movement in one joint will automatically necessitate movement at connecting joints. In standing with both feet on the floor, the lower extremities are in a closed kinematic chain. In this closed system, movement at one joint necessitates movement at all related joints. For example, when a person squats from a standing position, the flexion at the knee also causes hip flexion and ankle dorsiflexion. Open and closed kinematic chains in relation to human movement also describe nonweight-bearing or weight-bearing conditions. Simply stated, the open chain represents non-weight-bearing, whereas the closed chain is the weight-bearing position. In general, during most functional movement, the lower extremity is weight bearing and in a closed-chain position, providing stability, while the upper extremity is in an open-chain position, allowing freedom of movement of the hand to perform tasks (Hall, 1999; Levangie & Norkin, 2005; Steadman, 1982).

When analyzing and prescribing activities in therapy, it is important to note the type of kinematic chain needed. If a client has reduced balance and equilibrium reactions, it would be beneficial to begin with closed-chain activities. As the client progresses, open-chain activities can be incorporated to provide mobility superimposed on stability. This is a precursor to functional movement and activity, as many life activities require dynamic motion.

Open- and Close-Pack Joint Positions

Joints can also be positioned in an open-pack or close-pack position. These positions refer to the stability of the joint structure. Joint stability is often described as the ability of the joint to resist one bone end from sliding off the other bone end, or displacing. Many factors influence joint stability, such as muscles, tendons, and the shape of the joint. In addition, the position the joint is in affects its stability. Because articulating joint surfaces are not all symmetrical or of the exact same size, there is typically one position in which the joint fits together best, or in which the contact between both sides of the joint is optimal. When the fit is optimal, the two sides of the joint are in the closest contact possible over the greatest surface area. This optimal fit is referred to as the **close-pack position** and generally is the position that offers the most stability. The **open-pack position** is sometimes referred to as *loose packed*. In this position, the joint is not as stable because there is less total contact area of the joint surfaces. This position occurs any time the joint is not in the close-pack position. Some joints are shaped such that they have a greater amount of contact between articulating surfaces regardless of position and thus provide better stability overall. One such joint is the hip joint, due to the large and deep articulating surface of the acetabulum (Hall, 1999). Injury is more likely to occur in the open-pack position. Clipping, a common football injury, is caused when a player is stationary with knees bent and is hit with force on the side of the leg. In this flexed, open-pack position, the knee is relatively easily twisted or dislocated. Adding to the problem is the fact that the lower extremity is in a closed kinematic chain in this position. As such, the foot and ankle are planted or stabilized on the ground and do not move with the impact. The next joint in the kinematic chain is the knee, which suffers the force of the impact.

When considering functional movement for clients, kinematic chains and pack positions need to be analyzed and addressed. For example, if a client is unable to fully extend the knee during a standing pivot transfer, it is important to remember the knee will be less stable than if in the extended, close-pack position. The client would need to be educated about this, and precautions might be needed to avoid twisting the knee during the transfer. If the practitioner is aware of the effects of the kinematic chain or joint position, an activity or task can be modified to either enhance stability or enable mobility, depending on the need of the client. It is important to remember that all functional movement involves a combination of the positions discussed. The client must be able to fluidly move from open-pack to close-pack and vice versa, as well as change between an open and closed kinematic chain. The gait cycle offers a good example of this rapid and repeated changing of positions. Gait will be discussed further in Chapter 6.

Summary

Functional movement requires complex interactions of multiple factors in addition to the actual body components discussed in the previous chapter. Context, environment, and other related factors can enable or impede movement as well as participation in daily activities. Often, these factors have more influence on movement than the underlying body functions; therefore, it is essential that the OT practitioner consider these various factors when working with clients. Only through the unity of all factors is participation achieved.

APPLICATIONS

The following activities will help you apply knowledge of the factors influencing movement in real-life situations. Activities can be completed individually or in a small group to enhance learning.

1.   **Contextual Factors:** Contextual factors can greatly impact function or participation in activity. The purpose of this application is for the student to explore various ways in which contextual variables impact the individual.

      a.   Select two holiday traditions in which you engage. Analyze these traditions using the four contextual components, and determine how each component impacts the tradition. Examples are provided for you. Refer to Table 3-2 to complete this application.

      b.   Contextual factors can impair participation or enable it. This activity will help identify ways in which this can happen.

            i.   Select several significant events from different times in your life related to a specific activity or occupation. List these at the top of the columns

Table 3-2	Holiday Traditions		
		Holiday Traditions	
Contextual Factors	**Christmas—Opening Presents**	**Thanksgiving Dinner**	
Cultural	*My family gives gifts on Dec. 25.*	*Certain family members always arrive at least 1 hour late, to everyone else's dismay.*	
Personal	*I am usually somewhat sad after gifts are opened; there was so much anticipation and build-up to Christmas. Then, it is over in a short time. Additionally, I dislike the commercialism of Christmas.*	*The entire extended family is invited, and they often bring friends. Uncle Bob always brings sweet potato casserole. Although deceased, someone has to make Nana's favorite recipes.*	
Temporal	*We open gifts Christmas morning as soon as the children are awake.*	*We have dinner late in the day so people can eat the noon-time meal at the in-laws' home.*	
Virtual	*My parents always videotape the gift opening.*	*Phone calls, Facebook entries with pictures, and sometimes video greetings are sent to those far off who could not attend.*	

Table 3-3	**Significant Life Events**		
	Significant Life Events		
Contextual Factors	**Adoption of Foreign-Born Child**		
Cultural	*Enhance—diversity enriches all of our lives, travel to foreign country; Impede—some family and community members not accepting of child with different skin color*		
Personal	*Enhance—very much wanted child; Impede—want independence and ample time for self*		
Temporal	*Older parent Enhance—financially secure, more patience; Impede—no cohort group, "grandparent" age*		
Virtual	*Enhance—ability to access information such as vital records (birth, marriage) from other states; Impede—many online agencies not necessarily concerned about best interest of child (many are very responsible, however)*		

in Table 3-3. For each contextual area, try to list one component that interfered with this activity or occupation and one that enhanced it. A personal example is provided.

    ii.   Select a personal movement-related life event in which you were successful or pleased with the outcome. Determine the contextual factors that enabled this successful outcome. Next, imagine if the contextual factors were different, what the outcome might have been. An example is provided in Table 3-4. Complete the table with your own experience(s).

2.   **Accessibility, Negotiability, Universal Design:** The purpose of this activity is to raise awareness of the concepts of universal design and how they benefit all people. Certain structures or places may meet Americans with Disabilities Act legal requirements for accessibility but lack negotiability for the user. For this activity, you will need to borrow a wheelchair and visit several area attractions and public buildings (restaurants,

Table 3-4	Positive and Negative Potential Effects of Contextual Factors on Significant Movement-Related Life Events			
	Significant Life Event			
	High School Volleyball			
Contextual Factors	**Positive Attributes**	**Potential Negative Attributes**	**Positive Attributes**	**Potential Negative Attributes**
Cultural	*Peer group of athletes, family history of athleticism*	*Peers, family place little or no value on athleticism; time spent at home more important*		
Personal	*Role identity as athlete, competitive nature, pride in achieving personal goal*	*Unsure of self, question ability, half-hearted attempt at goal*		
Temporal	*Made team first year; young player/rookie on team*	*Young, uncoordinated, minimal skill set*		
Virtual	*Games on local TV, radio*	*Dislike attention to self, pictures of self*		
Effect of contextual factors on performance	*Increased desire to excel; to prove skill to family, self, older players*	*Did not try out for team, did not set goals for self, minimal identity of roles*		

playgrounds, museums, libraries, etc.). It is suggested to work in pairs or small groups with each pair or group assessing a different location. The information gathered can then be shared with the entire class.

    a.   Determine the accessibility of the location visited. It is suggested to print and use a checklist designed for this purpose. Accessibility checklists can be found in Appendix A.

    b.   Determine the negotiability of each location. Once you enter the area (accessibility), see if you can easily use it for the purposes it was created. For example, if the purpose of the location is dining, can you reach the table? Are the silverware and drinking glass easy to grasp and lift, and is the lighting ample to read the menu? Generate your own checklist for this, or list items that you discover are not negotiable during your visit. Remember to consider things such as ease of use of handles on doors and faucets, height and location of towel and toilet paper dispensers, weight of doors, weight of eating utensils or glasses, steepness or unevenness of terrain, and so forth.

    c.   Summarize your findings from a and b above. Make suggestions as to how the location could be made more accessible and negotiable. Discuss how designing new locations with these concepts in mind would support the concepts of universal design and access for all.

    d.   Consider sharing this information with the appropriate people at the location, with building associations, or with students in other programs as a community service. Perhaps some simple changes could be made that would enable more people to enjoy the location. (This information can be easily shared via PowerPoint presentations.)

3.   **Newton's Laws:** After this activity, you should be able to apply Newton's laws to everyday movements and motions. Review the three laws of motion. Decide which law best fits the activity or situation described. Complete Table 3-5.

4.   **Levers:** The goal of this exercise is to familiarize yourself with the three types of levers and their uses.

    a.   Find as many examples of levers in the environment as you can. Determine the class of lever the item is. Note the type of advantage the lever gives the user. This information can be recorded in Table 3-6. An example is provided.

    b.   Practice picking things up with a long-handled reacher.

        i.   Are items harder to pick up than they would be if you simply used your hand? Why or why not?

        ii.   How can you make an item easier to pick up?

            1.   Which arm are you changing, force or resistance?

        iii.   What recommendations would you make to a client who you are suggesting should use a reacher?

5.   **Active and Passive Insufficiency**: The following activities will increase understanding of the concepts of active and passive insufficiency and how they affect movement. These activities can be performed individually; however, you might want a partner to observe for subtle changes in movement.

    a.   **Active insufficiency**—First, define active insufficiency in your own words. Then, complete the activities that follow.

        i.   Stand holding onto something for support. Bend your knee and raise that same leg as far as you can. Notice how much hip flexion you have. Keeping your leg elevated, straighten your knee. Consider what happens.

Table 3-5	**Application of Newton's Laws of Motion**	
Activity or Motion	**Newton's Law**	**How Does This Law Impact Client Performance?**
Maintaining same speed while walking to dining hall	*Law of inertia*	*It is easier to move at same speed than to start and stop; it takes more energy to initiate movement or to stop movement*
Large bowling ball rolls slower than small one		
Needing more effort to push heavy person in wheelchair than light person		
Jumping on a trampoline		
Pushing off from starting blocks for a race		
Rising from a chair		
Sitting up in bed		
Propelling wheelchair on beach (compared to concrete)		
Wheelchair coming to abrupt stop		
Your example here		
Your example here		
Your example here		

Table 3-6	**Application Exercise: Levers**			
Lever/Item	**Class of Lever (1st, 2nd, 3rd)**	**Advantage of Lever (speed, range of motion, less force needed)**	**Uses for Lever**	**Label or Describe the Axis (A), Force (F), and Resistance (R)**
Crow bar	*1st*	*Requires less force or effort to move object*	*Moves large rocks, pries things open*	*A—pivot point that crow bar rests on and rotates over, may be smaller rock or stump* *F—your strength pushing down* *R—rock or item being moved*

1.   Does the amount of hip flexion you have change? How? Why do you think this occurs?
2.   Do you feel something in your anterior thigh? Describe the feeling.
3.   You are experiencing active insufficiency of what muscle group?

ii.   Lay in a prone position on a mat. Flex your knee as far as possible. Notice how much hip flexion you have. Keeping your knee flexed, flex your hip. Consider what happens.

1.   Does the amount of hip flexion you have change? How? Why do you think this occurs?
2.   Do you feel something in your anterior thigh? Describe the feeling.
3.   You are experiencing active insufficiency of what muscle group?

iii.   Is active insufficiency dependent on the muscle group used?
iv.   What muscle group does active insufficiency occur in?

b.   **Passive insufficiency**—First, define passive insufficiency in your own words. Then, complete the activities listed below.

i.   Squat and touch your toes. Notice how much hip and knee flexion you have. While keeping your hands on your toes, extend or straighten your knees as much as possible. Consider what happens.

1.   Does the amount of hip flexion you have change? How? Why do you think this occurs?
2.   Do you feel something in your posterior thigh? Describe the feeling.
3.   You are experiencing passive insufficiency of what muscle group?

ii.   Stand holding onto something for support. Flex your hip and knee on the same side. Hold your foot against your buttocks with your free hand. Notice how much knee flexion you have. Slowly move your hip into extension. Consider what happens.

1.   Can you achieve full hip extension if the knee maintains full flexion? Why or why not?
2.   What do you feel in your anterior thigh?
3.   You are experiencing passive insufficiency of what muscle group?

iii.   Rest your right elbow on the table with your hand pointing toward the ceiling. Now, relax your right wrist, and allow it to drop into flexion.

1.   Describe the position of your fingers when the wrist is in flexion.
2.   Using your left hand, manually extend the right wrist. Describe the position of your fingers.

6.   **Open and Closed Kinematic Chains:** Work with a partner or in small groups.

a.   Walk slowly across the floor while your partner or group observes. Determine when each leg is in a closed kinematic chain and when it switches to an open chain. Discuss the stability and mobility of these two positions.

b.   You may perform this next activity while eating. Begin with eating and drinking the way you usually do. Observe the ease and fluidity of your movements. In most cases, your upper extremities will be in an open kinematic chain. Now, support your upper body weight on your elbows, as if you had no trunk control and needed to hold yourself up. This places the upper portion of the arm in a closed chain. Eat and drink again.

     i. How did this closed-chain position affect your ability to cut your food, feed yourself, and drink? Note all differences or changes.

     ii. Referring to the differences or changes you noticed, why do you think these occurred?

     iii. Discuss how eating or performing oral motor hygiene in this position might impact a client with general weakness.

7. **Open- and Close-Pack Joint Positions**: Working with a partner, place your knee and elbow joints in varying positions. In each position, gently move your partner's joint in all directions.

    a. Determine which seems to be the most stable position. This is your close-packed position. Describe the close-pack position for the joint.

      i. Knee

      ii. Elbow

      iii. Interphalangeal joints of fingers

    b. Place your joint in an open-pack position. Describe how it feels when your partner tries to gently move your joint from side to side.

      i. Knee

      ii. Elbow

      iii. Interphalangeal joints of fingers

    c. Are there any similarities in between joints in the close-pack position? If so, list them.

    d. Was it easier to determine these two positions in certain joints? Why do you think this is? Review the bony structures of the joint, especially the articulating surfaces, for clues.

REFERENCES

American Occupational Therapy Association. (2008). Occupational therapy practice framework: Domain and process (2nd ed.). *American Journal of Occupational Therapy, 62*, 625–683.

Center for Universal Design, College of Design, North Carolina State University. (2008). Retrieved from http://www.design.ncsu.edu/cud/index.htm.

Cronin, A., & Mandich, M. (2005). *Human development and performance throughout the lifespan.* Clifton Park, NY: Thomson Delmar Learning.

Dail, N. W., Agnew, T. A., & Floyd, R. T. (2011). *Kinesiology for manual therapies.* New York, NY: McGraw-Hill.

Free Dictionary On-line. Retrieved from http://www.thefreedictionary.com

Hall, S. J. (1999). *Basic biomechanics* (3rd ed.). Boston, MA: WCB/McGraw-Hill.

Levangie, P. K., & Norkin, C. C. (2005). *Joint structure and function: A comprehensive analysis* (4th ed.). Philadelphia, PA: F. A. Davis Company.

Luttgens, K. E., & Hamilton, N. (1997). *Kinesiology: Scientific basis of human motion* (9th ed.). Dubuque, IA: Brown & Benchmark Publishers.

Mace, R. Center for Universal Design. (2008). Retrieved from http://www.design.ncsu.edu/cud/about_ud/about_ud.htm.

Merriam-Webster Online Dictionary. Retrieved from http://www.merriamwebster.com/dictionary.

Ravilious, K. (2010). *Isaac Newton: Who he was, why google apples are falling.* York, England for National Geographic News, January 4, 2010; Retrieved from http://news.nationalgeographic.com/news/2010/01/100104-isaac-newton-google-doodle-logo-apple.html.

Smith, L. K., Weiss, E. L., & Lehmkuhl, L. D. (1996). *Brunnstrom's clinical kinesiology* (5th ed.). Philadelphia, PA: F. A. Davis Company.

Steadman, T. (1982). *Steadman's Medical Dictionary* (24th ed.). Baltimore, MD: Williams and Wilkins.

World Health Organization. (2001). *International classification of functioning, disability and health* (ICF). Geneva, Switzerland: Author.

chapter 4

Introducing Movement Demands

Jeremy L. Keough, MSOT, OTR/L

HUMAN MOVEMENT FOR FUNCTION

Occupational Therapy Practice Framework, 2nd Edition

The *Occupational Therapy Practice Framework, 2nd Edition* (OTPF-2) is a good place to start in describing the overwhelming concept of human movement. As presented earlier in this text (Chapter 1), particular aspects of occupational therapy's domain have been identified that relate to kinesiology. The aspect of client factors that impact movement can include values, beliefs, spirituality, body structures, and body functions. **Body structures** responsible for movement refer to anatomical parts of the body, such as joints, bones, muscles, and structures of related body systems. Similarly, **body functions** are physiologic functions of the body and include a category called "neuromusculoskeletal and movement-related functions." Table 4-1 identifies some of the neuromusculoskeletal and movement-related functions listed in the OTPF-2. Occupational therapy (OT) realizes, though, that human movement is composed of much more than just minimization of movement to the smallest components of body structures and body functions. Within the OTPF-2, the domain aspect of performance skills provides another avenue to view human movement.

As previously mentioned in Chapter 1, **performance skills** are defined as the abilities clients demonstrate in the actions they perform. Body structures and body functions impact a client's performance skills as does context, specific activity demands, and multiple other factors. The OTPF-2 includes the category motor and praxis skills under performance skills. Table 4-2 provides the description of the motor and praxis skills category from the OTPF-2. This category provides an explanation of motor/muscular movements as well as **praxis**. Praxis is the ability to plan and perform purposeful movement. Examples provided include, but are not limited to, bending and reaching, pacing tempo of an activity/occupation, coordinating body movements, maintaining balance, manipulating objects, and adjusting/anticipating posture. Movement varies as it can include all of these actions as well as only some of these actions.

Body functions and performance skills have been introduced as one approach to describing movement. An example is presented in Figure 4-1, which displays David playing on a piano. Neuromusculoskeletal and movement-related body functions used by David to play the piano include range of motion to reach the playing keys, strength to lift up and maintain his arm against gravity, endurance to play a whole song, and possibly standing, his position during engagement in this activity.

- 85 -

Keough, J. L., Sain, S. J., Roller, C. L.
Kinesiology for the Occupational Therapy Assistant:
Essential Components of Function and Movement (pp. 85-112).
© 2012 SLACK Incorporated.

Table 4-1	**Neuromusculoskeletal and Movement-Related Functions**
Functions of Joints and Bones: (not intended to be an all-inclusive list)	
Joint mobility	Joint range of motion
Joint stability	Joint alignment (this refers to the physiological stability of the joint related to its structural integrity as compared to the motor skill of aligning the body while moving in relation to task objects)
Muscle power	Strength
Muscle tone	Degree of muscle tone (e.g., flaccidity, spasticity, fluctuating)
Muscle endurance	Endurance
Motor reflexes	Stretch, asymmetrical tonic neck, symmetrical tonic neck
Involuntary movement reactions	Righting and supporting
Control of voluntary movement	Eye-hand/foot coordination, bilateral integration, crossing the midline, fine and gross motor control, and oculomotor (e.g. saccades, pursuits, accommodation, binocularity)
Gait patterns	Walking patterns and impairments, such as asymmetric gait, stiff gait. (Note: Gait patterns are considered in relation to how they affect ability to engage in occupations in daily-life activities.)

Reprinted with permission of American Occupational Therapy Association. (2008). Occupational therapy practice framework: Domain and process (2nd ed.). *American Journal of Occupational Therapy, 62,* 636.

Table 4-2	**Performance Skills: Motor and Praxis Skills**	
Definition		**Examples**
Motor: Actions or behaviors a client uses to move and physically interact with tasks, objects, contexts, and environments (adapted from Fisher, 2006). Includes planning, sequencing, and executing new and novel movements. *Praxis:* Skilled purposeful movements (Heilman & Rothi, 1993). Ability to carry out sequential motor acts as part of an overall plan rather than individual acts (Liepmann, 1920). Ability to carry out learned motor activity, including following through on a verbal command, visual-spatial construction, ocular and oral-motor skills, imitation of a person or an object, and sequencing actions (Ayres, 1985; Filley, 2001). Organization of temporal sequences of actions within the spatial context, which form meaningful occupations (Blanche & Parham, 2002).		• *Bending* and reaching for a toy or tool in a storage bin. • *Pacing* tempo of movements to clean the room. • *Coordinating* body movements to complete a job task. • *Maintaining* balance while walking on an uneven surface or while showering. • *Anticipating or adjusting posture and body position* in response to environmental circumstances, such as obstacles. • *Manipulating* keys or lock to open the door.
(not intended to be an all-inclusive list)		

Reprinted with permission of American Occupational Therapy Association. (2008). Occupational therapy practice framework: Domain and process (2nd ed.). *American Journal of Occupational Therapy, 62,* 640.

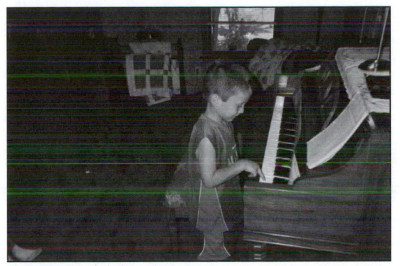

Figure 4-1. David playing on a piano.

Motor and praxis performance skills used by David to play the piano include tempo of movements to play the appropriate keys, coordinating his fingers and body to reach the keys, maintaining standing balance, manipulating the key cover board, and adjusting posture to weight shift demands. As can be seen, multiple aspects can affect human movement in engagement in a functional activity.

Quite often, within the medical model, OT practitioners address those specific aspects that enable or hinder movement for a client to maximize health and participation in life. While at times, these aspects are more readily noted, a skilled practitioner trained on how the body moves is necessary to provide the appropriate approach and treatment needed to achieve the optimal outcome. This vagueness is unavoidable without further clarification of the margins of human movement that this text is able to cover. In particular, this text emphasizes a kinematic view of human movement with emphasis on functional movement important to OT practitioners. Defining human motor behavior is essential.

Motor Behavior

Spaulding (2005) identifies **motor behavior** as observable and measurable movement. More specifically, Whiting and Rugg (2006) define motor behavior as a term that describes how the similar concepts of motor development, motor learning, and motor control combine to typify muscular control and movement. **Motor development** identifies the changes in movement behavior that occur as the client progresses through the lifespan from infancy until death (Whiting & Rugg, 2006). **Motor learning** is also defined as the acquisition and/or modification of learned movement patterns over time (Pendleton & Schultz-Krohn, 2006). Lastly, **motor control** is defined as the outcome of motor learning involving the ability to produce purposeful movements of the extremities and postural adjustments in response to activity and environment demands (Pendleton & Schultz-Krohn, 2006). Gold Box 4-1 represents how each concept relates over the lifespan. Each concept, while different, is important to understand in order to develop an understanding of human movement.

Whyte and Morrissey (1990, p. 45) identify **motor development** as "a process of continuous modification caused by neurologic growth and maturation, residual effects of previous experiences, and effects of new motor experiences." Motor development then continuously occurs during the time from birth to death. Motor development is often associated with motor milestones of the developmental sequence. The development sequence is beneficial to view the sequential attain-

Gold Box 4-1

Motor Behavior Areas

Motor development: Events that occur covering months, years, or decades.
Motor learning: Events that occur over hours, days, and weeks.
Motor control: Events that occur over short time intervals.

Whiting & Rugg (2006)

Table 4-3	**General Motor Stages of the Developmental Sequence**	
1. Prone	10. Pulls sit to stand	18. Rides tricycle
2. Reaches for objects	11. Walks with support	19. Skips on one foot
3. Sits with support	12. Stands alone	20. Hops on one foot
4. Rolls prone to supine	13. Climbs stairs holding railings	21. Climbs stairs with one foot per step
5. Wriggles and crawls	14. Climbs stairs alone	22. Skips on both feet
6. Palmar grasp	15. Jumps on both feet	23. Runs on toes
7. Rolls supine to prone	16. Walks on tips of toes	24. Walks heel to toe
8. Sits unsupported	17. Stands on one foot	25. Kicks, throws, climbs
9. Stands with support		

Adapted from Simon, C. J. & Daub, M. M. (1993). Human development across the life span. In H. Hopkins & H. Smith (Eds.), *Willard & Spackman's occupational therapy* (8th ed., pp. 95–130). Philadelphia, PA: J.B. Lippincott Co.; Whyte, J., & Morrissey, J. (1990). Motor learning and relearning. In M. B. Glenn and J. Whyte (Eds.), *The practical management of spasticity in children and adults* (pp. 44–69). Philadelphia, PA: Lea & Febiger.

ment of motor milestones; however, it does not explain motor development that follows through adulthood and later life. Table 4-3 identifies general motor stages of the developmental sequence. These stages help to view the sequential nature of the developmental sequence.

The developmental sequence is hierarchical, where one motor milestone builds on the development of the previous motor milestones. While they are sequential, there is no specific timeframe for acquisition of skills, and, at best, a range of typical motor behavior norms for milestone acquisition may be provided. The developmental sequence provides an explanation for how the human body develops motorically and provides information on the building blocks of skilled movement. Initially, responses of infants are reflexive and involuntary but later lead to voluntary controlled movement. Whyte and Morrissey (1990) identify that movement initially sequences from mobility to stability and then to controlled mobility to distal skilled movement with proximal stabilization. Other types of developmental sequences for motor development have been suggested to exist. They include proximal to distal development, cephalocaudal direction, and reflex-dominated activity to reflex-inhibited activities. The developmental sequence, while beneficial, may not be the only method for how the human body organizes motor movements throughout the lifespan.

Motor learning is defined as the acquisition and/or modification of learned movement patterns over time (Pendleton & Schultz-Krohn, 2006). Motor learning takes into consideration the client, task, and environment. Motor learning has provided valuable information on the development of treatment approaches, such as the task-oriented approach and constraint-induced movement therapy (Pendleton & Schultz-Krohn, 2006). Further description of motor learning is outside the focus of this text; however, it is again an important concept to understand human movement behavior.

Motor learning explains how people move and develop motor skills over time with practice and experience. **Motor skills** are defined as voluntary movements used to complete a desired task or achieve a specific goal (Whiting & Rugg, 2006). Motor skills are goal directed and observable as a client interacts with the environment and task. Examples may include writing your name, drinking from a cup, or turning a key. Motor skills may be synonymous with motor control; however, there are subtle differences in the definitions provided.

Motor control is the outcome of motor learning involving the ability to produce purposeful movements of the extremities and postural adjustments in response to activity and environment demands (Pendleton & Schultz-Krohn, 2006). The definition of motor skills includes "voluntary movements," which may exclude the use of reflexes and automatic reactions as motor skills. Motor control includes the term *purposeful movements* but also recognizes postural adjustments. In OT, reflexive and automatic reactions may be used to enable function or achieve a desired goal.

Steve, in Figure 4-2, illustrates another example of how the different concepts of motor behavior can influence movement. In Figure 4-2, Steve is playing the Wii (Nintendo, Redmond, WA) game system as a therapeutic activity. This is the first time Steve has played the Wii so he is using his motor control to provide the proper outcome with manipulating the game controllers. As Steve continuously uses the Wii over days and weeks, motor learning is occurring, which allows Steve to achieve improved outcomes for the desired movements required. Steve has to have integrated early reflexive patterns and progressed along the developmental sequence to sit upright or stand when needed to participate in the game. The developmental sequence would have started years earlier at birth. All three concepts of motor behavior collaborate to allow purposeful goal-directed motor behavior to occur.

Shumway-Cook and Woollacott (2001) identify key aspects of skilled movement to include the ability to adapt and move efficiently and consistently in a variety of environments. Motor control and motor skills are aspects that are important for the production of skilled movements. Both motor skills and motor control consider the person, activity, and context. Motor learning and motor development, while important, include topics outside the scope of this text and will be covered more in other courses. Developing an understanding of normal movement is essential to apply the concepts of motor behavior and OTPF-2 in OT.

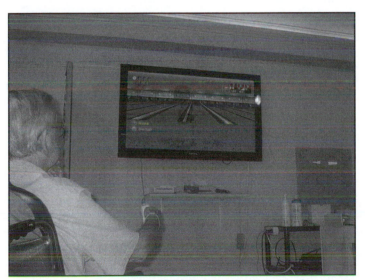

Figure 4-2. Steve is playing the Wii game system as a therapeutic activity during therapy.

Movement Characteristics

Martin (1977) describes human movement as a change in position and object that passes through a series of positions. Movement for the sake of movement is not functional and is not reflective of what consists of normal or typical motor behavior. Movement is inexplicably linked to function. *Merriam-Webster's Collegiate Dictionary* (1991, p. 498) describes function as "performing or being able to perform a regular function." It also includes "the normal and specific contribution of a body part to the economy of a living organism." As such, functional movement correlates well with the definitions already provided of motor control and motor skills. Functional movement, however, may not be synonymous with normal movement.

Normal movement may be a misnomer in that there may be a wide variation of movement that may be considered normal, and as cited in Latash and Anson (1996, p. 3), Sheridan identified varying movement as "normal," "normality," and "normal movement patterns." Spaulding (2005) supports this by stating that there are many different functional abilities in the well population as well as those with disabilities. People can often function at high levels without ever meeting optimum levels of ability, depending on the strategy used (Fisher & Yakura, 1993). The Functional Movement Continuum, as described in Table 4-4, was created to help characterize the variety of functional movement available.

The functional movement continuum is based on Latash and Anson's (1996, p. 2) presentation of "normal movement patterns to span a broad range of patterns from clumsy and impaired movements to uniquely specific movements." This continuum has been expanded upon to reflect function and those characteristics important in OT. The functional movement continuum describes adaptive motor behaviors that occur over the four common categories in the continuum. **Adaptive motor behaviors** are defined as follows

1.   Certain ways the body acts in a situation (Horak, 1987).
2.   Appropriate and efficient movement strategies used by the body (Horak, 1987).
3.   The body's ability to apply normal movement strategies to achieve functional goals (Landel & Fisher, 1993).

Adaptive motor behaviors reflect the body's ability to select and choose from a variety of movement options. These movement options may roughly be categorized into four groups:

1.   Abnormal atypical movement
2.   Normal atypical movement
3.   Normal typical movement
4.   Normal (enhanced) typical movement

Functional movement characteristics are provided for each category to reflect the functional capabilities and quality of movement that can be found in each section (Horak, 1987).

At one end of the continuum is **abnormal atypical movement**. This category is characterized by the inability to produce the desired movement strategy necessary to complete an activity within generally accepted parameters. Impairments that may prevent or limit movement strategies may include increased or decreased spasticity, pathological movement synergies, decreased interjoint coordination, incorrect timing of motor sequence, or muscle weakness (Roby-Brami et al., 2003). Abnormal postural adjustments, muscle weakness, and a lack of mobility may also limit movement strategies (Cirsea & Levin, 2000). Functional examples might include a person with severe rheumatoid arthritis who is no longer able to sit-to-stand from a commode or is no longer able to grasp due to severe ulnar deviation of the wrist. Another example might include a client with a high complete cervical injury who is no longer able to complete a functional task independently with adaptations. Individual impairments may affect movement patterns over time and lead to nonfunctional maladaptive movement behaviors.

The abnormal atypical movement category reflects a lack of movement options and significantly impaired motor movements that prevent the participation and completion of functional tasks even with adaptive approaches. Accepted parameters for performance may be individual or

Table 4-4	**Functional Movement Continuum**		
Adaptive Motor Behaviors			
Abnormal Atypical Movement	**Normal Atypical Movement**	**Normal Typical Movement**	**Normal (Enhanced) Typical Movement**
Motor Behavior Characteristics			
Inability to produce the desired movement strategies and characteristics necessary to complete an activity/occupation in generally accepted parameters.	Awkward Uncoordinated Inefficient Conscious thought Limited movement options Low complexity Increased time Low joint angle One joint motion Low velocity Low acceleration	Smooth Coordinated Efficient Automatic Variety of movement options High complexity Decreased time High joint angle Multiple joint motions High velocity High acceleration	Highly trained motor skills or motor control that allow for high efficiency, adaptability, and consistency in a variety of environments.
(not intended to be an all-inclusive list)			

environmental, depending on the task and context of movement application. An example might include that a client is able to self-dress completely; however, the task takes more than 2 hours to complete. Ultimately, there is a lack of movement strategies for the task and environment, which may lead to permanent disability if the activity cannot be completed adequately (Shumway-Cook & Woollacott, 2001).

Perhaps the majority of human motor behaviors can be characterized as either normal typical movement, or normal atypical movement. Fisher (1987) reported that normal typical movement may be reported by a person as being easier and feeling like the limb is lighter. **Normal typical movement/motor behavior** may be able to access and select from numerous movement possibilities to produce multiplanar, complex combinations of movement (Greene & Wolf, 1989). Movement may occur efficiently and effectively with no undue stress or injury production (Fisher & Yakura, 1993). Table 4-4 identified movement characteristics that might be found in normal typical movement. Examples of normal typical movement may include writing with your dominant hand, smiling at a joke, or bringing a utensil to the mouth during eating. Figure 4-3 demonstrates a child participating in self-feeding. He is initiating normal typical movement required in that context to eat.

Normal typical movement is different for each person. As each person's motor behavior has the capacity to adapt, normal typical movement is always changing. As a child loses his or her front baby teeth or has a loose tooth, the child adapts motor behavior for chewing. Another example of adaptation may include the multiple ways to wave hello. All may be correct depending on the person, task, and environment (or context). A focus on function and the task must be maintained due to the infinite number of movement combinations that may be considered normal and typical.

Normal atypical movement reflects the motor behavior response of a client/individual when typical movement strategies are temporarily or completely no longer feasible. Additionally, a new task may require novel or previously inexperienced motor behaviors, which may be characterized

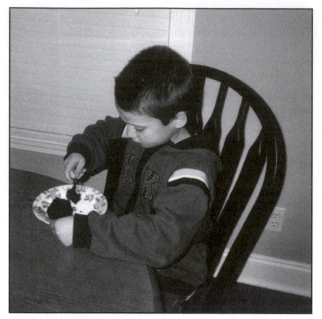

Figure 4-3. Child using normal typical movement to participate in self-feeding.

within this category. As motor development and motor learning occur, movement for the new task may adapt to be more reflective of normal typical movement. Movement characteristics, as presented in Table 4-4, change from the description of normal typical motor behavior possibly due to a lack of or loss in the repertoire of movement options available. McPherson et al. (1991) support this when they identified that individuals with cerebral palsy displayed a greater range of movement components in reaching as compared to individuals without cerebral palsy. There continues to be movement options available to complete a task; however, the number of movement options may be reduced.

An example of normal atypical movement may include a client with flaccid **hemiparesis** in the dominant upper extremity following a stroke. The individual may be able to use his or her non-dominant arm to enable self-feeding or use the flaccid dominant upper extremity as a second-ary assist to complete a functional task. Figures 4-4 and 4-5 display Johnny, who was diagnosed with a cerebrovascular accident (CVA) and left upper extremity weakness. Figure 4-4 illustrates Johnny writing with his nondominant right upper extremity, and Figure 4-5 illustrates Johnny engaging in functional mobility with a wheelchair. In each case, Johnny is not able to complete the purposeful activity of writing or ambulation as he would have prior to onset of the CVA. With adaptive motor behaviors, however, Johnny is still able to complete writing and functional mobility.

In the well population, an example of atypical normal movement may include learning to play video games on the Wii. Prior experience from playing video games on a Playstation (Sony Computer Entertainment America, LLC, Foster City, CA) game system is helpful with adapting motor behaviors; however, motor behavior with the Wii may be characterized as normal but atypical until mastered. Another example may include a fake smile versus a genuine smile and hitting or catching a ball with the nondominant upper extremity. Figures 4-6, 4-7, and 4-8 pres-ent a picture of a child with a real (normal typical) smile and a child with a fake (normal atypical) smile. While the quantity of muscles needed to smile can be argued, it surely can be accepted that different muscles are used with a normal typical smile versus a contrived smile. Can you identify which picture is the real smile and which is the contrived smile?

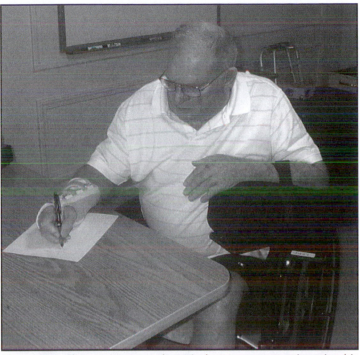

Figure 4-4. Client using normal atypical movement to write using his nondominant upper extremity.

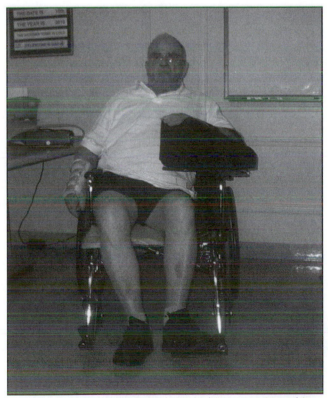

Figure 4-5. Client using normal atypical movement to achieve functional mobility.

Figure 4-6. Child purposefully not smiling.

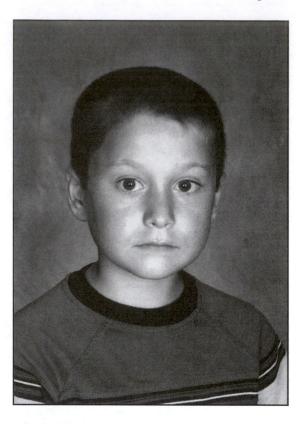

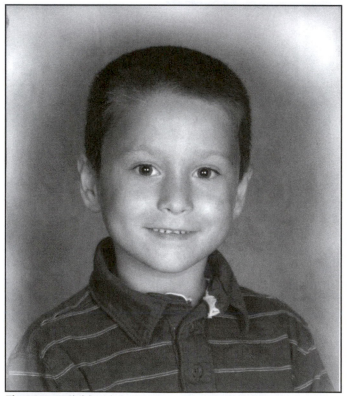

Figure 4-7. Child with a genuine normal typical smile.

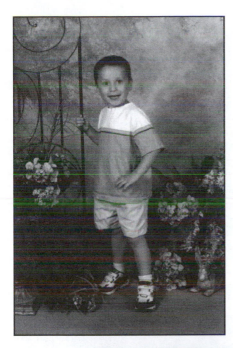

Figure 4-8. Child with a contrived, normal atypical smile.

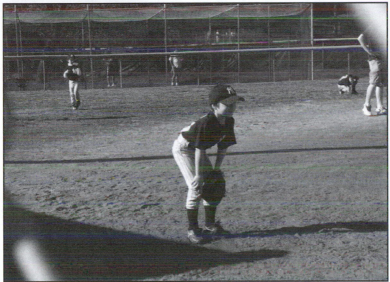

Figure 4-9. Baseball player in the ready position at third base demonstrating normal typical (enhanced) movement.

Lastly, **normal (enhanced) typical movement** is reflective of highly trained motor skills and motor control. This motor behavior allows for high efficiency, adaptability, and consistency in performance of a task in a variety of environments. Quite often, normal (enhanced) typical movement does not occur naturally. It is also very specific to the individual, task, and context and can be found in many different situations. One example might include a baseball player playing the position of pitcher or third base in the infield. While any person might be able to play these positions, by the end of the baseball season, a player may develop high efficiency and consistency with movements required above what may be accepted of any person. Figure 4-9 illustrates a baseball player in the ready position at third base in the infield. Figure 4-10 also illustrates a baseball player pitching the ball.

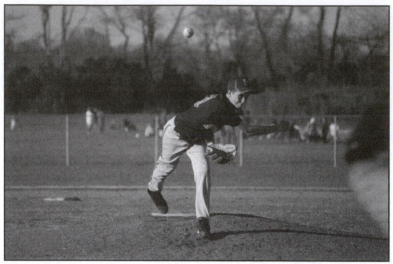

Figure 4-10. Baseball player pitching a baseball, demonstrating normal typical (enhanced) movement. (Reprinted with permission of Ryan Glass.)

<u>**Gold Box 4-2**</u>

Posture: "State of the body in relationship to gravity, the ground and to its body parts or extremities" (Martin, 1977).

Postural control: "The regulation of the body's position in space for the dual purpose of stability and orientation" (Shumway-Cook & Woollacott, 2001).

Anticipatory postural movements: "Reflect movements of the trunk or posture in response to changes in task or environmental demands" (Shumway-Cook & Woollacott, 2001).

Posture and Anticipatory Postural Movements

Functional movement occurs simultaneously with posture and anticipatory postural movements. Gold Box 4-2 presents definitions of **posture**, **postural control**, and **anticipatory postural movements**. Posture is a separate aspect of movement that can be typified by particular positions, such as static standing, squatting, static sitting, and lying. Posture has to change when the body moves in transitions (e.g., when moving from static sitting to dynamic sitting or static standing to dynamic standing). Postural control and anticipatory postural movements are descriptions of posture that more specifically relate to changes in position relative to the person, task, and environment or context.

Postural movements and changes are important because they do the following:
1.   Contribute to the development of motor ability (Kanbur, Düzgün, Derman, & Baltaci, 2005).
2.   Precede limb movement for increased function (Horak, 1987; Tyldesley & Grieve, 2002).
3.   Maintain stability, center of gravity, and base of support.
4.   Prepare the body for movement (Martin, 1977).

Anticipatory postural movements occur automatically and precede voluntary limb movement (Horak, 1987). Postural adjustments may occur in sequence and may be difficult to identify through observation, possibly due to their subtleness (Horak, 1987). Martin (1977) identifies that this difficulty may be attributed to the inability to identify when automatic behavior ends and becomes voluntary movement. Additionally, while postural adjustments may be similar for a particular movement, changes in the environment or context may require further adaptation for functional movement. An example may include standing on a sandy beach. Differing postural adjustments may be needed if you are standing in the surf as the sand washes away from around your feet. Another example occurs when a client sits on the edge of a mat or sits all the way back on a mat. Sitting on the edge of a mat requires much more trunk control and postural adjustments versus sitting comfortably on a mat, which is less challenging. Certainly, the inability to appropriately sequence, initiate, or adequately produce desired anticipatory postural movements can affect upper extremity movement and engagement in functional tasks.

Maintaining stability, base of support (BOS), and center of gravity (COG) are key aspects of posture. **Stability** refers to the ability to maintain the body in equilibrium. Stability is essential to movement to prevent falls and enable distal mobility of the extremities to occur. Tyldesley and Grieve (2002) identify that a stable equilibrium is created when the line of gravity lies within the BOS. COG refers to the balance point of an object where all sides are equal (Lippert, 2006). COG can include the body as a whole as well as parts of the body. Due to the differences in weight, height, and body distribution among clients, the COG is always moving and may not be the same among clients. Also, COG is always changing. **Line of gravity** (LOG) is the vertical line from the COG to the earth, and BOS is contained within the area of the body parts in contact with the ground (Lippert, 2006).

Gold Box 4-3 identifies six principles that demonstrate the relationship between balance, stability, and motion (Lippert, 2006). First, lowering the COG will result in increased stability. A person who is sitting is more stable than a person who is standing. Additionally, lying down has a lower COG and even more stability. The second principle states that the COG and LOG must reside in the BOS for stability. This can be seen when leaning forward in sitting or standing. At some point, you will have to stop leaning, increase the BOS, or risk falling and a loss of stability as the LOG moves outside the BOS. As a client engages in dynamic sitting balance activities and reaching, he or she may be at increased risk that the LOG will fall outside of the BOS.

The next principle states that the greater the mass, the greater the stability. An empty bottle of soda may fall over easier than a full bottle of soda. Again, this principle can be seen with clients sitting on the edge of a mat. The fourth principle identifies that increasing BOS will result in increased stability. Standing results in a small BOS. When a client moves from sitting to standing, his or her BOS decreases, which may increase his or her risk for falls. Holding a grab bar may increase BOS and stability. Another example can be placing hands on a mat or bedside table while sitting at the edge of the mat for increased stability. Lying down allows for a great range for BOS, which also provides for a great deal of stability.

The fifth principle identifies that increasing friction between the object and surface will result in increased stability. Examples can be seen when placing dycem on a wheelchair seat to prevent sliding or placing dycem under a client's feet in sitting or standing. Other examples include using nonskid strips in the shower to prevent falls or using nonskid socks when standing. The last principle identifies that by focusing on a stable object during standing or sitting, stability will be increased. This incorporates multiple functions of the body such as vision and attention span to enhance stability. Quite often, a person or object will incorporate multiple principles of stability into consideration when performing a functional task.

Gold Box 4-3

Principles of Stability

1. Lowering the center of gravity will increase stability.
2. Center of gravity and line of gravity must remain in the base of support for stability.
3. Increasing the mass will increase the stability.
4. Increasing the base of support will increase the stability.
5. Increasing friction between the object and surface will increase stability.
6. Focusing on a spot will increase stability.

Adapted from Lippert (2006)

Therapists cannot address movement or task alone in the context of a client's engagement in daily tasks of interest. Movement aspects were presented as they are described by the OTPF-2. Motor behavior and characteristics of movement were also presented to provide a basis for observing and facilitating movement during therapy. Lastly, posture and anticipatory postural movements were presented as key aspects of the body to allow for functional movement. Posture and anticipatory postural movements are essential to identify in order to facilitate human movement. Skilled observation by trained therapists is quite often used in the identification of human movement. While observation is beneficial, it alone does not provide the specifics necessary to fully assess, monitor change, and set movement goals.

RANGE OF MOTION AND MANUAL MUSCLE TESTING

Measuring Movement

The occupational therapy assistant (OTA) is quite often expected to identify functional movement during therapeutic intervention and grade therapeutic activities and exercises to maximize the benefit for the client. Examples can include training a client to use a reacher or shoe horn, increasing or decreasing resistance to an arm bike, or altering the reaching distance to an object. The occupational therapist may establish a movement goal through the OT evaluation and treatment planning process. OTAs can assist through documenting their observations of the client's performance as well as administering standardized evaluations for which the OTA has displayed "service competency." The OTA practitioner then can assist in the assessment of movement from the OT evaluation throughout treatment with the collaboration of the occupational therapist. As movement in function cannot be defined simply, one approach alone may not be adequate to identify appropriate movement demands.

Lieber and Bodine-Fowler (1993) recommended that each component of the system should be identified to evaluate the complex phenomenon of movement. Gentile identified three levels of goal-directed functional behaviors that can be evaluated, as described in Shumway-Cook and Woollacott (2001). They include action, movement, and neuromotor process. Action refers to the area of occupation that is being performed by the client. Ultimately, can the client complete an activity of daily living (ADL) task of interest to the client? Remember, functional movement includes the interaction of the individual, activity, and environment or context.

The second level of analysis, movement, refers to the movement strategies used to complete a functional task. This may include transitional movements, such as sitting to standing or supine to sitting, bed mobility, and reaching to complete a task. This level of analysis fits well with aspects found in the performance, motor, and praxis skills of the OTPF-2 (see Table 4-2). The motor activity log (MAL) is a good example of an assessment that identifies movement that fits in this category. The MAL is a structured interview used to assess a client's perception of movement strategies chosen to complete a task. Taub and colleagues (1993) created the MAL to assess movement changes following constraint-induced movement therapy. The MAL identifies the client's perceived amount of movement (AOM) and quality of movement (QOM) during a functional task. AOM is identified by the percentage of motion created from no movement to 100% of available movement. QOM is identified through a sequential scale from poor, fair, and normal quality of movement.

The neuromotor process is the last category for analysis. Shumway-Cook and Woollacott (2001) identify that this process includes sensation, perception, strength, and motor coordination. Body functions, such as neuromusculoskeletal and movement-related functions (see Table 4-1), provide more examples of components that can be analyzed by this process. Overall, many assessment

---

Gold Box 4-4

Assessment Tools for the Identification of Movement

Bennet Hand Tool Dexterity Test (H-TDT)

Berg Balance Scale

Bruinicks-Oseretsky Test of Motor Proficiency, 2nd edition (BOT-2)

Children's Handwriting Evaluation Scale (CHES)

Erhardt Developmental Prehension Assessment (EDPA)

Jebson-Hand Function Test

Box and Block Test

Nine-Hole Peg Test

Crawford Small Parts Dexterity Test (CSPDT)

Fine Dexterity Test

Fine Motor Task Assessment

Fugl-Meyer Evaluation of Physical Performance

Grooved Peg Board Test

Lincoln-Oseretsky Motor Development Scale

Minnesota Rate of Manipulation Test

Motor Activity Log

Purdue Peg Board

Range of Motion

Manual Muscle Testing

Adapted from Crepeau, Cohn, & Boyt-Schell (2009)

---

tools may be needed to provide specific information on functional movement. Some assessment tools that provide information on body functions and performance skills relative to movement are identified in Gold Box 4-4. Range of motion and manual muscle testing are two common assessment tools used by OT practitioners and will be covered in greater detail throughout this text.

Introduction to Gross Range of Motion

Range of motion (**ROM**) and **manual muscle testing** (**MMT**) are two of the most common assessments in the physical disability setting used by OT practitioners. During the OT evaluation, ROM and MMT help to identify problems with movement, assist in developing treatment goals, and aid in the overall analysis of occupational performance. During the intervention process, ROM and MMT aid in intervention planning, treatment implementation, and treatment review needed to modify the treatment plan as needed. Last, ROM and MMT are useful in identifying progress and achievement of OT goals and in providing a measurement for functional outcomes.

ROM is defined as the arc of motion through which a joint moves. Articles on ROM techniques and recommendations can be traced back to the first issues of the *American Journal of Occupational Therapy* in 1947 (Hurt, 1947a, 1947b, 1948).

ROM is used in many OT clinics to do the following:

1.   Determine available mobility and identify impairments.
2.   Establish a baseline.
3.   Document improvements in mobility.
4.   Aid in selecting effectiveness of interventions.

Active range of motion (**AROM**) and passive range of motion (PROM) are different types of measurements used by OT practitioners. AROM describes the joint movements as the client alone moves a joint through the available ROM. At times, **active assist range of motion** (AAROM) is used by the clinician. AAROM identifies that the therapist manually assisted the client to move the joint; however, the client also activated some joint motion. PROM, on the other hand, refers to joint movement created by the OTA moving the extremity. With PROM, the client relaxes muscles to not participate in joint motion. Sabari, Maltzev, Lubarsky, Liszkay, and Hanel (1998) identified that AROM measurements may be more reliable than PROM measurements due to the variability in force that can be applied by the examiner. This also means that PROM may be slightly more difficult to measure due to variations of force that can be applied at the end range of movement. **End feel**, or how the joint movement feels at the end of the ROM, influences the amount of force a clinician will use to identify the available ROM. Table 4-5 describes the different types of end feel that may be experienced.

Gajdosik and Bohannon (1987) stressed that identification of movement through visual observation is unreliable when precision and accuracy is needed. As such, assessing AROM and PROM in the clinic is most often achieved with the use of a goniometer. A goniometer is a tool used to measure joint movements and angles. A goniometer has a stable or stationary arm on one side that usually includes numbers around a circle on the central part of the arm. Like a protractor, the circular numbers represent degrees of angular measurement. The other arm of the goniometer is called the moving or movement arm. The moving arm rotates around the stationary arm of the goniometer at a central point called the fulcrum. As can be seen in Figure 4-11, many types of goniometers exist to increase the accuracy and ease of measuring different joints of the body.

Table 4-5	**Types of End Feel**	
End Feel: The feel experienced by a clinician at the end range of motion for a joint.		
Types of End Feel		**Examples**
Soft end feel: The feel experienced when two muscle groups are compressed.		- Knee flexion and elbow flexion
Firm end feel: The feel experienced when a normal joint or ligament is stretched.		- Wrist flexion or extension
Hard end feel: The feel experienced when two bones block motion.		- Elbow extension
Abnormal end feel: The feel experienced when the typical quality of feel is different.		- Spasticity, muscle guarding, or springy sensation

Adapted from Thomas, C. L. (Ed.) (1993). *Taber's cyclopedic medical dictionary* (17th ed.). Philadelphia, PA: F.A. Davis.

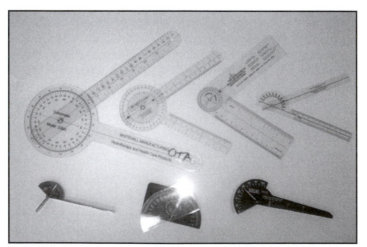

Figure 4-11. Assortment of different types of goniometers.

The goniometer measures joint angle changes in one plane. Wrist flexion is an example of a movement that occurs in one plane. A goniometer, however, does not measure joint movement in multiple planes. Wrist flexion and ulnar deviation, for example, could not be measured together or similarly, as these movements occur in different planes. A different joint axis would be needed due to the different planes. A joint axis is defined as the fixed center point from which the joint moves around. Usually, landmarks at the joint are used to align the fulcrum of the goniometer to the joint axis point to provide an accurate joint ROM measurement. Exceptions may have to occur due to obesity or when the landmark cannot be identified.

Range of motion is usually recorded using the neutral zero method (American Medical Association, 2008). The starting point for joint measurement is the neutral position or 0 degrees ending at the degree of available ROM. An example of the neutral zero measurement for the elbow joint might be 0 to 165 degrees. In this example, the client can move the elbow joint from full extension all the way to 165 degrees of elbow flexion. If the client is not able to reach the starting position, the measurement may be recorded differently. For example, a measurement of 20 to 165 degrees identifies that the elbow joint cannot reach the neutral position or starting point of zero. This can also be recorded as –20 degrees of elbow extension, meaning a loss of 20 degrees of ROM. Extension lag, or the sign (–), refers to the incomplete extension ability to return to the starting position (AMA, 2008). Additionally, some settings may also use the sign (+) to reflect a joint's ability to move into hyperextension. Often, the documentation will be determined by the setting, third-party requirements, and the experience of the therapists. ROM for each joint of the body can be found in Appendix B.

In assessing ROM, clinicians often first assess gross ROM. If a client appears to display atypical movement, the clinician then usually assesses formal AROM. PROM may be performed if impairments are noted with AROM. Collaborating with the occupational therapist may provide further insight into the causes of ROM impairments and their overall impact on occupational performance.

When assessing AROM, the clinician positions the client in the most supportive position to conduct ROM testing. Other joints may be stabilized while the joint being measured is isolated and moved to the neutral position for the start of goniometric testing. The fulcrum of the goniometer is placed over the landmark representing the axis of the joint being measured. The stationary arm is usually positioned proximal to the joint being measured and parallel to or along the plane being measured. The moving arm is usually placed distal to the joint being measured and again parallel to or along the plane being measured. Landmarks of the body will also be used for alignment of the goniometer arms. While maintaining the fulcrum of the goniometer over the joint axis, the moving arm follows the motion of the joint, and the stationary arm stays aligned proximal to the joint where no movement occurs. The client only moves the joint through the available ROM.

If impairments are noted with AROM, PROM may be required. In PROM, the clinician again positions the client in such a manner as to support and facilitate PROM testing. The fulcrum of the goniometer is placed over the landmark representing the axis of the joint being measured. The stable arm is usually positioned proximal to the joint being measured and parallel to or along the plane being measured. In positioning the stable arm, the clinician can provide stabilization proximal to the joint to eliminate compensatory movement and multiple joint motions. The moving arm is usually placed distal to the joint being measured and again parallel to or along the plane being measured. While positioning the moving arm of the goniometer, the clinician should be able to grasp just distal to the joint being measured to provide the force needed for joint movement. With PROM, the clinician provides the force needed for joint motion instead of the client.

While repeated measurements from the same therapist are most reliable, measurements from different therapists can be reliable if standardized procedures are followed (Rothstein, Miller, & Roettger, 1983). Table 4-6 provides measures to increase standardization for ROM by OT practitioners. Gajdosik and Bohannon (1987) also identified that one ROM measurement is just as effective

Table 4-6	Measures to Increase Standardization for Range of Motion

1. When possible, have the same clinician perform repeated ROM measurements or at least ensure the client performs the same procedures.
2. Use the same type and size of goniometer as prior measurements.
3. Practice using a goniometer to establish service competency with goniometer placement.
4. Control contextual considerations to limit impact on ROM measurements (i.e., the temperature of the room, effects of gravity).
5. Use the most appropriate goniometer for the size and shape of the joint being measured.
6. Select the client position that will not limit joint ROM.
7. Document any factors that may have influenced ROM measurements (i.e., pain, obesity, edema).
8. When possible, assess AROM first to identify need for PROM or isolated ROM measurements.
9. Observe and measure the unaffected extremity first to provide insight into the typical movement capability of the other arm.

as finding the average of repeated measurements. The upper extremity chapters in this text will allow for practice of ROM applications found in OT. One last consideration is that some clients may have contraindications or precautions with ROM. Possible contraindications and precautions for ROM and MMT are identified in Table 4-7.

Introduction to Gross Manual Muscle Testing

Quite often, MMT accompanies ROM testing within the clinical setting. While ROM tests for available joint range, MMT assesses the accompanying muscles' abilities to generate force. MMT is defined as a manual technique used to identify the relative strength of specific muscles (Thomas, 1993). Isolated MMT attempts to identify strength of individual muscles while gross MMT is used to assess the strength of muscle groups required to create a joint motion. This text focuses on allowing students to develop service competency with ROM and gross MMT. It is important to recognize, though, that particular OT settings may require the OTA practitioner to develop service competency with isolated MMT. In many settings, gross MMT techniques provide an adequate testing procedure to meet the needs of clients.

MMT is the most common method of testing muscle strength in the clinic (Bohannon, 2005; Dvir, 1997; Knepler & Bohannon, 1998). The purpose of MMT is the following:
1. Determine strength and identify impairments.
2. Establish a baseline.
3. Document improvements in strength.
4. Aid in selecting effectiveness of interventions.

As different testers may apply varying levels of resistance, MMT, like ROM testing, is most effective when the same therapist completes repeated tests. Other factors that can affect MMT include gender, strength of the tester, service competency level, and spasticity or fluctuating tone. Like ROM, MMT should be performed with precautions and contraindication in mind. Table 4-7 identifies ROM and MMT contraindications and precautions.

MMT is graded on a scale from 0 to 5 where the MMT grade of 0 is equivalent to no muscular contraction or movement and the MMT grade of 5 is equivalent to normal MMT strength. Table 4-8 displays the MMT scale, and it is important for each student to memorize. Of significance, isometric MMT grading techniques are used if the client demonstrates a minimal MMT strength grade of 3 or higher. Dvir (1997) identified that no more than 35% of maximal strength is required to support the arm in an antigravity position. Also, MMT grading techniques are

Table 4-7	Range of Motion and Manual Muscle Testing Contraindications and Precautions
Contraindications and Precautions of ROM and MMT	**Examples**
1. Inflammation	Significantly swollen hand or upper extremity
2. Pain	Pain with joint movement, to touch, or resistance
3. Recent surgery	Surgery for shunt placement or to treat a fracture
4. Myositis ossificans	Bony growth at the joint or bone affecting muscles
5. Bone cancer	Compromised bone function and structure
6. Osteoporosis	Compromised bone function and structure
7. Dementia	Inability to follow commands due to agitation/cognitive impairments
8. COPD	Shortness of breath, inability to move extremity adequately
9. Cardiovascular conditions	Recent heart surgery, cardiac precautions
10. Multiple sclerosis	Increased fatigue unwarranted
11. Arthritis	Compromised joint function and structure

Adapted from Latella, D., & Meriano, C. (2003). *Occupational therapy manual for evaluation of range of motion and muscle strength.* Clifton Park, NY: Delmar Cengage Learning.; Pendleton, H. M., & Schultz-Krohn, W. (2006). *Pedretti's occupational therapy: Practice skills for physical dysfunction* (6th ed.). St. Louis, MO: Mosby Elsevier.

conducted in the gravity-eliminated position if the client demonstrates a MMT strength grade of 2 or less. The gravity may be eliminated by positioning the joint perpendicular to the pull of gravity. Shoulder flexion in a gravity-eliminated position can be achieved in side lying, and shoulder abduction gravity can be eliminated when supine on a mat.

The steps of MMT include positioning the client and extremity to be tested, stabilizing the joint, palpating appropriate joint muscle groups, observing muscle contractions, resisting muscles, and grading strength (Killingsworth & Pedretti, 2006). If gravity-eliminated MMT is indicated, the clinician will follow the same steps; however, resistance is not applied, and the client will be positioned differently (i.e., the gravity-eliminated position). The OTA practitioner will follow these steps for gross MMT:

1. Positioning the client and extremity: First, the OTA will position the client in the optimum position to perform MMT. Quite often, the client will be positioned in a wheelchair. MMT can be performed if the client is supine in bed or lying on a mat; however, the effects of gravity may be different from that experienced in a sitting position. Quite often, it is useful to observe how the client moves. This may help to identify intact body structures and body functions and possible impairments. The OTA may also refer to the OT evaluation for a baseline status or rely upon prior OT treatment and observations.

    At this point, the OTA is able to identify if the client needs isometric testing or gravity-eliminated testing. In isometric testing, the joint is typically positioned at about half the available ROM, which allows the muscle to ideally be positioned to maximize the force production for joint movement. Muscles have lower force generation capability when there is a small joint angle as well as when the joint angle is closer to the available end range of movement.

2. Stabilizing the joint: The clinician needs to stabilize the joint being measured. The OTA will place one hand just proximal to the joint being measured to stabilize the joint. This is called the stabilizing hand. Positioning the client may also provide methods to

Table 4-8	Isometric Manual Muscle Testing Grades		
	Numerical Grade	Alternative Grading Scale	Description of Movement *(The Client...)*
Isometric Grading	5	Normal (N)	Maintains the testing position against gravity and maximal resistance.
	4	Good (G)	Maintains the testing position against gravity and moderate resistance.
	4-	Good- (G-)	Maintains the testing position against gravity and less-than-moderate resistance.
	3+	Fair+ (F+)	Maintains the testing position against gravity and minimal resistance.
Screening Test	3	Fair (F)	Moves the joint through full available ROM against gravity or maintains the testing position.
	3-	Fair- (F-)	Moves the joint through greater than half but less than full available ROM against gravity.
	2+	Poor+ (P+)	Moves the joint through less than half of the available ROM against gravity.
Gravity Eliminated	2	Poor (P)	Moves the joint through full ROM with gravity eliminated.
	2-	Poor- (P-)	Moves the joint through greater than half but less than full available ROM with gravity eliminated.
	1+	Trace+ (T+)	Moves the joint through less than half of the available ROM with gravity eliminated.
	1	Trace (T)	Demonstrates no joint movement, but there is a slight observable or palpable muscle contraction.
	0	Zero (0)	Demonstrates no joint movement and no palpable or observable muscle contraction.

stabilize other parts of the body and avoid compensatory movements or compensation. Compensation is defined as the use of other muscles by the client to achieve joint movement. While stabilizing the joint, the OTA can often palpate the muscles responsible for the joint movement.

3.   Palpating appropriate joint muscle groups: Many muscles may be able to be palpated due to their location close to the surface of the body. Muscle characteristics that may be observed include the size of the muscle contraction, muscle striations or directional pull of the muscles, response upon muscle activation, and response once resistance is applied. The skilled practitioner will feel for when the contraction begins and ends. Is there a smooth build-up in force or is the contraction an all or nothing response? What is the effect of hypotonicity, or decreased tone, if present? Additionally, in the case of increased tone, can the practitioner identify when the voluntary contraction ends and when the

involuntary movements begin? Hypotonicity and hypertonicity may provide inaccurate results for manual muscle testing. Care must also be provided to ensure that the muscle contraction is not impeded by palpation.

4. Observing muscle contractions: Observing muscle contractions may also provide evidence of muscle activation and joint movement. Quite often, observation of muscle contractions occurs simultaneously with palpation of the muscles, causing joint movement. Observing muscle movement occurs when the OTA first meets the client and observes functional movement. The first observations provide clues on movement and what adaptations to the approach need to be incorporated to standardize MMT. Observation of muscles during testing may also provide evidence of muscle contraction when palpation is not possible. Gold Box 4-5 provides a good suggestion to increase service competency with application of MMT.

Gold Box 4-5

By assessing MMT of the uninvolved intact extremity, the clinician will be able to gain information of typical normal movement that may be characteristic of the involved impaired extremity.

---

5. Resisting muscles: Resistance is only applied for isometric MMT. The OTA has already positioned the client, positioned the extremity, and stabilized the joint by placing a stabilizing hand just proximal to the joint. The OTA is also observing and palpating available muscle contractions. The OTA then places his or her other hand just distal to the joint being tested halfway to the next distal joint in the extremity. This is the location for placement of resistance and provides a standard location for repeated tests. The palmar surface of the hand provides a uniform application of force for the application of resistance. Use of fingertips for force application should be avoided due to discomfort to the client from poking the muscle and possible inconsistent application of force, not to mention poor ergonomics for the practitioner.

    The OTA asks the client to maintain his or her arm in the position of roughly half available ROM as force is applied to the arm to cause joint movement. Force is briefly applied in just enough time to assess resistance to the force produced by the therapist. The therapist builds up the application of force as the client provides resistance and in such a manner as to not surprise the client. It is important to remember precautions to MMT with force application. For example, arthritic joints and weak bones may not have the structure necessary to resist typical applications of force. Refer back to Table 4-7 for examples of precautions and contraindications of MMT.

6. Grading strength: The OTA will use the isometric MMT grades presented in Table 4-8 to assess muscle strength. Quite often, the OTA will first identify whether the client has a MMT strength grade of 3, or fair (F). The client will demonstrate this grade if the joint moves through the full available ROM against gravity or is able to maintain the testing position.

    If the client demonstrates MMT strength of at least a 3, or fair (F), the OTA will then perform the isometric grading test procedures. Resistance is applied for all muscle grades above 3, or fair (F). The amount of resistance determines the MMT strength grade.

    If the client demonstrates a MMT strength of less than 3, or fair (F), then the OTA will perform the gravity-eliminated grading test procedures. The MMT grade is determined by the amount of joint movement in the gravity-eliminated position. If joint movement is not possible in the gravity-eliminated position, then the MMT grade is determined by the presence or absence of a muscle contraction.

Table 4-9	Measures to Increase Standardization for Manual Muscle Testing

1. When possible, have the same clinician perform repeated MMT measures or at least ensure the client performs the same procedures.
2. Practice applying MMT to develop "Service Competency."
3. Control contextual considerations to limit impact on MMT (i.e., the temperature of the room, effects of gravity, temperature of mat or OTA's hands).
4. Document any factors that may have influenced MMT measurements (i.e., pain, dementia, edema, age, gender, weakness, command following).
5. Observe and measure the unaffected extremity first to provide insight into the typical movement capability of the other arm.
6. Gain information prior to the MMT through reviewing medical records, observing the client move and perform a functional task, and assessing the intact bilateral extremity first.
7. Minimize variations to MMT, and identify when variations exceed standardization to the point that accurate MMT may not be possible.

Summary

MMT can be a reliable and effective method of assessing strength in the clinic, especially when the OTA practitioner displays service competency. Like ROM, MMT assesses only one aspect of the numerous body functions affecting movement. The body functions of joint motion and strength are particularly needed for movement and have historically been widely assessed within the medical model. These body functions do not shed light on the numerous other body functions affecting movement. In addition, minimum needed ROM angles and MMT strength required to adequately be "within functional limits" (WFL) or "within normal limits" (WNL) are purposefully not stressed in this text. The redundancy of human movement and infinite ability to compensate or substitute motions can lead to infinite possibilities for acceptable functional movement to complete a task.

One of the focuses of this text is to aid the development of service competency for both ROM and MMT. Table 4-9 provides suggestions to increase service competency for MMT. In order to develop service competency, it is also important to memorize the isometric MMT grading scale to easily and appropriately apply muscle strength grades. This textbook only provides one norm for ROM and one scale for MMT; however, numerous different scales exist. The OT clinic protocols, service provider, and third-party payer requirements may determine which ROM norms and MMT scale will be used.

APPLICATIONS

The following activities will help you apply knowledge of movement in real-life applications. Activities can be completed individually or in a small group to enhance learning.

1.   **OTPF-2: Body Functions—Neuromusculoskeletal and Movement-Related Functions:** Many body functions affect movement. The purpose of Application #1 is to help the reader become more familiar with body functions identified in the OTPF-2 and how they impact function and movement. The body functions identified in the OTPF-2 and particularly involved in movement (i.e., neuromusculoskeletal and movement-related functions) are listed next. For Application #1, identify two activities and explain how each body function impacts the ability to participate in that functional activity.

Body Functions	Activity Example *(Getting Dressed)*	Activity #1	Activity #2
Joint ROM	*to doff and don clothes*		
Joint Alignment	*for pain-free smooth ROM*		
Strength	*for picking up clothes and body parts*		
Muscle Tone	*to activate UE reaching movements*		
Muscle Endurance	*to complete dressing in timely manner*		
Movement Reactions	*righting reactions, protective reactions*		
Walking Patterns	*needed to get clothes to wear*		

Questions:

A. Why do you think that ROM and MMT have historically been assessed more regularly in the clinic more so than the other body functions identified in the OTPF-2?

B. Are all body functions identified as important in each activity above? Why or why not?

C. Are all the body functions identified incorporated in the activities listed above? Minus a body function, can the activity still be performed?

2. **OTPF-2: Performance Skills—Motor and Praxis Skills:** Many performance skills in the OTPF-2 can also affect movement. The purpose of Application #2 is to help the reader become more familiar with the performance skills identified in the OTPF-2, particularly motor and praxis skills, and how they impact function and movement. The examples of the performance skills—motor and praxis skills identified in the OTPF-2—are listed below. For Application #2, use the same two activities from the previous application, and explain how each performance skill impacts the ability to participate in that functional activity.

Performance Skills	Activity Example *(Getting Dressed)*	Activity #1	Activity #2
Bending	*for socks and shoes, pick up items*		
Pacing	*timely sequence of arm in dressing*		
Coordinating	*UE; holding sleeve while putting other arm in sleeve*		
Maintaining	*balance on foot to put other leg in pants*		
Anticipating and Adjusting Posture	*i.e., changing body posture when needed like when standing on pants when pulling pants up*		
Manipulating	*to fasten pants or belt buckle*		

Questions:
A. When reflecting on performance skills, do you think that multiple body functions can influence how a performance skill is related to movement?
B. Are body functions more important than performance skills in enabling movement for the activities you've chosen? Explain your decision.
C. Are all of the performance skills identified incorporated in the activities listed previously?
D. Minus a performance skill, can the same activity be performed?

3. **Functional Movement Continuum:** Most functional movement may be described as normal atypical movement or normal typical movement. This application is designed to help accentuate both aspects of adaptive motor behaviors. At some point in your life, you have probably performed one of the following tasks listed below. For this application, refer back to that experience, and select one of the activities to answer the following questions.
Selected Activities:
- Dribble a basketball with your dominant arm.
- Throw a ball with your dominant arm.
- Brush your teeth, hair, or apply make-up with your dominant arm.
- Write a sentence with your dominant arm.
- Dribble a basketball with your nondominant arm.
- Throw a ball with your nondominant arm.
- Brush your teeth, hair, or apply make-up with your nondominant arm.
- Write a sentence with your nondominant arm.

Select an activity listed above: _____. For this activity, circle the descriptors below that best characterize the movement produced.

Normal Atypical Movement	Normal Typical Movement
Awkward	Smooth
Uncoordinated	Coordinated
Inefficient	Efficient
Conscious thought	Automatic
Limited movement options	Multiple movement options
Low complexity	High complexity
Increased time	Decreased time
Low joint angle	High joint angle
One joint motion	Multiple joint motions
Low velocity	High velocity
Low acceleration	High acceleration

Questions:
A. If the activity selected was with the dominant arm, are more characteristics circled under the column "Normal Typical Movement"?
B. Likewise, if the activity was performed with the nondominant arm, are more characteristics circled under the column "Normal Atypical Movement"? If not, why do you think this occurred?

4. **Motor Behavior:** The human body continuously learns and adapts movement to the activity being performed. First identify an activity. Next, identify the best descriptor of motor behavior (motor learning, motor control, or motor development) for each activity/task below. Try to give an example of each motor behavior.

Activity	Most applicable motor behavior
a.	
b.	
c.	
d.	
e.	
f.	

5. **ROM:** The purpose of this application is to gain experience using a goniometer to measure an angle. Choose an object in the room to find an example of an angle that you can measure. If you are not able to identify an object in the room, intersecting two lines on paper will create an angle that you can measure with a goniometer. An example might include a hardcover book standing on its end. Align the goniometer arms along the top edge of the front and back cover of the book. The fulcrum of the goniometer may not be directly over the spine of the book but that is ok. Appropriately aligning the goniometer arms will center the fulcrum of the goniometer in the proper position that is parallel to the apex of the angle produced by the open book. For your example, identify the following items:

   □   What are you trying to measure?
   □   What is the apex of the angle?
   □   Were the goniometer arms aligned?
   □   What is the joint angle measurement?

6. **MMT Grade Scale:** Match the MMT grade to its description of movement:

MMT Grades		Description of MMT Grade Movement
5 ____	a.	Maintains testing position against gravity and minimal resistance
4 ____	b.	Moves the joint through full ROM with gravity eliminated
4- ____	c.	Moves joint through less than half of available ROM and no gravity
3+ ____	d.	Moves joint through less than half of available ROM and gravity
3 ____	e.	No joint movement and no palpable muscle contraction
3- ____	f.	Maintains testing position against gravity and maximal resistance
2+ ____	g.	Moves joint through full available ROM against gravity
2 ____	h.	No joint movement but slight observable muscle contraction
2- ____	i.	Maintains testing position against gravity and moderate resistance
1+ ____	j.	Moves joint through more than half ROM but less than full ROM in gravity
1 ____	k.	Moves joint through more than half ROM but less than full ROM, no gravity
0 ____	l.	Maintains test position against gravity and less than moderate resistance

Questions:
A. What MMT grades are included in isometric grading?
B. What MMT grades are included in antigravity testing?
C. What MMT grades are not included in either isometric grading or antigravity testing?

7. **Palpating Muscles:** Using anatomical pictures of muscles, muscle models, and other materials, attempt to see how many different muscles you can palpate on the upper extremity individually or in groups. Identify the muscle, location, and joint motion it produces.

Palpable Muscle	Location	Motion and Joint
1. *i.e., biceps brachii*	*anterior surface upper arm*	*elbow flexion*
2.		
3.		
4.		
5.		

REFERENCES

American Medical Association. (2008). *Guides to the evaluation of permanent impairment* (6th ed.). Chicago, IL: Author.

Ayres, A. J. (1985). *Developmental dyspraxia and adult onset apaxia.* Torrance, CA: Sensory Integration International.

Blanch, E. I., & Parham, L. D. (2002). Praxis and organization of behavior in time and space. In S. Smith Roley, E. I. Blanch & R. C. Schaaf (Eds.), *Understanding the nature of sensory integration with diverse populations* (pp. 183-200). San Antonio, TX: Therapy Skill Builders.

Bohannon, R. W. (2005). Manual muscle testing: Does it meet the standards of an adequate screening test? *Clinical Rehabilitation, 19*, 662–667.

Cirsea, M. C., & Levin, M. F. (2000). Compensatory strategies for reaching in stroke. *Brain, 123*, 940-953.

Crepeau, E. B., Cohn, E. S., & Boyt-Schell, B. A. (2009). *Willard & Spackman's occupational therapy* (11th ed.). Philadelphia, PA: Lippincott Williams & Wilkins.

Dvir, Z. (1997). Grade 4 in manual muscle testing: The problem with submaximal strength assessment. *Clinical Rehabilitation, 11*, 36–41.

Filley, C. M., (2001). *Neurobehavioral anatomy.* Boulder, CO: University Press of Colorado

Fisher, A. (2006). Overview of performance skills and client factors. In H. Pendleton & W. Schultz-Krohn (Eds.), *Pedretti's occupational therapy: Practice skills for physical dysfunction* (pp. 372–402). St. Louis, MO: Mosby Elsevier.

Fisher, B. (1987). Effect of trunk control and alignment on limb function. *Journal of Head Trauma Rehabilitation, 2*(2), 72–79.

Fisher, B., & Yakura, J. (1993). Movement analysis: A different perspective. *Orthopaedic Clinics of North America*, March, 1–14.

Gajdosik, L., & Bohannon, R. W. (1987). Clinical measurement of range of motion: Summary of goniometry emphasizing reliability and validity. *Physical Therapy, 67*(12), 1867–1872.

Greene, B. L., & Wolf, S. L. (1989). Upper extremity joint movement: Comparison of two measurement devices. *Archives of Physical Medicine & Rehabilitation, 70*, 288–290.

Heilman, K. M., & Roth, L. J. G. (1993). *Clinical neuropsychology* (3rd ed.). New York, NY, Oxford University Press

Horak, R. (1987). Clinical management of postural control in adults. *Physical Therapy, 67*(12), 1881–1885.

Hurt, S. P. (1947a). Joint measurement. *American Journal of Occupational Therapy, 1*(4), 209–214.

Hurt, S. P. (1947b). Joint measurement: Part II. *American Journal of Occupational Therapy, 1*(5), 281–285.

Hurt, S. P. (1948). Joint measurement: Part III. *American Journal of Occupational Therapy, 2*(1), 13–15.

Kanbur, N. Ö., Düzgün, I., Derman, O., & Baltaci, G. (2005). Do sexual maturation stages affect flexibility in adolescent boys aged 14 years? *Journal of Sports Medicine and Physical Fitness, 45*(1), 53–57.

Killingsworth, A. P., & Pedretti, L. W. (2006). Evaluation of muscle strength. In H. Pendleton and W. Schultz-Krohn (Eds.), *Pedretti's occupational therapy: Practice skills for physical dysfunction* (pp. 469–512). St. Louis, MO: Mosby Elsevier.

Knepler, C., & Bohannon, R. W. (1998). Subjectivity of forces associated with manual muscle testing grades of 3+, 4-, and 4. *Perceptual and Motor Skills, 87*, 1123–1128.

Landel, R., & Fisher, B. (1993). Musculoskeletal considerations in the neurologically impaired patient. *Orthopaedic Physical Therapy Clinics of North America, 2*(1), 15–24.

Latash, M. L., & Anson, J. G. (1996). What are "normal movements" in atypical populations? [unedited preprint]. *Behavioral and Brain Sciences, 19*(1), 55–106. Retrieved from http://www.bbsonline.org/Preprints/OldArchive/bbs.latash.html.

Lieber, R. L., & Bodine-Fowler, S. C. (1993). Skeletal muscle mechanics: Implications for rehabilitation. *Physical Therapy, 73*(12), 844–856.

Liepman, H. (1920). Apraxie. *Ergebnisse der Gesamten Medizin, 1,* 516–543

Lippert, L. S. (2006). *Clinical kinesiology and anatomy* (4th ed.). Philadelphia, PA: F. A. Davis Company.

Martin, J. P. (1977). A short essay on posture and movement. *Journal of Neurology Neurosurgery and Psychiatry, 40,* 25–29.

McPherson, J. J., Schild, R., Spaulding, S. J., Barsamian, P., Transon, C., & White, S. (1991). Analysis of upper extremity movement in four sitting positions: A comparison of persons with and without cerebral palsy. *American Journal of Occupational Therapy, 42*(2), 123–129.

Merriam-Webster's collegiate dictionary (9th ed.) (1991). Springfield, MA: Merriam-Webster.

Pendleton, H. M., & Schultz-Krohn, W. (2006). *Pedretti's occupational therapy: Practice skills for physical dysfunction* (6th ed.). St. Louis, MO: Mosby Elsevier.

Roby-Brami, A., Feydy, A., Combeaud, M., Biryokova, E. V., Bussel, B., & Levin, M. F. (2003). Motor compensation and recovery for reaching in stroke patients. *ACTA Neurologica Scandinavica, 107,* 369–381.

Rothstein, J. M., Miller, P. J., & Roettger, R. F. (1983). Goniometric reliability in a clinical setting. *Physical Therapy, 63*(10), 1611–1615.

Sabari, J. S., Maltzev, I., Lubarsky, D., Liszkay, E., & Hanel, P. (1998). Goniometric assessment of shoulder range of motion: Comparison of testing in supine and sitting positions. *Archives of Physical Medicine & Rehabilitation, 79,* 647–651.

Shumway-Cook, A., & Woollacott, M. H. (2001). *Motor control: Theory and practical applications* (2nd ed.). Philadelphia, PA: Lippincott Williams & Wilkins.

Spaulding, S. J. (2005). *Meaningful motion: Biomechanics for occupational therapists.* New York, NY: Elsevier Churchill Livingston.

Taub, E., Miller, N. E., Novak, T. A., Cook III, E. W., Fleming, W. C., Nepomuceno, C. S.,. . .Crago, J. E. (1993). Technique to improve chronic motor deficit after stroke. *Archives of Medicine & Rehabilitation, 74,* 347–354

Thomas, C. L. (Ed.) (1993). *Taber's cyclopedic medical dictionary* (17th ed.). Philadelphia, PA: F.A. Davis.

Tyldesley, B., & Grieve, J. (2002). *Muscles, nerves and movement in human occupation* (3rd ed.). Malden, MA: Blackwell Publishing Co.

Whiting, W. C., & Rugg, S. (2006). *Dynatomy: Dynamic human anatomy.* Champaign, IL: Human Kinetics.

Whyte, J., & Morrissey, J. (1990). Motor learning and relearning. In M. B. Glenn and J. Whyte (Eds.), *The practical management of spasticity in children and adults* (pp. 44–69). Philadelphia, PA: Lea & Febiger.

chapter 5

Function and Movement of the Trunk and Neck

Teresa Plummer, PhD, MSOT, OTR/L, ATP

The following occupational profile is provided to demonstrate how posture, positioning, and stability are all related to occupational performance. Terrence, the client in the following occupational profile, will be referred to in this chapter in order to apply the kinesiological and anatomical principles involved with sitting posture and trunk movements. During the occupational therapy (OT) evaluation, the following data were gathered:

Subjective: Terrence states that he has difficulty raising his arms overhead while sitting in his wheelchair. Additionally, the occupational therapist identifies that Terrence has difficulty with swallowing and seems short of breath. Terrence has used a manual wheelchair since his admission to an assisted-living facility 6 years ago. Terrence reports a decrease in his ability to perform any overhead activity (recently increased trouble combing his hair and retrieving items above him in the refrigerator). Recently, Terrence has been experiencing increased fatigue and difficulty swallowing, especially when drinking from a cup or glass.

Terrence is able to propel his lightweight manual wheelchair to the dining area approximately 50 feet from his apartment. He states, however, that this has been more difficult than usual as he feels tired by the time he gets to the dining area. He has not been able to finish his meal without needing frequent rest breaks. Terrence also reports difficulty raising his glass and tilting his head back to finish his beverages. Due to fatigue, Terrence has to return to his room after meals rather than staying in the lobby to read the newspaper with his friends.

Terrence moved to the assisted-living apartment 6 years ago from his downtown apartment after his retirement from the university where he taught economics for nearly 25 years. He was diagnosed with secondary-progressive multiple sclerosis 14 years ago. Terrence enjoys reading, playing chess, listening to music, playing the piano, and engaging in social groups at the university as well as the assisted-living center. He uses a rolling walker in his apartment, but states that his arms are very tired after walking to the bathroom from his living room. He spends much of his day napping to recuperate from the activities that he has completed. He states that he is afraid of falling, especially in the bathroom, and as a result he has learned to limit his fluid intake to avoid unnecessary trips to the bathroom.

Objective: Terrence has no complaint of pain at rest but does state that his endurance is more limited than it was 3 months ago. He was recently evaluated for a power wheelchair for mobility and positioning. The areas addressed during the wheelchair assessment included the following:

Keough, J. L., Sain, S. J., Roller, C. L.
*Kinesiology for the Occupational Therapy Assistant:
Essential Components of Function and Movement* (pp. 113-140).

- Skin integrity
- Spine and pelvis mobility
- Presence of orthopedic deformities and whether each is flexible or fixed
- Presence of abnormal tone
- Adequate joint range of motion (ROM) for the seated posture
- Adequate ROM and strength for the mode of propulsion or drive control
- Balance and the presence of asymmetries and orthopedic deformities (Davis, 2007).

An improper wheelchair may create limitations in mobility, health issues, and/or decreased participation in activities of daily living (Bolin, Bodin, & Kreuter, 2000; Brubaker, 1986; Guerraz, Blouin, & Vercher, 2003; Herman & Lange, 1999).

The evaluation highlighted the following:

Functional skills: Terrence is unable to ambulate more than 10 feet without fatigue and shortness of breath. He uses a manual wheelchair for distances greater than 10 feet, but fatigues when propelling the wheelchair to the dining room and other areas within the assisted-living facility. Terrence is independent with activities of daily living (ADL) tasks. He utilizes a grab bar, tub bench, and hand-held shower for bathing. Terrence requires moderate assistance for instrumental activities of daily living (IADL) tasks and eats two of his three meals in the dining room at the assisted-living facility. He is able to complete simple meal prep for breakfast, but requires assistance for shopping as he is unable to propel his wheelchair to the local grocery store two blocks away. He is independent for modified stand pivot transfer using his walker but complains of anxiety when performing transfers due to a fear of falling. He schedules his day to limit the number of times he gets into and out of his manual wheelchair. Additionally, he limits the number of times per day that he uses the restroom and the number of days per week that he takes a shower due to a fear of falling. He has recently developed a urinary tract infection and is on medication.

Range of motion: Active range of motion (AROM) is grossly within normal limits with the following exceptions.

- Glenohumeral (GH) joint flexion: Right: 0 to 75 degrees; Left: 0 to 70 degrees
- GH joint abduction: Right: 0 to 60 degrees; Left: 0 to 65 degrees
- GH joint external rotation: Right: 0 to 25 degrees; Left: 0 to 45 degrees
- GH joint internal rotation: Right: 0 to 35 degrees; Left: 0 to 40 degrees
- Hip extension: Right: 0 to 20 degrees; Left: 0 to 25 degrees
- Hip flexion: Right: 0 to 80 degrees; Left: 0 to 80 degrees
- Knee extension: Right: 0 to 20 degrees; Left: 0 to 15 degrees

Strength: Strength is 4/5 (Good) with the following exceptions:
- GH joint flexion: Right: 3/5; Left: 3/5
- GH joint abduction: Right: 3-/5; Left: 3-/5
- GH joint external rotation: Right: 3/5; Left: 3/5
- GH joint internal rotation: Right: 3/5; Left: 3/5
- Hip extension: Right: 2+/5; Left: 2+/5
- Hip flexion: Right: 2+/5; Left: 2+/5
- Knee extension: Right: 3/5; Left: 3/5

Balance: Static sitting balance is fair, and dynamic sitting balance is poor. Static standing balance is fair, and dynamic standing balance is poor.

Posture: The client sits with a flexible posterior pelvic tilt, slight obliquity (tilt) to the right, and minimal rotation on the right side. He exhibits mild thoracic kyphosis and mild cervical hyperextension.

Assessment: The client is at risk for falls, pressure ulcer development, and impaired orthopedic limitations. A power wheelchair is recommended with the following features:
- Tilt and recline, seat elevator and elevating leg rest, and angle adjustable foot plates
- Seat cushion with good pressure-relieving attributes
- High-contour back with headrest attached

- Pelvic positioning belt
- Joystick control—retractable swing away
- Height-adjustable desk-length arm rest

Short-Term Goals:
1. Client will demonstrate safe and independent use of power seat functions of tilt, recline, elevator, and leg elevation by 2 weeks.
2. Client will demonstrate safe and proficient use of power mobility device including on/off, steering, navigating doorways, and areas where furniture is in close proximity by 2 weeks.
3. Client will be safe and independent in sit-to-stand transfers using the seat elevator to assist by 2 weeks.
4. Client will demonstrate improved endurance with use of power mobility device by 2 weeks.

Long-Term Goals:
1. Client will be independent in pressure relief with power wheelchair features after instruction by 4 weeks.
2. Client will be independent and safe in sit-to-stand transfers using appropriately placed grab bars in the bathroom by discharge.
3. Client will demonstrate improved respiration with appropriate use of tilt and recline position by 4 weeks.
4. Client will demonstrate improved social interactions secondary to improved endurance and improved posture by 4 weeks.
5. Client will prevent the development of pressure ulcers and orthopedic deformities by discharge.

BODY FUNCTIONS OF THE TRUNK AND NECK

According to the U.S. Census Bureau's Survey of Income and Program Participation, an estimated 2.8 million people living outside of institutions use a wheelchair for mobility (LaPlante & Kaye, 2010). A wheelchair that is ill fitting to an individual may lead to negative consequences, such as injuries, pressure ulcers, and even death (Batavia, Batavia, & Friedman, 2001). The process of providing a wheelchair to an individual requires the occupational therapy assistant (OTA) to consider many factors. Among these factors, it is necessary to consider a client's anatomical characteristics to include orthopedic abnormalities, motor and sensory processes, functional skills, and individual needs. It is also necessary to consider a client's posture, skin integrity, and ability to perform movements and occupational tasks.

This chapter reviews many of these concepts as well as provides an in-depth presentation of kinesiological principles of the trunk and head. Joint motions, spinal curves, and movement characteristics will also be identified in the following sections. Their relationship to posture, movement, and function will be presented in subsequent sections. Finally, common problems associated with orthopedic deformities will be presented.

Motions of the Trunk and Neck

The vertebral column is considered a triaxial joint, which allows for movement in the three planes (sagittal, frontal, and horizontal). To understand how the spine moves, it is helpful to visualize the body as a two-dimensional plane. As a review from Chapter 2, Table 5-1 identifies the planes that help to visualize movement of the body. Flexion, extension, and hyperextension occur in the sagittal plane around multiple axes along the spine. Lateral flexion occurs in the frontal plane around a sagittal axis and involves some degree of rotation. Rotation occurs in the horizontal plane around a vertical axis. Rotation involves some degree of lateral flexion of the spine. Rotation specifically does not occur at the joint of C1 and the skull.

Table 5-1	The Planes of the Body and Their Location
Plane	**Meaning**
Sagittal or median plane	Divides the left and right sides of the entire body.
Frontal or coronal plane	Divides the front and back halves of the entire body.
Horizontal or transverse plane	Divides the body at the waist (top and bottom halves of the body).

Motions of the pelvic girdle are also integral to the motions of the trunk. The pelvic girdle unites the sacrum and the two hip bones at several different joints. The posterior joints include the right and left sacroiliac joint, and the anterior joint is called the pubic symphysis. The pelvic girdle also unites with the vertebrae at the lumbosacral joint. The lumbosacral joint is the most important articulation in the pelvic girdle, as all pelvic movements involve this joint. Every pelvic movement then involves the vertebral column. As such, every pelvic motion also impacts all functional movement and the ability to perform daily life tasks. Gold Box 5-1 supports the importance of the pelvis in functional movements. The following section discusses these typical movement patterns.

Gold Box 5-1

Reaching Tasks

The ability to perform reaching tasks while seated is fundamental to occupational performance, self-care, independence, and quality of life.

Dean, Shepherd, & Adams (1999)

Visual Observation for Function

Posture is a combined activity requiring many anatomical body parts, such as the pelvis, spine, feet, head, and neck. Additionally, posture is dependent upon the sensory system. In particular, the visual and vestibular systems are linked to posture and postural adjustments. Head orientation also affects haptic perception (Guerraz et al., 2003). As defined by Steadman (1982, p. 620), *haptics* refers to the "science concerned with the tactile sense." In other words, haptic perception refers to a person's ability to control his or her hand movements as related to the orientation of his or her head over the trunk. Tilting the head may influence the ability to write or control fine motor movements. The position of the head can also influence functional tasks, such as swallowing, reading, and eye contact. Considering the relationship of the head and trunk is a critical aspect of a visual observation for function.

Table 5-2	Vertebral Segments		
Segment	**Number**	**Anterior Curve**	**Fixed or Flexible**
Cervical	7	Convex	Moveable/flexible
Thoracic	12	Concave	Moveable/flexible
Lumbar	5	Convex	Moveable/flexible
Sacral fused with the coccyx	5 and the coccyx	Concave	Fixed
Adapted from Lippert, L. S. (2006). *Clinical kinesiology and anatomy* (4th ed.). Philadelphia, PA: FA Davis Company.			

Observation of the Vertebral Curves

The vertebrae are referred to by their location and are referred to as either cervical, thoracic, lumbar, sacral, or coccygeal vertebrae. The vertebral column is divided into segments and is arranged to form anterior/posterior (concave/convex) curves in the vertebral column. A concave curve refers to a curve that extends inward or anteriorly. A bowl or cup has a concave curve. A convex curve refers to a curve that extends outward or in relation to the body, posteriorly. A ball has a convex curve. In a healthy spine, the three curves occur at the cervical, thoracic, and lumbar vertebrae. The cervical curve is considered convex as it projects anteriorly at your neck. The thoracic curve projects posteriorly or is concave and is located in the middle section of your back. Finally the lumbar curve in the lower back is once again convex or in an anterior orientation. The change from concave to convex and back again to concave adds to the structural support, stability, and strength of the vertebral column. Other purposes of the spinal curves are to provide for balance, movement, shock absorption, and an upright posture. While there is movement between each of the spinal segments or curves, the vertebral curves also move in unison with the vertebra near them. Table 5-2 summarizes the vertebral segments.

Observation of the Trunk and Pelvic Girdle

People move in positions that include all of the pelvic motions. In addition to a neutral pelvic tilt, the pelvic motions include anterior and posterior pelvic tilt, pelvic rotation, and pelvic obliquity (also called lateral tilt). In a seated posture, the neutral pelvic tilt is accompanied by an erect spine and allows a person to move weight from behind the ischial tuberosities (ITs) to in front of the ITs with trunk extension. This allows people to reach out in front of them without falling forward. A lack of trunk extension during reaching can cause a person to fall. Additionally, during a lateral reach, a person must be able to maintain the pelvis in a stable way while shifting weight to one of the ITs, while at the same time elongating the weight-bearing side. This lateral weight shift with trunk elongation allows people to functionally access their environment. The motions of the pelvic girdle will be discussed throughout this chapter as well as in Chapter 6 due to the importance of the pelvic girdle in lower extremity function. Further information will be provided on neutral pelvic tilt, anterior pelvic tilt, and posterior pelvic tilt due to their importance.

A **neutral pelvic tilt** is characterized as equal weight distribution across the femurs in a sitting position. The natural and functional position for activity participation when sitting is usually a neutral pelvic tilt with trunk extension. This position allows weight shifting across a stable base of support offered by the ITs and the large muscle groups attached to the pelvis. Figure 5-1 shows a neutral pelvic tilt with accompanying trunk extension.

An **anterior pelvic tilt** is characterized as the pelvis "dipping" forward, lifting the buttocks upward and creating a hyperlordosis in the lumbar spine. A hyperlordosis in the lumbar spine is a more exacerbated curve than typical. Anterior pelvic tilt is illustrated in Figure 5-2. This movement is observed in women who are pregnant or in people who carry excessive weight in the

Figure 5-1. Neutral pelvic tilt. (Reprinted with permission of Michael Babinec.)

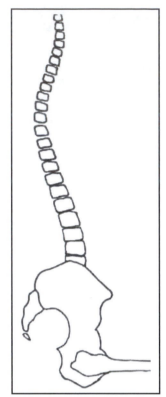

Figure 5-2. Anterior pelvic tilt. (Reprinted with permission of Michael Babinec.)

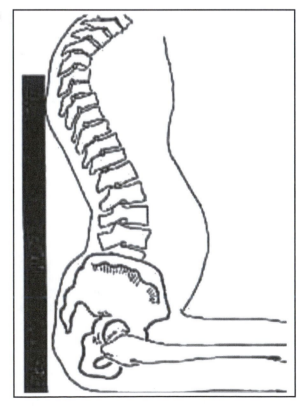

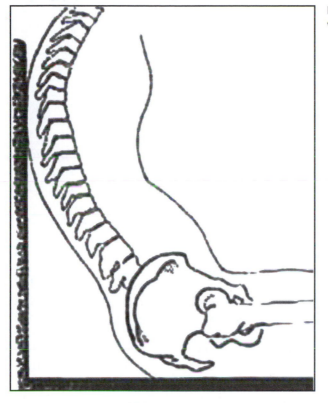

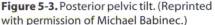
Figure 5-3. Posterior pelvic tilt. (Reprinted with permission of Michael Babinec.)

abdomen. This weight imbalance also causes the center of gravity to shift forward. Another common cause of an anterior pelvic tilt is a muscle imbalance in the abdomen, lower limb, and pelvis.

A **posterior pelvic tilt** is the opposite of an anterior pelvic tilt and is characterized by the tailbone tucking beneath the body or the posterior superior iliac spine (PSIS) shifting backward. Posterior pelvic tilt is illustrated in Figure 5-3. This movement will cause the lumbar spine to flatten and the thoracic spine to flex or become kyphotic. The term *kyphosis*, as defined by Steadman (1982, p. 752), is a "deformity of the spine characterized by extension." Kyphotic refers to an orthopedic deformity caused by maintaining an abnormal posture for a long period of time. Orthopedic abnormalities will be covered in further detail in a subsequent section of this chapter. Often, kyphosis also results in cervical hyperextension if the individual is in a seated posture, such as a wheelchair.

Observation of Sitting Balance

An observation of the trunk, pelvic girdle, and neck is often performed during sitting. One important component of sitting is termed **sitting balance**, which involves the ability to maintain a seated posture without falling but it also refers to the ability to reach. In other words, a person moves his or her upper extremity over a base of support during functional activities that require reaching. The base of support is provided by the pelvis, the thighs, and the feet (Dean et al., 1999). The ability to reach and maintain balance is essential to independence. Individuals with movement disorders or trunk weakness have difficulty with coordinating the movements of the extremities while also maintaining balance. Poor trunk balance has also been associated with poor functional outcomes of rehabilitation efforts (Dean et al., 1999). Gold Box 5-2 describes why a seated posture may provide a more stable position for clients to use during functional activities.

Gold Box 5-2

Stability in Sitting Versus Standing

In sitting, the center of gravity is lower and the base of support is greater than that of standing. The increased stability of the body with proper support for the buttocks, the feet, and the back will increase one's ability to perform fine motor activities with the hands.

Zacharkow (1988)

Sitting balance, or postural control in sitting, is a complex interaction of coordinating numerous factors involving the central nervous system. Kyvelidou et al. (2009) suggest that postural control can be explained using a dynamic system theory (DST). According to DST, the development of postural control is a product of cognitive information as well as the synergistic organization of the neuromuscular system and morphologic, biomechanical, and environmental information. Postural control also requires the integration of several processes. Westcott and Burtner (2004) describe these processes as motor processes, sensory processes, and musculoskeletal components. Motor processes include the emergence of neuromuscular response synergies to maintain the stability of the neck, trunk, and legs. Sensory processes include the visual, vestibular, and somatosensory systems, as well as the central sensory strategies of limb orientation. Musculoskeletal components consist of things such as soft tissue, muscle strength, and ROM. Additionally, sensory processes incorporate proprioception, which was first described in 1906 by Sherrington as sensations arising from deep areas of the body that contribute to conscious sensations, postural equilibrium, and joint stability (Hagert, Persson, Werner, & Ljung, 2009). In sitting postures, proprioceptive input is generated at the pelvic region. The proprioceptive input to the hip helps to elicit a muscular response from the trunk extensors to improve trunk posture. Therefore, it is helpful to allow some freedom of movement for an individual who maintains a seated posture for long periods of time, such as an individual in a wheelchair.

Postural control is an on-going skill for infants. The development of head and trunk control begins very early in infancy and continues to develop into adolescent years (Sveistrup, Schneiberg, McKinley, McFadyen, & Levin, 2007). Gold Box 5-3 further points out the relationship between postural control and function.

Gold Box 5-3

Coordination of Movements

The coordination between head, trunk, and arm movements, such as self-feeding in children, is dependent on adequate postural control.

Sveistrup et al. (2007)

Stabilization of the head in space is an important aspect of postural stability. Head stabilization provides a stable gravitational reference for the vestibular system and facilitates visual information (Allum, Bloem, Carpenter, Hullinger, & Hadders-Algra 1998). As mentioned previously, it is important to consider head alignment during activities. Additionally, when individuals use a wheelchair as a means of mobility, it is essential to consider their posture and balance, recognizing the importance of head alignment as it relates to vision.

It is helpful to understand what parts of the vertebral column move when considering sitting posture, sitting balance, and postural control as they relate to functional abilities. Additionally, the amount and type of motion available in each of the various sections of the vertebral column is important to note. Table 5-3 provides an outline of the ROM of each section of the vertebral column.

Table 5-3	Range of Motion of the Vertebral Column			
	Flexion	**Extension**	**Lateral Flexion**	**Rotation**
Cervical	40 degrees	75 degrees	35 to 45 degrees	45 to 50 degrees
Thoracic			20 degrees	35 degrees
Lumbar			20 degrees	5 degrees
Thoracolumbar	105 degrees	60 degrees		

Adapted from Gillen, G., & Burkhardt, A. (2004). *Stroke rehabilitation: A function-based approach* (2nd ed.). St. Louis, MO: Mosby

Common Problems With the Trunk and Neck

Orthopedic Abnormalities of the Spine and Pelvis

Occupational performance and all movement require an extensive array of movement capabilities of the trunk, pelvis, and head. When an individual experiences an orthopedic alignment problem in any aspect of the spine or pelvis, it will influence his or her ability to perform functional movements. An individual's ability to move the distal segments, such as the hands or lower extremities, is greatly influenced by pelvic and spinal alignment. This is an important consideration in wheelchair positioning. For example, if a client is unable to shift weight from one IT to the other due to a fixed posterior pelvic tilt or pelvic obliquity, the client will have difficulty elongating the trunk on the weight-bearing side to allow for balance. In the occupational profile of Terrence, his ability to comb his hair, drink from a glass, and reach for items in his environment were all affected by his motion and positioning of his pelvis. Some of these issues were the result of orthopedic abnormalities. Several orthopedic abnormalities will be presented.

A pelvic rotation abnormality refers to the position of one anterior superior iliac spine (ASIS) in relationship to the other ASIS. Figure 5-4 illustrates pelvic rotation. A pelvic rotation abnormality refers to a deviation in the frontal plane. If one ASIS is situated further back from or posterior to the other ASIS, then the pelvis is rotated. A pelvic rotation abnormality does not describe the typical movement of pelvic rotation. In a sitting position, this may look like one leg is longer than the other. This is not always the situation; a leg may appear longer due to misalignment of the pelvis.

A pelvic obliquity abnormality is characterized by one side of the hip being higher than the other as illustrated in Figure 5-5. Pelvic obliquity, or lateral tilt of the pelvis, is a deviation of the pelvis in the frontal plane. Lateral pelvic tilting may be accompanied by rib cage displacement and lateral spinal flexion. A pelvic obliquity may be caused by, or accompany, scoliosis. Typically, when a person has a pelvic obliquity, the spine will curve, creating scoliosis.

Scoliosis is a spinal deformity in the frontal plane characterized by a lateral curvature of the vertebra. Scoliosis may result from congenital anomalies, neuromuscular disorders, neurofibromatosis, connective tissue disorders, skeletal dysplasia, or iatrogenic causes (Harrop, Birknes, & Shaffrey, 2008). An iatrogenic problem is caused by an unfavorable response to therapy itself (Steadman, 1982). Scoliosis can be either structural or nonstructural.

A structural or irreversible scoliosis is a lateral curve of the spine with fixed rotation of the vertebrae. Compression of the ribs will result in the concave side of the curve and separation of the ribs on the opposite side. The vertebral bodies will rotate toward the convex side of the curve, and the spinous processes will rotate in the opposite direction. In addition to the lateral curvature of the spine, the ribs and scapula protrude from the posterior aspect of the back when the client bends forward. The nucleus pulposus may have lateral displacement in the disk space. Structural scoliosis cannot be corrected by positioning or voluntary effort. Depending on the severity of the

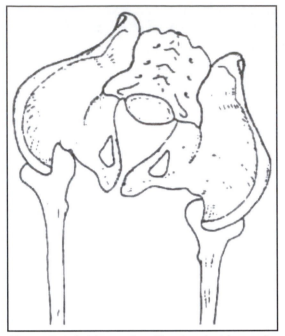

Figure 5-4. Pelvic rotation. (Reprinted with permission of Michael Babinec.)

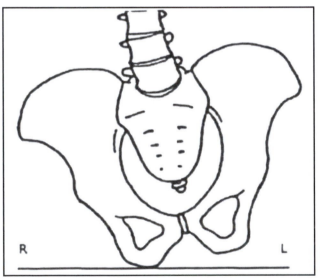

Figure 5-5. Pelvic obliquity. (Reprinted with permission of Michael Babinec.)

structural changes, scoliosis may have a huge negative impact on functioning. As the curvature and rotation increases, the internal organs decline in their ability to function normally. This occurs primarily in the thorax, affecting organs such as the lungs and heart. Scoliosis can become so severe that it impedes proper respiratory and circulatory functioning and can lead to death.

A nonstructural scoliosis is a reversible lateral curve of the vertebral spine. Nonstructural scoliosis may be corrected if adequate support and muscle re-education are provided. Most pelvic obliquities will present with some degree of scoliosis as illustrated in Figure 5-6.

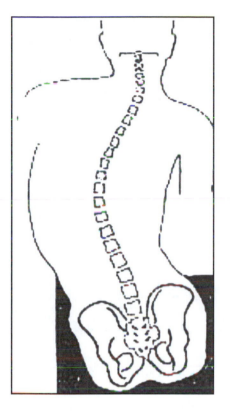

Figure 5-6. Scoliosis. (Reprinted with permission of Michael Babinec.)

Kyphosis is a spinal deformity and refers to an excessive curvature in the thoracic spine. Often, sitting in a posterior pelvic tilt will create kyphosis in the thoracic spine. The trunk flexes where the rib cage ends and the thoracic spine forms a C-shaped bend. Kyphosis is often seen in elderly women. Kyphosis may also be present in the lumbar spine in children with spina bifida.

As previously mentioned, a lumbar lordosis is an exacerbated curvature of the lumbar spine. As noted earlier in Figure 5-2, when the pelvis is in an excessive anterior pelvic tilt, the spine forms a lumbar lordosis. The abdomen appears to protrude forward, and the lumbar spine is barely in contact with the seat back. This may also be referred to as sway back.

In the occupational profile presented at the beginning of this chapter, Terrence demonstrates a sitting posture of posterior pelvic tilt, with a mild thoracic kyphosis, pelvic obliquity to the right side, slight rotation of the right pelvis, and mild cervical hyperextension. When sitting in a posterior pelvic tilt, the body attempts to correct this misalignment by altering the placement of the spine and attempting to place the head and center of vision in line with the horizon. This is an effort to keep vision functional. In other words, if a person sits in a posterior pelvic tilt with thoracic kyphosis, the eyes will face downward onto his or her lap. To correct this, a person may hyperextend the neck in order to see the environment. Again, the optimal seated posture is one of neutral pelvic tilt with trunk extension and cervical extension.

BODY STRUCTURES OF THE TRUNK AND NECK

Body Structure of the Spine and Rib Cage

The spine is formed by 33 bones. These bones are called the vertebrae, and their combined structure is referred to as the vertebral column. The vertebral column is additionally divided into five areas: cervical, thoracic, lumbar, sacral, and coccygeal areas. The purpose of the vertebral column is to maintain the longitudinal axis of the body. The vertebral column also serves as a

Figure 5-7. Thoracic spine with nerve roots. (A) Spinal cord. (B) Nerve root. (Reprinted with permission of Susan Sain.)

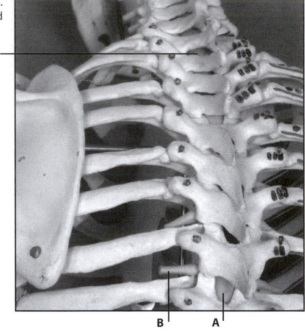

protective covering for the spinal cord, which is composed of nerves. The spinal cord is located in the center of the vertebral column also known as the vertebral foramen. Additionally, the vertebral column serves to provide a pivot point for the head and neck and an anchor point onto the pelvis. These combined purposes allow for both stability and mobility. The combination of stability of the trunk and mobility of the extremities allows for a multitude of motions that create functional movement patterns. Figure 5-7 illustrates most of the thoracic portion of the vertebral column. The spinal cord (A) is in the middle of the vertebral column, while the nerve roots (B) exit between the vertebrae.

The skull, sometimes referred to as the cranium, sits on the top aspect of the vertebral column. The skull provides a covering for the brain and is composed of cranial bones. The nerves that innervate the sense organs of hearing, sight, taste, smell, and vestibular responses are located in the cranium. Movement at the base of the skull is necessary for normal sensory information to enter the brain.

Between each of the 33 vertebrae is a flat, plate-like structure made of fibrocartilage that separates each disk. This protective layer of fibrocartilage is called the intervertebral disk. There are 23 disks that function to absorb and transmit shock, as well as maintain spinal flexibility. The intervertebral disk is one of the strongest aspects of the spine. The disks are held in place by ligaments that allow for flexible movement yet also provide adequate strength to prevent the dislocation of the vertebrae. The external portion of the disk is made of a fibrocartilaginous ring and is called the annulus fibrosus, and the inner aspect is the nucleus pulposus. A common form of damage in the intervertebral disk is known as a "slipped disk," "herniated disk," or "disk prolapse." Such a condition causes the soft nucleus pulposus to bulge out through a weak area of the annulus fibrosus. This may compress a spinal nerve root, causing pain and muscle weakness in the legs.

The Cervical Vertebrae

The neck region of the spine includes the cervical vertebrae. The seven cervical vertebrae are the smallest vertebrae in the spine. The first cervical vertebra (C1) is called the atlas and supports the cranium. Though it does not have a body, it does have a shortened spinous process and a long transverse process. The superior surface contains two large concavities that articulate with the

Table 5-4	Definitions of Vertebral Structures
Body	A cylindrical mass of cancellous bone. This is the anterior and weight-bearing portion of the vertebrae. It is not palpable on the back. C1 does not have a body.
Facet or facet joint	A small, flat, smooth surface on a bone. The facet is the articulation between the superior articular process of the vertebrae below and the corresponding inferior articular process of the vertebrae above. A facet also refers to the articulation of the thoracic vertebrae and the rib bone.
Foramen	An opening.
Intervertebral foramen	The opening formed by the inferior vertebral notch and the superior vertebral notch.
Lamina	Portion of the vertebrae that connects the spinous process to the transverse process.
Neural arch	The posterior portion of the vertebrae.
Pedicle	The portion of the vertebral arch. It lies posterior to the body and anterior to the lamina.
Spinous process	The posterior projection found on the neural arch. It also is an attachment point for muscles and ligaments. The seventh cervical vertebra, also known as the vertebrae prominens, has an unusually long spinous process. One can easily palpate this aspect. This is where the cervical and thoracic area conjoin.
Transverse process	The union of the lamina and pedicle, where the ligaments and muscle attach to the spine.
Vertebral foramen	The opening formed by the joining of the bodies of the vertebrae.

Adapted from Lippert, L. S. (2006). *Clinical kinesiology and anatomy* (4th ed.). Philadelphia, PA: FA Davis Company.

occipital condyles of the skull. The articulation between the head and C1 (atlas) is the atlanto-occipital joint. This joint allows for flexion and extension. Rotation does not occur at this joint.

The second cervical vertebra is the **axis**, which is characterized by a short protrusion known as the odontoid process or the dens. The dens extends into the vertebral foramen of the first vertebra (C1) and is the pivot point of the cervical spine and head. This joint, the atlantoaxial joint, allows for rotation of the head. Together, the axis and atlas enable the head to turn right and left. In addition to rotation, this joint also allows for a nodding-type movement. Most of the head movements occur at the C1 and C2 joints. The neck joints also allow for other movements, such as tucking your chin. The combined movement of neck flexion at C1 and neck extension of the joints of C2 through C7 is referred to as axial extension or cervical retraction. An upright posture encourages cervical retraction as opposed to cervical hyperextension.

With the exception of the first two cervical vertebrae, known as C1 and C2, or the atlas and the axis, the moveable vertebrae all have similar structures. The moveable vertebrae are shaped like a ring. The vertebrae are composed of the following parts: body, facet, foramen, intervertebral foramen, lamina, neural arch, pedicle, spinous process, transverse process, and vertebral foramen. These structures are defined in Table 5-4.

The Thoracic Vertebrae

The thoracic vertebrae occur below, or inferior to, the cervical spine. These 12 vertebrae make up the most stable aspect of the spine. Many aspects of the thoracic vertebrae are similar to the cervical vertebrae. One significant difference, however, is the presence of facet joints. Facet joints are the articulation of the spine to the ribs. The articulation of the ribs on the thoracic spine limits the ability for flexion and lateral flexion. This in turn provides for stability of the thoracic spine. The ribs also protect many internal organs. The facet joints and the intercostal muscles allow for the ribs to expand during respiration. Additionally, the thoracic spine differs from other vertebrae as the spinous processes point inferiorly. This projection limits the thoracic spine from hyperextension.

The Lumbar Vertebrae

The lumbar vertebrae of the spine have five vertebrae, numbered L1 through L5. The lumbar vertebrae support the weight of the body, thus they are the largest of the moveable vertebrae. ROM is limited in the lumbar spine because the articular processes are more pronounced. One exception is at the largest of the lumbar vertebrae, the fifth lumbar vertebrae, which articulates with the sacrum. This articulation has the greatest amount of ROM in the lumbar spine. The lumbar facet joints allow for flexion and extension but limit rotation. The lumbar spine has more available ROM than the thoracic spine but less than the cervical spine. The lumbar spine is the most frequently injured, most likely due to the fact that it supports the weight of the body.

Table 5-5 provides characteristics for the different types of cervical, thoracic, and lumbar vertebrae.

The Sacral Vertebrae

The sacrum represents the fusion of the five sacral vertebrae. The sacrum is posterior to the pelvis. Sacral vertebrae S1 through S5 fuse together into a triangular shape and fit between the two hip bones. The last lumbar vertebra, L5, articulates with the sacrum at the lumbosacral joint. The last vertebra in the sacrum articulates with the coccyx or the tailbone.

The Coccygeal Vertebrae

The coccyx, or tailbone, is formed of four rudimentary vertebrae. No movement occurs at these vertebrae. The most common cause of injury to the tailbone is falling down on a hard surface.

Rib Cage

The rib cage is composed of the sternum, the dorsal aspect of the 12 thoracic vertebrae, and the 12 ribs. The rib cage encloses the heart and lungs. All of the ribs articulate with the vertebrae but only seven pairs attach to the sternum. These are referred to as true ribs, while the three pairs of ribs that attach only to the vertebra and not the sternum are called the false ribs. These sets of ribs all interdigitate or interlock with connective tissue called costal cartilage. The last two pairs of ribs are called the floating ribs and do not attach to the sternum, nor do they attach to the costal cartilage. Between the ribs are the intercostal muscles, which move the ribs up and down during respiration.

In addition to protecting the heart and lungs, the rib cage also provides support for the upper extremities and assists in respiration. Upon inhalation, the intercostal muscles lift the rib cage, allowing the lungs room to expand. Upon exhalation, the rib cage moves down, forcing air out of the lungs. During trunk extension, the rib cage lifts and migrates anteriorly. During spinal flexion, the rib cage moves posteriorly, depressing the ribs. Most of the available spinal flexion occurs at the point where the rib cage ends. Thus, in a sitting position, maintaining thoracic extension is important to hold the rib cage upright, which will also allow for proper breathing. During spinal flexion while sitting, the rib cage compresses the diaphragm, making it difficult to breathe.

Table 5-5 Characteristics of the Vertebrae

	Size	Body Shape	Vertebral Foramen	Transverse Process	Spinous Process	Superior Articular Process	Vertebral Notches
Cervical	Smallest	Small, oval	Large, triangular	Foramen for vertebral artery	Short, stout	Faces medially	Equal in depth
Thoracic	Intermediate	Heart-shaped, with facets that articulate with ribs	Smallest	Facets that connect with ribs are long, thick, and point posterior and laterally	Long, slender, and point inferiorly	Faces posterior and laterally	Deeper inferior notches
Lumbar	Largest	Large, oval	Intermediate	No foramen and no articulation	Thick, points posterior	Faces posterior	Deeper inferior notches

Reprinted with permission of Lippert, L. S. (2006). *Clinical kinesiology and anatomy* (4th ed.). Philadelphia, PA: FA Davis Company.

Body Structures of the Pelvic Girdle

The pelvic girdle is comprised of three bones: two iliac bones and the sacrum. There are three joints of the sacrum, including two sacroiliac joints and the symphysis pubis. These joints will be discussed in this section. The hip bones are formed by the intersection of the pubis, ilium, and ischium. In the front (anteriorly), the hip bones are bound together by the symphysis pubis and in the back (posteriorly) by the sacroiliac articulation known as the sacroiliac joint (SI joint). The SI joint is part synovial and part **syndesmosis**. Syndesmosis indicates a fibrous joint where the ligaments provide the stability. Movement at this joint is limited because it is a nonaxial joint with cartilage in between the bony aspects of the joint. The addition of ligaments at this joint limits the amount of mobility, thus providing quite a bit of stability.

Each of the iliac bones comes together in the front at the symphysis pubis. The symphysis pubis is a cartilaginous joint with two ligaments providing additional support. These are the superior pubic and arcuate pubic ligaments. The acetabulum is the fossa where the femoral head articulates to form the hip joint. The ITs are the prominent protuberances of the hip bones. ITs support the weight of the body in a seated position and are particularly vulnerable to pressure ulcers. A person is able to sit on these bony prominences as the gluteus maximus covers them, adding cushioning. The ITs are also covered by a fluid-filled bursa to help reduce friction as the gluteus maximus crosses over the ITs in a seated position. It is necessary to provide adequate support and cushioning for individuals who sit for long periods of time. For individuals who use wheelchairs, pressure relief cushions and repositioning are essential to prevent pressure ulcer development. Gold Box 5-4 provides a definition for pressure ulcers or decubiti.

Gold Box 5-4

Pressure Ulcer Definition

A pressure ulcer is a localized injury to the skin and/or underlying tissue usually over a bony prominence, as a result of pressure, or pressure in combination with shear force and/or friction. A number of contributing or confounding factors are also associated with pressure ulcers. The significance of these factors is yet to be elucidated.

National Pressure Ulcer Advisory Panel (NPUAP) (2010)

The pelvis is the base of support for the rest of the body in sitting. "The position of the pelvis dictates body position throughout the seating arrangement" (Taylor, 1987, p. 713). The pelvis, in conjunction with the trunk, provides for a more stable support system to allow for functional movement. Therefore, proper measurement of the hips and pelvis is a key component for providing the appropriate seating. Additionally, accurate measurements for the seating system are crucial for optimal functional mobility (Pederson, 2000).

A client such as Terrence is at risk of pressure ulcer development. Thus, the wheelchair assessment completed by the occupational therapist must take into consideration the skin integrity of the client and ensure that proper measurements were taken for the prescribed wheelchair. Figure 5-8 shows what a pressure ulcer may look like.

Wheelchair research indicates that improper alignment and an inappropriate sitting surface in which the client is unable to efficiently relieve pressure are two of the main causes of pressure ulcers. According to Cron and Sprigle (1993, p. 141), to protect against "pressure ulcers from a seated position, a wheelchair cushion and a properly fitted wheelchair are equally important." Additionally, between 36% and 50% of pressure ulcer formation among the elderly was attributed to sitting in a wheelchair for an extended period of time (Aissaoui, Boucher, Bourbonnais, Lacoste, & Dansereau, 2001).

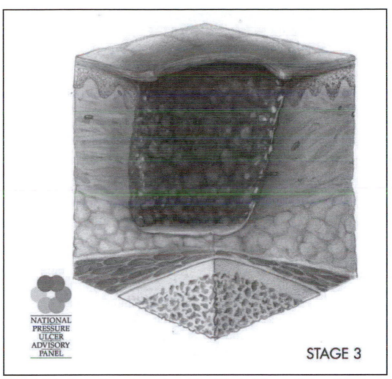

Figure 5-8. Stage 3 pressure ulcer. (Reprinted with permission of National Pressure Ulcer Advisory Panel.)

Ligaments

The strength of the trunk and neck is a result of muscular activity as well as ligamentous structures. There are two types of ligaments in the vertebral column. These ligaments are named intrasegmental and intratransverse. The intrasegmental ligaments hold the individual vertebrae together. The intrasegmental ligaments include the ligamentum flavum, the interspinous, and the intertransverse ligament.

The intersegmental ligaments include the anterior longitudinal ligament, posterior longitudinal ligament, supraspinatus ligament, and the nuchal ligament. The anterior longitudinal ligament covers the vertebral column on the anterior surface of the vertebral bodies. This ligament helps to prevent excessive hyperextension of the spine. The posterior longitudinal ligament covers the vertebral bodies posteriorly inside the vertebral foramen. These ligaments limit excessive flexion. The supraspinatus ligament extends from the seventh cranial vertebrae to the sacrum and runs posteriorly over the tips of the spinous processes. The supraspinatus ligament works with the posterior longitudinal ligament to limit forward flexion of the trunk. The nuchal ligament, which takes the place of the supraspinatus and interspinal ligaments in the cervical region, extends from the external occipital protuberance to the spinous process of the seventh cervical vertebrae. In addition to limiting flexion, this ligament serves as an attachment for the trapezius and splenius capitis muscles, which will be covered in the following section.

Muscles of the Trunk and Neck

The muscles of the neck and trunk are divided into those muscles that lie on the anterior portion and those on the posterior portion of the body. In general, anterior muscles cause flexion, whereas posterior muscles cause extension. Most muscles of the trunk are paired, one on each side of the vertebral column, or vertical axis, of the body. These pairs of muscles will cause different movements if they are contracted simultaneously, or bilaterally, as compared to a unilateral muscle contraction. For the most part, bilateral contractions cause flexion or extension, while unilateral contractions lead to rotation or lateral bending.

The two sides of the rectus abdominus span the front aspect of the trunk. They connect in the center at a point called the linea alba. The rectus abdominus flexes the trunk and aids in respiration. It also enables compression of the internal organs.

The external oblique muscles are large, thin muscles, that, when acting together, assist in trunk flexion. When contracted bilaterally, they also compress the abdomen and aid in exhalation. When one side contracts, unilateral contraction, the muscle laterally bends the trunk to the same side while it rotates the trunk toward the opposite side of the body. In other words, the left external oblique rotates the left side of the trunk toward the midline of the body or, stated another way, toward the right. The external oblique muscle originates on the lower ribs, runs inferiorly and medially to insert on the iliac crest and at the midline onto the linea alba via an abdominal aponeurosis.

The internal oblique muscle originates on the inguinal ligament, iliac crest, and the thoracolumbar fascia. The internal oblique muscle performs two major functions. It acts as an antagonist to the diaphragm during exhalation. In other words, when the diaphragm contracts, it pulls the lower chest cavity down, which allows the lungs to expand. When the internal obliques contract, they compress the abdomen and the internal organs, pushing them up into the diaphragm and forcing air out of the lungs. Second, the internal obliques rotate and laterally bend the trunk by pulling the rib cage toward the hip on the same side. Thus, they are "same-side" rotators, and the external obliques are "opposite-side" rotators. The internal obliques run deep to, and perpendicular to, the external oblique muscles.

The internal and external obliques can work together to strengthen trunk flexion or rotation. Contracting unilaterally, the left internal oblique and the right external oblique contract as the trunk rotates to bring the right shoulder toward the left side of the body. Contracting bilaterally, these muscles work together to enhance trunk flexion and compression of the abdominal contents.

The transverse abdominus muscle is the deepest of the abdominal muscles. The fibers of this muscle run horizontally, hence the name transverse. This muscle originates from the lateral portion of the inguinal ligament, the last six ribs, the iliac crest, and the thoracolumbar fascia. It inserts on the abdominal aponeurosis and the linea alba. Because of its horizontal line of pull, it does not have any influence on trunk movement. It does, however, play a significant role in pelvic and trunk stability. Additionally, it is important in the **Valsalva maneuver.** The Valsalva maneuver is an involuntary action that occurs during activities such as defecation, child birth, lifting, vomiting, and sneezing.

Muscles on the posterior aspect of the trunk include the erector spinae group, which includes the transverse spinal group, the latissimus dorsi, and the quadratus lumborum. The back muscles can be best understood by viewing them layer by layer. Beginning with the deepest layer, the deep or intrinsic muscles are divided into two groups: the transverse spinal muscles and the erector spinal muscles.

The deepest of the intrinsic back muscles include a group of three muscles called the transverse spinal muscle group. Their combined actions result in rotation and extension of the vertebral column. They attach on the transverse process of one vertebra and run somewhat diagonally to the transverse process of another vertebra. Thus, when contracted unilaterally, they are effective in rotation. Back extension is caused by bilateral contraction of these muscles.

Still deep in the intrinsic muscles of the back are the erector spinal muscles. The erector spinal muscles, sometimes called the sacrospinal muscles, extend from the base of the skull to the sacrum. The erector spinal muscles' function is not well understood (Andersson, Oddsson, Grundstrom, Nilsson, & Thorstensson, 1996). Electromyographic evidence demonstrates that the erector spinal muscles are involved in flexion and extension of the vertebral column. The involvement of the individual deep muscles of the lumbar spine is dependent on the task performed and the position of the upper body and pelvis (Andersson et al., 1996). The erector spinal muscles include the iliocostalis (lateral), longissimus (medial), and spinalis (most medial).

The quadratus lumborum muscle is a deep muscle originating from the iliac crest and inserting onto the last rib and transverse processes of the lumbar vertebrae. The quadratus lumborum is one of the primary muscles that contribute to low back pain. Its role is to balance postural distortions by realigning the pelvis. Its main function is pelvic elevation, or hip-hiking.

While the psoas and iliacus muscles are an aspect of the lower extremity, their role in spinal stabilization is important. Research by Andersson and colleagues (1996) suggests that the psoas and iliacus muscles play an important role in the stability of the lumbar spine, pelvis, and hip in sitting as compared to standing. The psoas and iliacus muscles are often referred to as one, the iliopsoas muscle. Additionally, when working with individuals who sit in wheelchairs for extended periods of time, the iliopsoas may become shortened or contracted. This may result in a contracture of this muscle group, limiting one's ability to extend the lower extremity.

The latissimus dorsi, although an arm mover, is also important in sitting postures. Because of its location, it has great influence on the trunk. It attaches on the axial spine from the sixth vertebrae of the thoracic spine, the dorsolumbar fascia, and crosses over the lateral aspect of the ribs and the inferior angle of the scapula. Additionally, it connects to the external oblique muscles. Because of its great size and relationship with the anterior trunk, posture affects the actions of this muscle. When one sits in posterior pelvic tilt, the latissimus dorsi becomes overly stretched, exerting force onto its insertion (the intertubular groove of the humerus). This results in internal rotation of the humerus. Try the following activity. Sit at the edge of your seat with your feet on the floor. Slouch your back into a posterior pelvic tilt. Now, try to raise your arms above your shoulders slowly. When you have raised your arms to a comfortable position, move your pelvis into an anterior pelvic tilt. Note that your arm moves more easily above your head and easily moves into external rotation. This is an important point to remember when asking a client to raise his or her arms or when performing ROM exercises. It is essential to have a person sit in neutral or anterior pelvic tilt when raising his or her arms overhead. Additionally, clients who sit in wheelchairs for extended periods of time in posterior pelvic tilt may experience limitations in external rotation due to the overstretching of the latissimus dorsi. Muscles of the pelvis that act on the trunk are identified in Table 5-6.

Maintaining an upright posture requires a careful balance of muscle activity around the pelvis, trunk, and abdomen. All of the muscles that support these structures work in unison or synergy to create upright trunk postures in both sitting and standing positions. When any one group of these muscles is weak, it will affect the other muscles. If the antagonist is stronger than the agonist, it will create a muscle imbalance. Such an imbalance influences the orthopedic alignment of the individual. As discussed earlier, these postures may be referred to as anterior pelvic tilt or posterior pelvic tilt. While these are not orthopedic deformities in and of themselves, a lack of movement may create a contracture of the muscles, leading to an orthopedic deformity.

Sometimes, a person's tendency to stay in a specific pelvic posture is due to concomitant factors, such as increased weight or girth around the abdomen, as during pregnancy. Approximately 50% to 80% of women who are pregnant report symptoms of low back pain (Sabino & Grauer, 2008). While not entirely related to increased abdominal girth, low back pain can be problematic for a pregnant woman. Additionally, posterior pelvic tilt may be associated with prolonged seated postures if the seat surface is not adequate. For instance, in children with cerebral palsy, the increased muscle tone around the pelvis and lower extremity may result in posterior pelvic tilt and an unstable trunk. Lacoste, Therrien, and Prince (2009) found that a high percentage of children with cerebral palsy demonstrated increased muscle tone around the pelvis with decreased tone (hypotonicity) of the trunk. These postures contribute to pelvic obliquity, posterior pelvic tilt, and pelvic rotation.

Muscle balance around the trunk, pelvis, and abdomen contribute to a stable base of support for trunk stability and upper extremity control. Additionally, muscular balance decreases the chance of developing an orthopedic deformity. Table 5-7 illustrates the various muscles that contribute to pelvic postures.

Table 5-6   Muscles of the Pelvis that Act on the Trunk

Muscle	Nerve	Trunk Flexion	Trunk Stability	Pelvic Stability	Anterior Pelvic Tilt	Posterior Pelvic Tilt	Other
Psoas Major	Anterior rami, T12 to L5	x	x	x			Maintains disk space
Hip flexors (rectus femoris)	Femoral nerve, L2 to L4					x	
Iliacus	Femoral nerve and branches of lumbar plexus						Lifts trunk from supine
Latissimus dorsi	Thoracodorsal nerve	Lateral			x		
Gluteus minimus, medius	Superior gluteal, L4, L5, and S1			x		x	

Adapted from Lippert, L. S. (2006). *Clinical kinesiology and anatomy* (4th ed.). Philadelphia, PA: FA Davis Company.; Stone, R. J. & Stone, J. A. (2003). *Atlas of skeletal muscles* (4th ed.). New York, NY: McGraw Hill.

Table 5-7	**Muscles That Contribute to Pelvic Position**	
Neutral Pelvic Tilt		
Muscle	**Origin**	**Insertion**
Hip extensors (gluteus maximus)	Ilium and sacrum	Gluteal tuberosity and iliotibial band
Oblique abdominals	Lower eight ribs	ASIS, pubic crest
Hip abductors	Gluteal surface of ilium	Greater trochanter of the femur
Hip adductors	Pubis	Medial and posterior surface of the femur
Posterior Pelvic Tilt		
Muscle	**Origin**	**Insertion**
Hip extensors	Ilium and sacrum	Gluteal tuberosity and iliotibial band
Hip abductors (gluteus medius and minimus)	Gluteal surface of ilium	Greater trochanter of the femur
Rectus abdominus	Pubis	Costal cartilage ribs of 5 to 7, xiphoid process of sternum
Iliotibial band with hip external rotation	Supracondylar tubercle of the femur	Tibia and patella
Anterior Pelvic Tilt		
Muscle	**Origin**	**Insertion**
Spinal extensors: Iliocostalis, longissimus, spinalis muscles	Sacrum and vertebrae	Runs parallel to the vertebral column
Iliopsoas	Transverse process of lumbar vertebrae	Lesser trochanter of the femur
Hip adductors	Pubis	Medial and posterior surface of the femur
Rectus femoris	ASIS	Patella and tibial tuberosity
Iliotibial band with hip internal rotation	Supracondylar tubercle of the femur	Tibia and patella

Muscles of the cervical spine are presented next. Muscles causing neck flexion include the sternocleidomastoid muscle, the scalene muscles, and the prevertebral muscles. The sternocleidomastoid muscle is the largest neck flexor. It has two heads. One head originates on the clavicle and is referred to as the clavicular head. The other head originates on the sternum and is thus referred to as the sternal head. Both heads insert on the mastoid process of the temporal bone. When the sternocleidomastoid muscle contracts bilaterally, it flexes the neck. When it contracts unilaterally, it laterally flexes to the same side and rotates the head toward the opposite side. That is, when you contract your left sternocleidomastoid muscle, you would be looking over your right shoulder. Of interest is the attachment on the nuchal line; this allows this muscle to hyperextend the neck as it contracts.

Deep below the sternocleidomastoid muscle are three scalene muscles. The anterior scalene muscle originates on the transverse process of C2 to C6 and inserts on the first rib. The middle scalene muscle originates on the transverse process of C2 to C7 and also inserts on the first rib. The posterior scalene muscle originates on C5 to C7 and inserts on the second rib. The scalene muscles as a group assist the sternocleidomastoid to perform elevation of the ribs, tilting of the neck, and rotation.

There is also a group of small muscles that are located on the anterior aspect of the cervical vertebrae called the prevertebral muscles. These small muscles are capable of flexion of the head, but, most importantly, they tuck the chin and help the body maintain postural control by making slight head motions. Individually, these muscles include the rectus capitus lateralis, the rectus capitus anterior, the longus capitus, and the longus colli. Table 5-8 outlines the various muscles of the neck.

APPLICATIONS

The following activities will help you apply knowledge of the lower extremity in real-life applications. Activities can be completed individually or in a small group to enhance learning.

1. **Standing Posture:** Understanding the body structures and functions is foundational to understanding how body structures and body functions influence occupational performance. It is helpful to relate these anatomical and kinesiology principles to postures in regard to the pelvis, trunk, and head. Let's first examine a standing posture. Maintaining an upright body position over a very small base of support, like the feet, requires an intricate balance anterior to posterior and left to right. In other words, one must balance the weight of the body over the small space that the feet occupy.

    To illustrate, work with a partner. Place a long string with a weight on the bottom of it from the ceiling and allow it to dangle almost to the floor. Begin by standing next to the string so it is close to your shoulder and elbow beside you, rather than in front of you. Try to align your body with the string, but do not touch the string. It may be necessary to have cueing from your partner. Ask your partner how to position certain aspects or joints of your body to be in line with the string. When you feel that you are balanced, note the location of your body in relationship to the string. Your upright and erect posture should demonstrate that the string follows these points on the body:
    - The mastoid process or slightly in front of your ear lobe.
    - A point slightly in front of the glenohumeral joint.
    - A point just behind the center of the hip joints.
    - A point just in front of your patella (knee joint).
    - A point approximately 2 to 2.5 inches in front of your ankle joint (Zacharkow, 1988).

    Questions:
    A. Can you align your body to the string as described above? Why or why not?
    B. Is it possible to move your body to align to the string? Explain what you have to do.

2. **Static Standing Posture:** Additionally, it is important to note that we rely on our vision to maintain postural stability. Lauren et al. (2010) found that a stationary environment stabilizes posture and limits the amount of postural sway associated with standing postures. This may be helpful in designing treatment interventions for clients who have difficulty maintaining upright postures. That is, having a fixed-in-space stationary visual object to look at during static standing may help the client to maintain an erect posture. More will be discussed in Chapter 6.

    Try standing upright on both feet while scanning the room. Most likely, you will not lose your balance. Now, try scanning the room while only one foot is on the ground. Fixating on a nonmoving object should help you to maintain your balance. A balance board may help to accentuate this point.

    Questions:
    A. Was it easier to maintain your balance while fixating on an object or scanning the room?

Table 5-8 Muscles of the Neck

Muscle	Nerve	Extension	Flexion	Lateral Flexion	Tilts the Neck	Rotation	Rotation Same Side	Respiration	Elevates Ribs
Sternocleidomastoid muscle	Cranial nerve XI, (accessory nerve), 2nd and 3rd cervical nerves	x	x	x		x			
Scalene muscles	Lower cervical nerves				x	x			x
Prevertebral muscles	Ventral primary rami of the cervical nerves		x						

Adapted from Lippert, L. S. (2006). *Clinical kinesiology and anatomy* (4th ed.). Philadelphia, PA: FA Davis Company.; Stone, R. J. & Stone, J. A. (2003). *Atlas of skeletal muscles* (4th ed.). New York, NY: McGraw Hill.

B. Do you think your base of support or center of gravity has any influence? Why or why not?

3. **Sitting Posture:** In a standing posture, the base of support is small. Sitting is a more stable position, because the base of support is larger than that of standing. In a sitting posture, the base of support extends from the feet to the most posterior aspect of the seated surface of the buttocks. In the case where there is a back support, an increase in stability may be noted. In fact, approximately 82% of the bodyweight is supported across the femurs and the remainder of the weight through the feet while sitting (Dean et al., 1999). However, if an individual is in a wheelchair and the femurs are not adequately supported, his or her sitting posture may be affected.

Try this: While seated in a wheelchair, flex your knees and place them on the footplates. This positions the knees above the angle of the hips. Where do you feel the weight of your legs? You should feel more weight on the posterior aspect of the femurs. Thus, it places increased pressure on the ITs.

Recall from the previous section that the ITs are bony prominences on the pelvis. Excessive pressure on the bony prominences and infrequent movement in a seated posture may contribute to increased risk of pressure-ulcer development. Thus, when working with individuals who sit for long periods of time, it is essential to provide education on proper sitting posture and pressure redistribution.

Questions/Activity:

A. Create a handout that describes proper sitting posture for a client. Include pictures or diagrams of proper positioning. Also, include a section related to skin breakdown, decubiti, and distribution of pressure. Remember to write this using vocabulary your client will understand. If you are unfamiliar with this topic, a good resource is the NPUAP. Patient education materials may also be found on their Web site.

B. Modify a wheelchair for yourself or a student in the classroom. Try to achieve a neutral pelvic tilt, hips at about 90 degrees flexion, knees at about 90 degrees flexion, and ankles in a neutral position supported on the leg rests. Again, try to support the femurs on the wheelchair.

4. **Sitting Posture:** Sit in a firm chair with your feet directly under your knees and on the ground so that your knees are in 90 degrees of flexion. Flex your right shoulder 90 degrees, or so that your arm is at shoulder level outstretched to the front with your elbow fully extended. Have your partner hold the tip of a yardstick beginning at your fingertips. Now, reach out in front of you as far as you can while maintaining your trunk positioning and your hand at shoulder level. Have your partner write down how far you were able to reach. Repeat this activity. This time, extend your legs by straightening your knee so that your feet are far out in front of you and your knees are not bent. Reach out in front of you with your trunk maintaining the same position as you did before. Have your partner record how far you were able to reach with your knees extended.

Questions:

A. If these numbers varied, explain why you think this would occur?

B. Reach sideways and diagonally, and complete the same measurements. Were they the same? Explain why or why not?

C. What are the implications of this to occupational performance, particularly for an individual in a wheelchair?

5. **Anatomical Considerations for Sitting:** Review the anatomical considerations for sitting. First, sit in a solid seat chair with your feet on the ground. Do not have your back resting against the seat back. Slump your back, and assume a posterior pelvic tilt posture. Think of moving your belly button toward your spine and really reach it back there. Now, raise your arms in front of you. Note that the end range is about at your shoulder level. Holding this arm position, move your pelvis into anterior pelvic tilt. Note how your arms

suddenly feel lighter and automatically move above your shoulders. You may also note that your humerus bone moves into an externally rotated position.

Questions:

A. Can you reach the same height with shoulder flexion? Why or why not?

B. Can you explain why these actions occurred?

6. **Body Structures of Trunk Muscles:** Work with a partner to review the origin and insertion of a few key trunk muscles. Think specifically about the latissimus dorsi and the trapezius muscles. When muscles are overly stretched, they cannot exert adequate strength to overcome the effects of gravity.

Questions:

A. In an upright trunk posture, is the latissimus dorsi active?

B. What role does this muscle play in sitting?

7. **Body Structures of Trunk Muscles:** While lying supine, without lifting your shoulder, lean your head to your left shoulder.

Questions:

A. What joint motion is occurring in the cervical spine?

B. What is the normal ROM for this aspect of the spine?

C. What is the name of this movement?

D. What muscles are the prime movers for this motion?

8 **Body Structures of Trunk Muscles:** Lie supine on a mat with your knees bent and your feet firmly placed on the mat. Clasp your hands together, and place them under your head. Move your right shoulder toward your left knee, as if attempting to do a sit-up.

Questions:

A. What trunk motions are occurring?

B. What muscles cause these trunk motions to occur?

9. **Body Structures of Neck Muscles:** Lying prone on a mat with your arms extended at your sides and your face on the mat, raise your trunk off the mat. Be sure to keep your head in neutral alignment, and do not rotate or laterally flex to either side. As you raise yourself off the mat, determine how far you can move.

Questions:

A. What aspect of the spine is moving (cervical, thoracic, or lumbar)? It may vary depending on how far you can raise yourself up off of the mat.

B. What muscle groups are involved in this activity?

C. If you keep your head in neutral alignment, what neck muscles must remain active?

10. **OTPF-2 Activity Demands:** Activity demands include all aspects of the actual activity, which also include the objects being used. Underlying required actions, body functions, and body structures are all considered. The purpose of this activity is to be more mindful of the life demands that impact what appears to be a simple activity. This activity should raise your awareness of what is really involved in completing an activity. It is important to realize that you have control over many of these demands and can modify or change them to enhance your overall success in performing the activity. Identify an activity and area of occupation that is relevant in your life. Place this item in the left hand column of Table 5-9. Next, list the associated activity demands. An example has been done for you.

Questions:

A. Are there activity demands that interfere with your completion of an activity? Identify these with a negative sign (–). Identify activity demands that might promote your activity with a positive sign (+).

B. Is there an example in class where one student identified a negative activity demand and another student identified that same activity demand as positive? Discuss why this might have occurred.

C. What activity demands do you feel are out of your ability to control? How can you change any of the activity demands with a negative sign to enable your engagement in the activity?

Table 5-9 *Occupational Therapy Practice Framework, 2nd Edition Activity Demands*

Activity and Areas of Occupation	Objects Used	Space Demands	Time Demands	Sequencing and Timing	Required Actions	Required Body Functions	Required Body Structures
Reaching items in the refrigerator; area of occupation is instrumental self-care	*Refrigerator, wheelchair*	*18 inches to the side of the refrigerator to allow door to open*	*Several times per day to allow one to secure beverage or food*	*Move self to side of door, open door, retrieve item, close door, carry item to a table*	*Trunk extension with shoulder movement to reach item in refrigerator, ability to weight shift and maintain trunk extension*	*Cognitive, motor, sensory*	*Nerves, muscles, skeletal alignment*
Your example here							

REFERENCES

Aissaoui, R., Boucher, C., Bourbonnais, D., Lacoste, M., & Dansereau, J. (2001). Effect of seat cushion on dynamic stability in sitting during a reaching task in wheelchair users with paraplegia. *Archives of Physical Medicine & Rehabilitation, 82,* 274–281.

Allum, J. H. J., Bloem, B. R., Carpenter, M. G., Hullinger, M., & Hadders-Algra, M. (1998). Proprioceptive control of posture: A review of new concepts. *Gait and Posture, 8,* 21–242.

Andersson, E. A., Oddsson, L. I. E., Grundstrom, H., Nilsson, J., & Thorstensson, A. (1996). EMG activities of the quadrates lumborum and erector spinae muscles during flexion-relaxation and other motor tasks. *Clinical Biomechanics, 11*(7), 392–400.

Batavia, M., Batavia, A. I., & Friedman, R. (2001). Changing chairs: Anticipating problems in prescribing wheelchairs. *Disability and Rehabilitation, 23,* 539–548.

Bolin, I., Bodin, P., & Kreuter, M. (2000). Sitting position: Posture and performance in C5-C6 tetraplegia. *Spinal Cord, 28,* 425–434.

Brubaker, C. E. (1986). Wheelchair prescription: An analysis of factors that affect mobility and performance. *Journal of Rehabilitation Research and Development, 23*(4), 19–26.

Cron, L., & Sprigle, S. (1993). Clinical evaluation of the hemi wheelchair cushion. *American Journal of Occupational Therapy, 47*(2), 141–144.

Davis, K. (2007, June). Seating and wheeled mobility evaluation. National Public Website on Assistive Technology. Retrieved from http://atwiki.assistivetech.net/index.php/Seating_and_wheeled_mobility_evaluation.

Dean, C., Shepherd, R., & Adams, R. (1999). Sitting balance I: Trunk-arm coordination and the contribution of the lower limbs during self-paced reaching in sitting. *Gait and Posture, 10,* 135–146.

Guerraz, M., Blouin, J., & Vercher, J.-L. (2003). From head orientation to hand control: Evidence of both neck and vestibular involvement in hand drawing. *Experimental Brain Research, 150,* 40–49.

Hagert, E., Persson, J., Werner, M., & Ljung, B.-O. (2009). Evidence of wrist proprioceptive reflexes elicited after stimulation of the scapholunate interosseous ligament. *American Society for Surgery of the Hand, 34A,* 642–651.

Harrop, J., Birknes, J., & Shaffrey, C. (2008). Noninvasive measurement and screening techniques for spinal deformities. *Neurosurgery, 63*(3), a46–a53.

Herman, J. H., & Lange, M. L. (1999). Seating and positioning to manage spasticity after brain injury. *NeuroRehabilitation, 12,* 105–117.

Kyvelidou, A., Stuberg, W., Harbourne, R., Deffeyes, J., Blanke, D., & Stergiou, N. (2009). Development of upper body coordination during sitting in typically developing infants. *Pediatric Research, 65,* 553–558.

Lacoste, M., Therrien, M., & Prince, F. (2009). Stability of children with cerebral palsy in their wheelchair seating: Perceptions of parents and therapists. *Disability and Rehabilitation: Assistive Technology, 4,* 143–150.

LaPlante, M., & Kaye, H. S. (2010). Demographics and trends in wheeled mobility equipment use and accessibility in the community. *Assistive Technology, 22,* 3–17.

Lauren, J., Awai, L., Bockisch, C. J., Hegemann, S., van Hedel, H. J. A., Dietz, V., & Straumann, D. (2010). Visual contribution to postural stability: Interaction between target fixation or tracking and static or dynamic large-field stimulus. *Gait and Posture, 31,* 37–41.

National Pressure Ulcer Advisory Panel. (2010) Pressure ulcer stages. Retrieved from http://www.npuap.org.

Pederson, J. P. (December, 2000). Functional impact of seating modifications for older adults: An occupational therapist perspective. *Wound Care and Seating, 16*(2), 73–85.

Sabino, J., & Grauer, J. (2008). Pregnancy and low back pain. *Current Review of Musculoskeletal Medicine, 1,* 137–141.

Steadman, T. (1982). *Steadman's Medical Dictionary* (24th ed.). Baltimore, MD: Williams and Wilkins.

Sveistrup, H., Schneiberg, S., McKinley, P. A., McFadyen, B. J., & Levin, M. F. (2007). Head, arm and trunk coordination during reaching in children. *Experimental Brain Research, 188,* 237–247.

Taylor, S. J. (1987). Evaluating the client with physical disabilities for wheelchair seating. *American Journal of Occupational Therapy, 41*(11), 711–716.

Westcott, S., & Burtner, P. (2004). Postural control in children: Implications for pediatric practice. *Occupational and Physical Therapy in Pediatrics, 24*(1/2), 5–55.

Zacharkow, D. (1988). *Posture: Sitting, standing, chair design and exercise.* Springfield, IL: Charles Thomas Publisher.

chapter 6

The Essential Functions of the Lower Extremity

Jeremy L. Keough, MSOT, OTR/L

OCCUPATIONAL PROFILE

The following occupational profile is provided to demonstrate how body functions and body structures are related to function and movement of the lower extremity. Through the client, Sarah, this occupational profile will show how occupational therapy incorporates knowledge of function and movement in the lower extremity. References to Sarah will be made throughout this chapter.

Sarah is a 68-year-old widow and retired Certified Nursing Assistant (CNA) who is receiving skilled occupational therapy (OT) at a long-term care facility. Sarah was diagnosed with a right cerebrovascular accident (CVA) with left hemiparesis 1.5 months ago.

During the OT evaluation, the following data were gathered:

Subjective: Sarah reports living in a two-bedroom, one-level home with five steps to enter. She has lived alone during the past year following her husband passing away. Sarah has no children, but has a good support system of neighbors and friends from church. Sarah belongs to a ladies' golf league and enjoys bridge and watching talk shows. Sarah states that she was driving and was able to complete all activities of daily living (ADL) and instrumental activities of daily living (IADL) tasks independently with no adaptive equipment prior to onset. Sarah enjoys going to church when she can and volunteering 2 to 3 days a week at the long-term care facility where she previously worked. Sarah expressed that her goals are to eventually drive again, increase functional ability with her dominant left upper extremity, return home within the next couple of months, and return to independent living. Sarah states that she is thankful that the doctor said she only had a mild stroke.

Objective: Upon admission to the facility, Sarah demonstrated the following ADL abilities:

- Self-feeding: Independent
- Grooming: Independent
- Upper extremity (UE) bathing: Set-up assistance
- Lower extremity (LE) bathing: Moderate assistance
- UE dressing: Supervision for static sitting balance and set-up assistance
- LE dressing: Moderate assistance
- Toileting: Dependent assistance
- Toilet transfer: Moderate assistance
- Tub transfer: Moderate assistance

Gold Box 6-1 identifies the general categories of an ADL scale that identify a client's performance in self-care tasks.

Keough, J. L., Sain, S. J., Roller, C. L.
Kinesiology for the Occupational Therapy Assistant:
Essential Components of Function and Movement (pp. 141-174).
© 2012 SLACK Incorporated.

Gold Box 6-1

General Categories of an Activities of Daily Living (ADL) Scale:

Independence	Client completes 100% of task typically by self.
Modified Independence	Client completes ADL task with adaptations.
Supervision	Client requires assistance of someone present to complete a task. This may include stand by assistance or standing next to the person.
Minimum Assistance	Client requires less than 20% assistance. Contact Guard Assistance may also be included in this category.
Moderate Assistance	Client requires between 20% to 50% assistance for ADL tasks.
Maximum Assistance	Client requires between 50% to 80% assistance for ADL tasks.
Dependent Assistance	Client requires between 80% to 100% assistance for ADL tasks.

Adapted from Foti & Kanazawa (2006)

UE Observations: Sarah is left-hand dominant and displays left UE weakness. Sarah cannot use her left UE alone to complete functional tasks due to weakness and impaired initiation of muscle activation for controlled movement. She is able to use her left UE as a secondary assist in functional activities. Sarah displays slight, increased spasticity in her left UE during functional tasks, further increasing the difficulty regaining use of the arm. She demonstrates left UE active range of motion (AROM) grossly within functional limits except for having only 0 to 60 degrees of shoulder flexion. Manual muscle testing (MMT) strength of the left UE is grossly 3+/5, except for shoulder MMT strength grossly 2/5. Left UE shoulder strength was identified by observation of functional movement because of the inability to separate when voluntary movement becomes involuntary due to spasticity. Sarah has full active/passive ROM with her right UE and 4/5 MMT strength grossly.

LE Observations: Sarah displays "foot drop" impairment with the affected left LE and no increased tone during left LE AROM movements. During standing and stand pivot transfers, Sarah is observed hyperextending her left knee and displays difficulty transferring her weight onto the affected left LE in standing. Sarah currently uses a rolling walker for stand pivot functional transfers as recorded in the physical therapy evaluation and the physical therapy recommended assistive mobility device. Sarah was later advanced to a quad cane for functional mobility by physical therapy. Sarah can also use grab bars for UE support with transferring to the commode. As per the physical therapy evaluation, Sarah displays AROM left LE grossly within functional limits (WFL) except for less than half AROM left ankle dorsiflexion. She also displays MMT strength of the left LE to include trace AROM left ankle, 3+/5 left knee, and 3+/5 left hip muscles grossly. AROM and MMT strength of the intact right LE are grossly WFL and 4+/5 MMT strength.

Sensory/Perception/Cognition: Sarah reports no visual or sensory impairments. Sarah demonstrates intact proprioception and sensation bilaterally. Sarah is alert and oriented x4 (person/place/date and situation) and is able to follow three-step commands.

OT goals were established by the occupational therapist in collaboration with Sarah and the interdisciplinary team and are presented below:

Short-Term Goals:
1. Client will be educated in, and demonstrate independence with, a home exercise program for increased left UE functional ability within 1 week.
2. Client will demonstrate supervision with stand pivot transfers using adaptive equipment appropriately by 2 weeks.
3. Client will demonstrate supervision with standing balance to sweep floors by 2 weeks.
4. Client will demonstrate modified independence to supervision with all ADL tasks by 2 weeks.

Long-Term Goals:

1.   Client will demonstrate modified independence with all functional stand pivot transfers by discharge.

2.   Client will demonstrate modified independence with self-care tasks using bilateral UE by discharge.

3.   Client will demonstrate MMT and grip pinch strength within functional limits in the left UE by discharge.

4.   Client will demonstrate modified independence with simple home management tasks by discharge.

The outcome of Sarah's OT intervention along with treatment techniques and goals achieved can be found in Appendix C.

BODY FUNCTIONS OF THE LOWER EXTREMITY

The LE has many functional purposes. Primarily, the LE enables an upright posture in standing, which increases a person's ability to engage in the environment. The LE also significantly participates in maintaining sitting and standing balance and equilibrium and supports the weight of the body (Greene & Roberts, 2005). Whenever the body leans away from the center of gravity, the LE adjusts to help maintain balance. Equilibrium is maintained through sensory receptors throughout the body as well as the LE. The LE provides support for the weight of the body in standing and shock absorption as the foot comes in contact with the ground. It also is involved with pushing up off the ground during walking.

The LE enables movement through gait or ambulation for mobility. Gait is defined as a manner of walking or moving on foot. There are multiple types or examples of gait patterns, both functional and impaired (*Merriam-Webster Collegiate Dictionary*, 1991; Thomas, 1997). Ambulation is defined as the process of moving from place to place by walking. For the purpose of this text, gait and ambulation will be used interchangeably. Functional mobility in the home is often referred to when a client can ambulate distances greater than 50 feet with or without assistive devices. An example might include the client being able to walk across the home from one side to the other. Functional mobility in the community is achieved when a client can ambulate distances greater than 150 feet with or without assistive devices. An example might include a client's ability to walk from a car in a parking lot to a grocery store entrance. A greater review of gait will be provided in this chapter.

Role of Occupational Therapy and the Lower Extremity

OT is not defined or constrained to the treatment of the UE as may be inaccurately expressed. Typically, however, OT is not the primary treatment for LE injuries and impairments. Physical therapy is often prescribed for LE injuries and impairments due to the emphasis on gait and LE function. As OT treats the whole body, therapists cannot just ignore the trunk and LE, because they significantly influence function. Specifically, OT practitioners may collaborate with physical therapy to reinforce physical therapy intervention in standing balance and safety; functional mobility using appropriate adaptive equipment; functional transfer techniques; ROM; and observation of clinical factors, precautions, and contraindications. It is important to recognize that these approaches should also support and target OT treatment plan and goals, ideally incorporating the client and interdisciplinary team.

Examples of OT incorporating the LE in treatment include but are not limited to the following:

1.   An occupational therapy assistant (OTA) walking a client to the commode during ADL retraining using a rolling walker. The OTA ensures safe use of the walker, avoidance of knee hyperextension, and ankle injury by proper foot placement. Sarah (in the

occupational profile) could use a rolling walker to transfer to the commode during toileting self-care retraining. The OTA would ensure that Sarah always keeps her rolling walker to her front, her body remains within the frame of the walker, all four legs of the rolling walker are kept in contact with the ground, and she makes small turns with the rolling walker.

2. An OTA collaborating with physical therapy and reinforcing functional safe transfer techniques by the client. The OTA may aid in the progression of transfer training, such as knowing when to move from a sliding board transfer to a lateral pivot transfer or even a stand pivot transfer. Additionally, the OTA student may need to educate the client on proper transfer techniques as well as ensure that proper transitional movements are being used. Refer to Gold Box 6-2 for a definition of transitional movements. As with Sarah in the occupational profile, the OTA can collaborate with physical therapy for when to advance Sarah from the rolling walker to a quad cane or standard cane. Additionally, the proper sequence of sit to stand can be reinforced, such as ensuring that Sarah pushes up from the armrests on the wheelchair versus pulling herself up by the handholds on the walker.

Gold Box 6-2

Transitional movements: Change or movement from one position to another.
Static balance: Balance where no movement is occurring; can describe a position in sitting or standing. The ability to maintain a steady position of the head and body in relation to gravity.
Dynamic balance: Balance with movement occurring; can describe movement in sitting or standing. Opposite of static balance. The ability to maintain a controlled position of the head and body during movement in relation to gravity.

Merriam-Webster Collegiate Dictionary (1991); Thomas (1997)

---

3. An OTA adapting and grading static or dynamic standing and sitting balance while looking at the base of support (BOS); muscle activation; and sequence of LE movement, trunk posture, and weight shifting as they influence UE functional reaching. Refer to Gold Box 6-2 for a definition of static and dynamic balance. In the case of Sarah, the OTA can monitor sitting balance at the edge of the bed when reaching during upper or lower body dressing. Another example may include standing to complete IADL tasks.

4. An OTA reaching into a kitchen cabinet for a plate using appropriate adaptive equipment and safety while monitoring static and dynamic standing balance. An example would include Sarah using a quad cane to help maintain her balance while reaching into a cabinet or standing at the kitchen counter. Figure 6-1 illustrates Sarah reaching into a kitchen cabinet.

5. Aiding a patient diagnosed with spinal cord injury to perform circle sitting for the self-care task of dressing. In this example, Sarah most likely would not need to learn to circle sit due to her intact trunk and LE function. Adaptive approaches, PROM, and impaired balance response may be appropriate for a client with a spinal cord injury who could benefit from circle sitting to increase independent ability.

OT is not limited to these examples. A common factor in all of these examples includes the use of therapeutic activities and engagement in occupations. It is important to note that a client is not standing for the sake of standing, but a client stands during the participation in an occupational role. Standing can be used in occupation-based interventions, purposeful activities, and preparatory methods in OT treatment. Transitional movements are also important to consider. Transitional movements occur between different positions or postures. Examples may include rolling from supine to prone, moving from sitting to standing, or moving from supine to sitting.

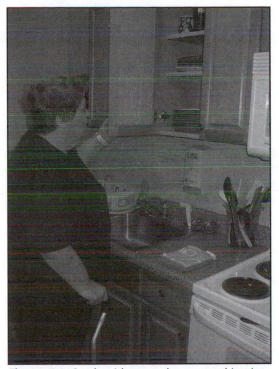

Figure 6-1. Sarah with a quad cane reaching into the cabinets.

Transitional movements are obviously very important during functional transfers. Quite often, the OTA is not selecting or initiating LE adaptive equipment, and certainly the OTA is not duplicating treatment performed by physical therapy. No one, though, should inaccurately describe OT as just treating the UE.

OTA practitioners should also be familiar with adaptive equipment used to increase the safety and efficiency of gait or standing as well as adaptive equipment used to correct and prevent deformity or impairment. Equipment used to increase the safety or efficiency of gait or standing may include (but is not limited to) crutches, cane, quad cane, hemi-walker, standard walker, and rolling walker. Usually, physical therapy practitioners determine which equipment is most advantageous for the client. A standard wheelchair or powered mobility device may also be used to enable functional mobility as well. Depending on the facility, training, and role expectations within the facility, OT or physical therapy practitioners may assume the primary responsibility for determining wheelchair and seating client needs. This responsibility may also be a shared expectation between OT and physical therapy practitioners. Due to the complexity involved with wheelchair seating and positioning, some information is provided in Chapter 5; however, in-depth discussion is outside the scope of this course and will be covered in other treatment courses.

Equipment used to correct or prevent deformity or impairments may include ankle-foot orthoses (AFO), casts, air splints, and various types and sizes of ankle and knee braces. Again, physical therapy practitioners often assess and issue this equipment. Service competency should be achieved as the OTA learns to appropriately don and doff splints and orthotic devices with clients. The OTA may need to instruct a client or educate caregivers on how to don and doff a splint/orthotic device as part of LE dressing. As in the occupational profile with Sarah, physical therapy may decide that an AFO or ankle air cast is appropriate due to the decreased ability to produce ankle dorsiflexion. In certain cases, physical therapy may recommend knee braces to prevent hyperextension or uncontrolled knee flexion. Part of lower body dressing may include independently donning or doffing these devices to enable a return to safe independent living at home.

Motions of the Lower Extremity

The LE includes the motions of the pelvic girdle, hip, knee, ankle, and foot. Typically, movements of the LE are generally described by these joint motions; however, variations at each joint increase the complexity and specificity for describing the specific movement at each joint. It is important for the OTA to be able to identify the most common joint movements of the LE and how each joint influences function. The pelvic girdle is a good place to start, because it is the most proximal body structure and connects the appendicular skeleton to the axial skeleton.

The pelvic girdle may appear to be part of the trunk due to its location proximal to the hip joint; however, the pelvic girdle is considered part of the appendicular skeleton. As presented in Chapter 5, the pelvic girdle is important as it influences posture and sitting balance and establishes stability for reaching with the UE. The pelvic girdle is also important to the LE because it influences posture and curvature of the spine in standing, provides stabilization needed for standing balance, and enables mobility to allow for movement of the LE as in gait. Movements of the pelvic girdle often occur in combination with movements in the LE to achieve functional goals. For example, all movements of the pelvic girdle occur during walking. The movements of the pelvic girdle include left lateral tilt (Figure 6-2), right lateral tilt (Figure 6-3), forward rotation (Figure 6-4), backward rotation (Figure 6-4), anterior pelvic tilt (Figure 6-5), and posterior pelvic tilt (Figure 6-6). Due to the importance of the pelvic girdle in LE movement, pictures of the movements of the pelvic girdle are illustrated in Figures 6-2 to 6-6.

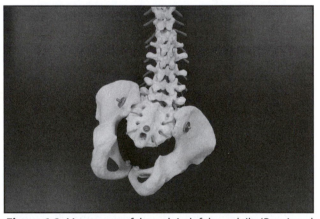

Figure 6-2. Movement of the pelvis: left lateral tilt. (Reprinted with permission of Carolyn Roller.)

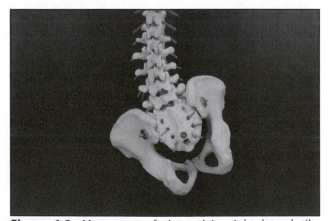

Figure 6-3. Movement of the pelvis: right lateral tilt. (Reprinted with permission of Carolyn Roller.)

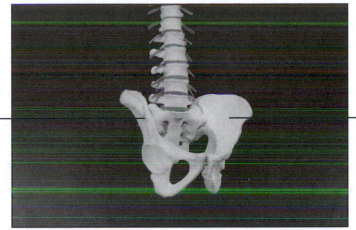

Figure 6-4. Movement of the pelvis. (A) Forward rotation: right ASIS rotating forward from the stationary left ASIS. (B) Backward rotation: left ASIS rotating backward from stationary right ASIS. (Reprinted with permission of Carolyn Roller.)

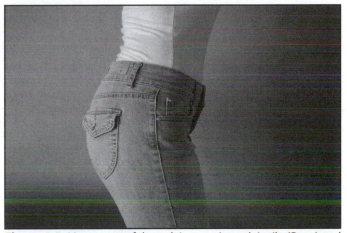

Figure 6-5. Movement of the pelvis: anterior pelvic tilt. (Reprinted with permission of Carolyn Roller.)

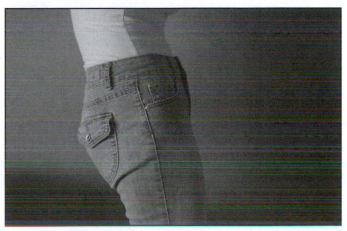

Figure 6-6. Movement of the pelvis: posterior pelvic tilt. (Reprinted with permission of Carolyn Roller.)

The reference points for pelvic girdle motions are the anterior superior iliac spine (ASIS) landmarks, which are located on each pelvic bone.

The hip joint has three degrees of freedom and thus can move in three planes of movement, which is typical for a triaxial joint. Structurally, the hip joint provides for greater stability as compared to the glenohumeral joint. With this greater stability comes lesser mobility as compared to the glenohumeral joint. The motions of the hip joint include flexion (Figure 6-7), extension (Figure 6-8), abduction (Figure 6-9), adduction (Figure 6-10), internal rotation (Figure 6-11), and external rotation (Figure 6-12).

Figure 6-7. Movement of the hip joint: flexion. (Reprinted with permission of Carolyn Roller.)

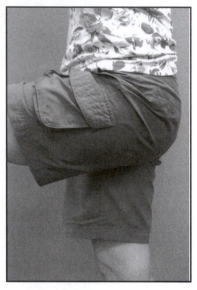

Figure 6-8. Movement of the hip joint: extension. (Reprinted with permission of Carolyn Roller.)

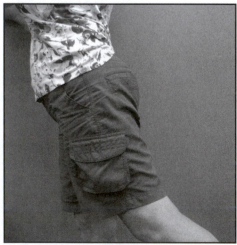

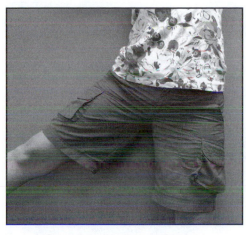

Figure 6-9. Movement of the hip joint: abduction. (Reprinted with permission of Carolyn Roller.)

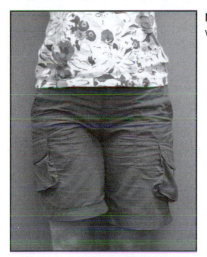

Figure 6-10. Movement of the hip joint: adduction. (Reprinted with permission of Carolyn Roller.)

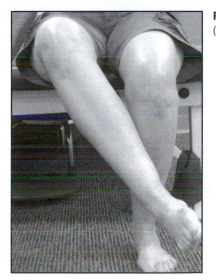

Figure 6-11. Movement of the hip joint: internal rotation. (Reprinted with permission of Carolyn Roller.)

Figure 6-12. Movement of the hip joint: external rotation. (Reprinted with permission of Carolyn Roller.)

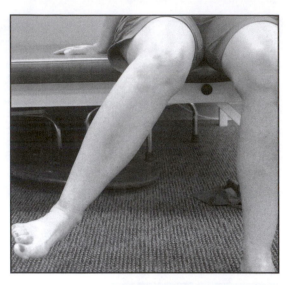

Figure 6-13. Movement of the knee joint: flexion. (Reprinted with permission of Carolyn Roller.)

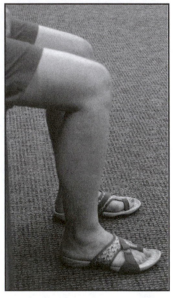

The knee and then the ankle are the next joints following the appendicular skeleton. The primary motion of the knee joint is flexion and extension. The knee is a combination of three articulations that enable movement. Due to the three articulations of the knee, a rotary movement also occurs to a lesser degree. The OTA is primarily concerned with the main joint motions of knee flexion (Figure 6-13) and extension (Figure 6-14).

The ankle joint also includes multiple articulations. The motions of the ankle can be referred to by different terms depending on the source. For this text, the primary motions of the ankle will be referred to as plantarflexion (Figure 6-15), dorsiflexion (Figure 6-16), eversion (Figure 6-17), and inversion (Figure 6-18). Greene and Roberts (2005) identify inversion and eversion as important, because these movements are used when the body shifts weight. They also provide better balance when on uneven ground. Dorsiflexion and plantarflexion are important movements as they allow the foot to clear the ground during walking and enable proper foot placement when the foot comes back in touch with the ground.

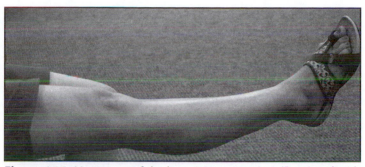

Figure 6-14. Movement of the knee joint: extension. (Reprinted with permission of Carolyn Roller.)

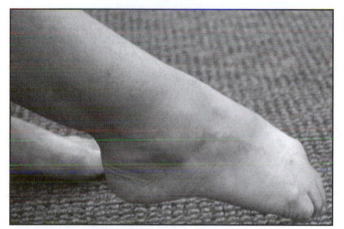

Figure 6-15. Movement of the ankle joint: plantarflexion. (Reprinted with permission of Carolyn Roller.)

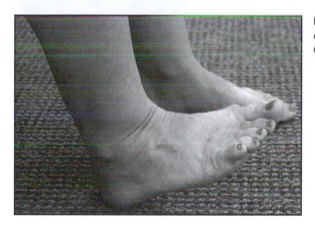

Figure 6-16. Movement of the ankle joint: dorsiflexion. (Reprinted with permission of Carolyn Roller.)

In addition to the motions already mentioned for the LE, there are also joints and motions that occur distal to the ankle joint. ROM and strength of the toes influence standing balance and push off during gait when the foot lifts off the ground. The OTA primarily will need to be aware of the motions at the pelvic girdle, hip, knee, and ankle as they are involved in functional tasks

Figure 6-17. Movement of the ankle joint: eversion. (Reprinted with permission of Carolyn Roller.)

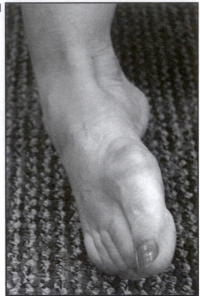

Figure 6-18. Movement of the ankle joint: inversion. (Reprinted with permission of Carolyn Roller.)

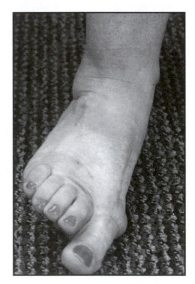

during sitting or standing. Table 6-1 identifies the joint, motion, landmark for joint measurement, and available ROM for each joint of the LE. Complicating the analysis of the LE is that most or all joints will be simultaneously involved in a functional activity and require observation of their movement. Consultation with physical therapy should be performed if more specific analysis of movement is needed or if variations exist to typical joint movement.

Table 6-1	Joints, Motions, Landmarks, and Range of Motion of the Lower Extremity	
Joint and Motion	**Landmark***	**Available ROM****
Hip flexion	Lateral aspect of greater trochanter	0 to 100 degrees
Hip extension		0 to 30 degrees*
Hip abduction	Over ASIS	0 to 25 degrees
Hip adduction		Adduction is the return to 0 degrees
Hip internal rotation	Over midpoint of the patella	0 to 20 degrees
Hip external rotation		0 to 30 degrees
Knee flexion	Over the lateral epicondyle of the femur	0 to 110 degrees
Knee extension		Extension is the return to 0 degrees
Ankle plantarflexion	Lateral aspect of the lateral malleolus	0 to 20 degrees
Ankle dorsiflexion		0 to 10 degrees
Ankle eversion	Over the anterior aspect of the ankle midway between malleoli	0 to 10 degrees
Ankle inversion		0 to 20 degrees

*Adapted from Latella, D., & Meriano, C. (2003). *Occupational therapy manual for evaluation of range of motion and muscle strength.* Clifton Park, NY: Delmar Cengage Learning.

**Adapted from American Medical Association. (2008). *Guides to the evaluation of permanent impairment* (6th ed.). Chicago, IL: Author.

Occupation-Based Mobility: The Visual Observation of Gait

The Occupational Therapy Practice Framework, 2nd Edition (OTPF-2), as displayed in Gold Box 6-3, identifies gait patterns, also called walking patterns, as a body function commonly considered by OT practitioners (American Occupational Therapy Association, 2008). Traditionally, physical therapy is able to analyze and detail the strengths and weaknesses associated with LE function and ambulation. While physical therapy may provide an in-depth evaluation of gait, OTA practitioners need to be able to provide observational gait analysis during treatment and occupational roles. Observational gait analysis can reflect distance traveled and the absence or presence of common characteristics of gait. This observational analysis can be used to ensure safety, prevent injury, reinforce carryover of physical therapy treatment, and facilitate progress toward OT goals. The OTA should also be able to communicate what he or she sees with physical therapy practitioners. Knowledge of gait and walking patterns as well as common terminology are needed to enable this communication with physical therapy and the rehabilitation team.

Gold Box 6-3

The *Occupational Therapy Practice Framework, 2nd Edition* (OTPF-2) identifies **gait patterns,** also called **walking patterns**, as a body function commonly considered by occupational therapy practitioners.

AOTA (2008)

While every person may have slightly different gait patterns, gait patterns have been broken down into common components called the **gait cycle**. The gait cycle describes the movement from the heel strike of one leg to the heel strike of the same leg on the ground. The gait cycle must be able to accommodate changes in the level of the ground, dodging obstacles, or increased distances. The gait cycle may also be referred to as stride. The distance traveled for one stride is called the stride length. Each stride length has two step lengths, to include a step with the right leg and a step with the left leg. Figure 6-19A illustrates a client at the start of the gait cycle taking a step with his right leg. Figure 6-19B illustrates the client halfway through the gait cycle as the left leg advances forward. Last, Figure 6-19C illustrates the client at the end of the gait cycle as the right foot again touches the ground.

The gait cycle can also be broken down into two phases, the stance phase and the swing phase. Gold Box 6-4 identifies the ROM needed in the LE for gait. The stance phase occurs when the leg is in contact with the ground and is about 60% of the gait cycle. Skinner, Antonelli, Perry, and Lester (1985) identify that the limb must demonstrate weight bearing, stability, progressional mobility,

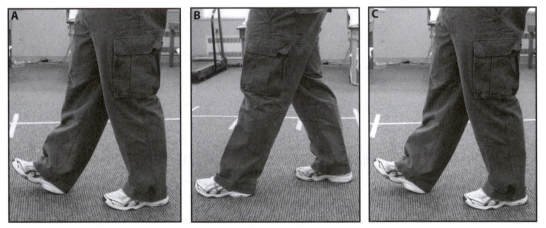

Figure 6-19. Gait cycle. (A) Step with right foot; left foot in contact with the ground. (B) Step with left foot; right foot in contact with the ground. (C) Step with right foot; left foot in contact with the ground. (Reprinted with permission of Carolyn Roller.)

Gold Box 6-4

Range of Motion Needed During Gait

	Stance phase	Swing phase
Hip flexion	0 to 30 degrees	0 to 30 degrees
Hip extension	0 to 20 degrees	0 to 20 degrees
Knee flexion	0 to 40 degrees	0 to 60 degrees
Knee extension	0 degrees	0 degrees
Plantarflexion	0 to 20 degrees	0 to 10 degrees
Dorsiflexion	0 to 10 degrees	0 degrees
Subtalar joint inversion	0 to 35 degrees	
Subtalar joint eversion	0 to 15 degrees	

Loudon, Swift, & Bell (2008)

and shock absorption during stance phase. The following are the traditional phases of the stance phase:

1.   Heel strike, also initial contact
2.   Foot flat, also loading response
3.   Midstance
4.   Heel off, also terminal stance
5.   Toe off, also pre-swing

Heel strike identifies when the heel comes in contact with the ground. Foot flat describes when the bottom of the foot is in contact with the ground. Midstance occurs when the body passes over the foot that is in contact with the ground. Next, heel off explains when the heel begins to lift off the ground, and toe off portrays when the toes push off the ground to propel the foot forward (Lippert, 2006). The traditional phases of the stance phase are illustrated in Figures 6-20 to 6-24.

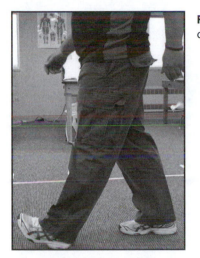

Figure 6-20. Stance phase: heel strike. (Reprinted with permission of Carolyn Roller.)

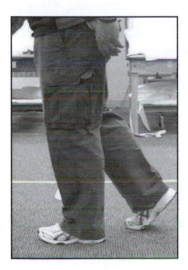

Figure 6-21. Stance phase: foot flat. (Reprinted with permission of Carolyn Roller.)

Figure 6-22. Stance phase: midstance. (Reprinted with permission of Carolyn Roller.)

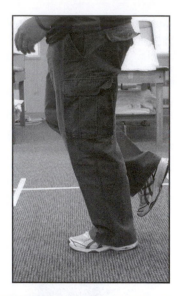

Figure 6-23. Stance phase: heel off. (Reprinted with permission of Carolyn Roller.)

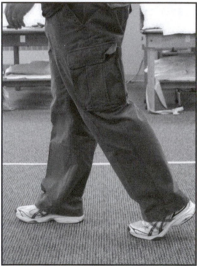

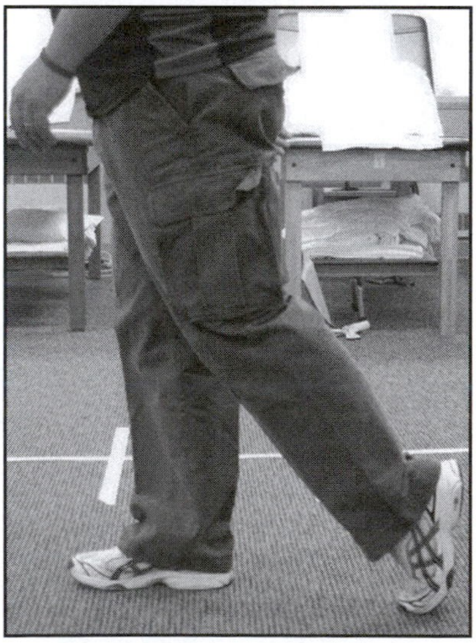

Figure 6-24. Stance phase: toe off. (Reprinted with permission of Carolyn Roller.)

The swing phase occurs when the foot leaves the ground, but before it again comes in contact with the ground and accounts for 40% of the gait cycle. The traditional phases of the swing phase include the following:

1. Acceleration, also called initial swing
2. Mid-swing
3. Deceleration, also called terminal swing

Acceleration occurs when the foot lifts off the ground, is behind the body, and is moving forward. Mid-swing describes the phase when the toes pass over the ground and the foot moves ahead of the weight-bearing leg. Finally, deceleration occurs when the toes point upward and the heel of the foot gets ready to strike the ground (Lippert, 2006). The traditional phases of the swing phase are illustrated in Figures 6-25 to 6-27.

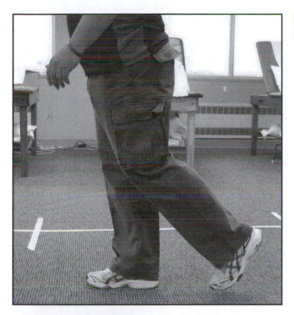

Figure 6-25. Swing phase: acceleration. (Reprinted with permission of Carolyn Roller.)

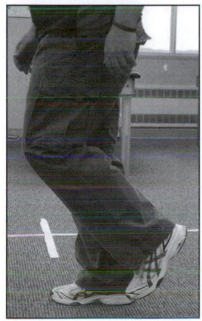

Figure 6-26. Swing phase: midswing. (Reprinted with permission of Carolyn Roller.)

Figure 6-27. Swing phase: deceleration. (Reprinted with permission of Carolyn Roller.)

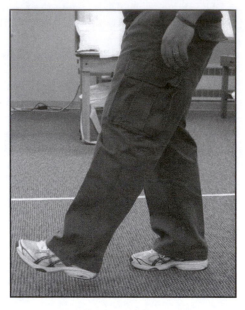

There are additional aspects that can be highlighted to describe ambulation. First is the number of feet in contact with the ground. **Single support** describes the part of the gait cycle when only one leg is in contact with the ground. **Double support** describes when both legs are in contact with the ground. During ambulation, the gait cycle is usually in either single support or double support. In addition to the number of legs in contact with the ground, the distance between both feet is called the step width. Typically, people do not step directly in front of each foot. Lippert (2006) identifies that step width may range from 2 to 4 inches during ambulation.

Functional ambulation can be identified by several different factors. As mentioned previously, distance traversed is quite often used to identify independence with ambulation. The use of adaptive equipment may also be important to identify functional ambulation. Adaptive equipment may increase the speed of walking as well as improve weight bearing on the targeted LE. The goal may be to maximize safe independence with mobility using the least amount of restrictive device. Overall quality of movement should be important to meet individual goals.

Another consideration for functional ambulation is the excursion of the center of gravity during gait. Excursion refers to the wandering from usual course of the center of gravity during gait. All three planes of pelvic movement are needed for typical excursion of the line of progression (Yavuzer & Süreyya, 2002). During ambulation, the center of gravity displaces up to 2 inches vertically and 2 inches horizontally as the body and pelvis move (Lippert, 2006). This vertical and horizontal displacement is called the line of progression and should typically be constant with stable variables. Increasing the excursion of the line of progression will increase energy expenditure and decrease stability and efficiency of walking.

Common Problems of the Lower Extremity

Foot Drop

Foot drop is a common disorder in neurological conditions where a person has an inability, or difficulty, in creating ankle dorsiflexion. The foot, toes, and ankle have difficulty pointing up in the air, deriving the name *foot drop*. Reduced knee function, hip flexion, and ankle dorsiflexion all may complicate toe clearance during swing phase. While neurological damage, either central nervous system (CNS) or peripheral nervous system (PNS), is most often associated with this disorder,

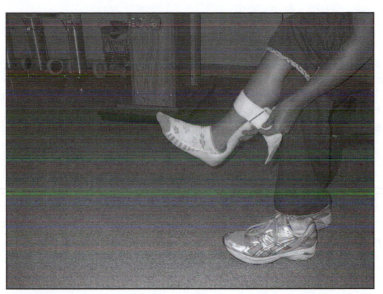

Figure 6-28. Sarah donning her AFO. (Reprinted with permission of Carolyn Roller.)

muscle damage, anatomical deviations, diabetes mellitus, tumors, motor neuron disease, multiple sclerosis, and adverse reactions to drugs and alcohol can also lead to this disorder (Hayes, 2004; Pritchett & Porembski, 2010).

In foot drop, the common peroneal nerve is often affected as it innervates the anterior tibialis muscle, which is the main muscle associated with picking up the foot, also called dorsiflexion. The common peroneal nerve branches off of the sciatic nerve, lumbosacral plexus, and the L5 nerve root proximally. Functionally, foot drop can significantly and negatively affect function. Foot drop does not allow for the normal gait pattern where the heel first comes in contact with the ground. Additionally, clients may have trouble clearing the foot and toes from the ground as they advance the foot forward. If untreated, the client can incorporate nonfunctional gait patterns that limit functional mobility and recovery. Additionally, the client can also be at risk for increased falls and further functional decline.

An example of a nonfunctional gait pattern is a circumducted gait, which is where the pelvis hikes while the hip abducts on the unsupported side. The leg then advances in a circular motion out to the side, swinging forward toward midline where the foot strikes the ground. This type of gait pattern can decrease safety, increase energy expenditure, and decrease movement options for the development of more functional gait patterns.

Treatment approaches will depend on the source of injury. Quite often, an AFO can be used maintain the position of the ankle through compensation, which allows improved function. Remedial approaches by physical therapy may include the use of modalities or exercises to strengthen the tibialis anterior. The OT practitioner typically does not provide the direct treatment for foot drop. Sarah in the occupational profile presents with foot drop. In Sarah's case, the physical therapy practitioner is using both electrical stimulation and exercises to strengthen and improve coordination of the affected LE. Physical therapy practitioners are also using an AFO during gait training to prevent injury, increase safety, decrease risk for falls, and increase functional mobility. The OTA ensures that the AFO is donned correctly whenever the client is up out of bed and incorporates treatment of donning and doffing the AFO in lower body dressing training. By ensuring that the AFO is donned correctly, the OTA is also helping to prevent further injury and deformity, facilitating the recovery process. Figure 6-28 illustrates Sarah as she dons her AFO.

Cerebrovascular Accident

A CVA, also called stroke, is one of the most common medical/health conditions among clients being treated by OT. A CVA quite often involves a blockage in the supply of blood to the brain, resulting in wide array of impairments, activity limitations, and participation restrictions depending on the severity of the injury. As a CVA affects the brain, it is a condition that affects the CNS. While the whole body may be affected by a CVA, impairments and activity limitations of the LE will be focused on. Specifically, a study by Neckel, Nichols, and Hidler (2010) identified that the impaired legs and unimpaired legs of clients who were diagnosed with CVA could not match the movement synergies of healthy subjects. Distinctive characteristics and patterns of movement can be found in clients who have had a CVA.

Foot drop, as mentioned earlier, can be an impairment caused by a CVA. Specifically, Cruz and Dhaher (2007) identified that reduced knee flexion, hip flexion, and ankle dorsiflexion can affect toe clearance during the swing phase of walking. As a result, the client can compensate by hiking the hip or circumducting gait to allow the clearance needed to advance the foot forward. Lippert (2006) identifies circumducted gait as the leg swinging out to the side during swing phase and returning toward the midline for the heel strike. Hemiplegic gait more readily describes the full movement synergy of a client who has been diagnosed with a CVA.

Hemiplegic gait typically describes the involved LE gait pattern of a client who has experienced a stroke. Lippert (2006) describes this synergy of movement or pattern as hip adduction, hip extension, hip medial rotation, knee extension, ankle plantarflexion, and ankle inversion. Yavuzer and Süreyya (2002) described characteristics of hemiplegic gait, including slow speed, short stance phase, poorly coordinated movements, and decreased weight bearing on the affected extremity.

Additional kinematic characteristics have been identified in the gait cycle. Moseley, Wales, Herbert, Schurr, and Moore (1993) identified common stance phase kinematic deviations to include the following:
- Decreased peak hip extension in late stance phase
- Decreased peak lateral pelvic displacement in stance phase
- Increased peak lateral pelvic displacement in stance phase
- Decreased knee flexion (or hyperextension) in stance phase
- Increased knee flexion in stance phase
- Decreased ankle plantarflexion at toe off

In addition, Moore, Schurr, Wales, Moseley, and Herbert (1993) identified common swing phase kinematic deviations to include the following:
- Decreased peak hip flexion in swing phase
- Decreased peak knee flexion in early swing phase
- Decreased knee extension prior to heel strike
- Decreased dorsiflexion in swing phase

The UE and trunk also affect gait in a client who has experienced a stroke. The client may not be able to produce a reciprocal arm swing due to weakness in the involved UE. A client may not swing the uninvolved limb in order to maintain balance, which will affect a typical LE gait cycle. Due to compensatory movements and weakness, the trunk also may not be able to maintain the alignment of the shoulders with the pelvis as well as eliminate all unnecessary or excessive movements to maintain the body over the BOS. Interestingly, holding onto an object or even slightly touching an object with a fingertip can decrease postural sway (Jeka, 1997). Postural sway is the natural anterior/posterior movement of the body in standing caused by movement at the ankles (Lippert, 2006). As can be seen, multiple factors in the LE and UE combine to influence functional mobility.

Unfortunately, the characteristics of neurological gait patterns can increase energy expenditure and prevent functional progress. These movement patterns can also limit functional recovery and movement potential. Clients may dislike their new movement repertoire for walking because it differs from their prior ability, while others may be able to visually perceive this difference during walking. Ultimately, deviations from normal gait following a stroke can be caused by multiple factors important to both OT and physical therapy practitioners.

BODY STRUCTURES OF THE LOWER EXTREMITY

Body Structures of the Hip

The hip joint is a ball and socket joint. Unlike the shoulder joint, the hip joint sacrifices some ROM in order to attain more stability. The hip joint is a triaxial joint, which means that it has movement in three planes. Logically, location of muscle groups can identify its function. Muscles on the anterior side can be associated with hip flexion, while muscles on the posterior side are associated with extension. Muscles located on the lateral side of the hip can be associated with muscles that create hip abduction.

Table 6-2 presents the muscles, nerves, spinal root levels, and actions of muscles of the hip joint.

The ligaments of the hip increase stability and limit mobility. The ligaments of the hip include the following:

- Iliofemoral ligament: Anterior ligament that resists loss of balance posteriorly, limiting hyperextension.
- Pubofemoral ligament: Limits hyperextension and limits abduction.
- Ischiofemoral ligament: Limits hyperextension and medial rotation.
- Ligamentum teres: Helps to stabilize the head of the femur to the acetabulum and may provide some blood supply to the head of the femur.

Body Structures of the Knee

The knee, also called the tibiofemoral joint, is made up of the distal end of the femur, patella, and the proximal end of the tibia. The knee is a synovial hinge joint, the largest joint in the body, and the joint most prone to injury. The fibula is not specifically included in consideration with the knee joint as a whole as it does not come in contact with the femur. The patella sits over the anterior surface of the knee in the quadriceps muscle tendon. This is called the patellofemoral joint. The patella provides a mechanical advantage for improved quadriceps function.

The knee muscles primarily produce knee extension or knee flexion. The knee also produces slight medial and lateral rotation. The knee flexors can be grouped together, called the hamstring group, and the knee extensors can be grouped together, called the quadriceps group. Quite often, treatment may focus more on strengthening the quadriceps group to decrease contracture formation and counter the powerful hamstring group. Table 6-3 identifies the muscles, nerves, spinal root levels, and actions for the muscles of the knee.

The ligaments of the knee increase stability, limit mobility, and protect the articular capsule. The ligaments of the knee include the following:

- Medial collateral ligament (MCL): Contributes to knee stability, specifically medial stability.
- Lateral collateral ligament (LCL): Contributes to knee stability, specifically lateral stability.
- Anterior cruciate ligament (ACL): Prevents anterior displacement of the tibia in relation to the femur. It is the most common injury in sports and occurs during twisting and bending of the knee.
- Posterior cruciate ligament (PCL): Prevents posterior displacement of the tibia in relation to the femur. The PCL is not commonly injured.
- Transverse ligament: Attaches to the anterior horns of the medial and lateral menisci.
- Patellar ligament: Helps the patella to create its mechanical advantage.

Table 6-2 Muscles, Nerves, Spinal Root Level, and Actions of Muscles of the Hip Joint

Muscle	Nerve	Spinal Nerve Root							Hip Flexion	Hip Extension	Hip Abduction	Hip Adduction	Hip Internal Rotation	Hip External Rotation
		L2	L3	L4	L5	S1	S2	S3						
Iliopsoas: psoas major iliacus	Lumbar plexus femoral nerve	x x	x x						x x					
Piriformis	Anterior rami					x	x							x
Obturator internus	Nerve from sacral plexus				x	x	x	x						x
Gemellus superior	Nerve to obturator internus				x	x								x
Gemellus inferior	Nerve to quadratus femoris				x	x								x
Obturator externus	Obturator nerve		x	x										x
Quadratus femoris	Branch from sacral plexus				x	x								x
Gluteus maximus	Inferior gluteal nerve				x	x	x			x	x			x
Gluteus medius	Superior gluteal nerve			x	x	x					x		x	
Gluteus minimus	Superior gluteal nerve			x	x	x					x		x	
Sartorius	Femoral nerve	x	x						x		x			x

(continued)

Table 6-2 Muscles, Nerves, Spinal Root Level, and Actions of Muscles of the Hip Joint (continued)

Muscle	Nerve	Spinal Nerve Root							Hip Flexion	Hip Extension	Hip Abduction	Hip Adduction	Hip Internal Rotation	Hip External Rotation
		L2	L3	L4	L5	S1	S2	S3						
Tensor fasciae latae	Superior gluteal nerve			x	x	x			x		x			
Rectus femoris	Femoral nerve	x	x	x					x					
Biceps femoris: long head	Sciatic nerve				x	x	x	x		x				
short head	Sciatic nerve				x	x	x							
Pectineus	Femoral nerve	x	x	x					x			x		
Gracilis	Obturator nerve		x	x								x		
Adductor longus	Obturator nerve		x	x					x			x		
Adductor brevis	Obturator nerve		x	x								x		
Adductor magnus	Obturator nerve		x	x								x		
Semi-tendinosus	Sciatic nerve				x	x	x			x				
Semi-membranosus	Sciatic nerve				x	x	x			x				

Adapted from Lippert, L. S. (2006). *Clinical kinesiology for physical therapy assistants* (3rd ed.). Philadelphia, PA: F. A. Davis Company.; Stone, R. I., & Stone, J. A. (2003). *Atlas of skeletal muscles* (4th ed.). New York, NY: McGraw Hill.

Table 6-3 — Muscles, Nerves, Spinal Root Level, and Actions of the Knee

	Muscle	Nerve	Spinal Nerve Root							Knee Flexion	Knee Extension
			L2	L3	L4	L5	S1	S2	S3		
Quadriceps Group	Rectus femoris	Femoral nerve	x	x	x						x
	Vastus lateralis	Femoral nerve	x	x	x						x
	Vastus intermedialis	Femoral nerve	x	x	x						x
	Vastus medialis	Femoral nerve	x	x	x						x
	Popliteus	Tibial nerve			x	x	x			x	
	Semitendinosus	Sciatic nerve				x	x	x		x	
Hamstring Group	Semimembranosus	Sciatic nerve				x	x	x		x	
	Biceps femoris Long head and	Sciatic nerve					x	x	x	x	
	Short head	Common peroneal nerve				x	x	x			
	Gastrocnemius	Tibial nerve					x	x		x	

Adapted from Lippert, L. S. (2006). *Clinical kinesiology for physical therapy assistants* (3rd ed.). Philadelphia, PA: F. A. Davis Company.; Stone, R. J., & Stone, J. A. (2003). *Atlas of skeletal muscles* (4th ed.). New York, NY: McGraw Hill.

Body Structures of the Ankle

The primary joint of the ankle is called the talocrural joint, which is also called the talotibial or true ankle joint. The subtalar joint, alternatively called the talocalcaneal joint, and the transverse tarsal joint are also closely situated near the ankle; however, they have limited participation in ankle movement. The talocrural joint is a synovial hinge joint that connects the tibia and fibula to the talus bone. Ankle muscles can be grouped by the motions they create. The ankle muscles primarily produce movements of plantarflexion, dorsiflexion, inversion, and eversion. Additional ways that the ankle muscles can be grouped include those muscles that act on the ankle alone and those muscles that act on the ankle and joints distal to the ankle. Just like the hand, there are intrinsic and extrinsic muscles of the foot that enable functional movement. For the purpose of this text, only muscles of the ankle will be illustrated. Table 6-4 presents the muscles, nerves, spinal root level, and actions of muscles of the ankle joint.

The ligaments of the ankle increase stability and limit mobility. The ligaments of the ankle include the following:

- Deltoid ligament: Supports the medial side of the ankle joint and helps to maintain the medial longitudinal arch of the foot.
- Three lateral ligaments:
    - Anterior talofibular ligament: Supports the lateral side of the ankle joint.
    - Posterior talofibular ligament: Supports the lateral side of the ankle joint.
    - Calcaneofibular ligament: Supports the lateral side of the ankle joint.

Quite often, physical therapy will focus on strengthening the dorsiflexion muscles due to the easier tendency to plantarflex the ankle. Interestingly, the ankle is also more stable in dorsiflexion. The anterior talofibular ligament is the weakest of the three lateral ligaments and is most often associated with a sprained ankle. There are additional ligaments, bones, and joints of the foot distal to the ankle that will not be addressed in this text.

APPLICATIONS

The following activities will help you apply knowledge of the LE in real-life applications. Activities can be completed individually or in a small group to enhance learning.

1. **Transitional Movements Sitting to Standing:** Transitional movements refer to changes of body position. Quite often, OTA practitioners reinforce certain transitional movements as part of transfer training and ADL retraining. Frequent transitional movements of concern to OT include moving from supine to sitting, sitting to supine, sitting to standing, and standing to sitting. This application is designed to increase your awareness of the sequence of movements required to complete these transitional movements. Select one of the transitional movements below and identify the sequence of movements that occur. Practicing the transitional movement yourself may give you insight into what muscles and joints are activated during the movement. Movements of the UE and trunk also occur during transitional movements; however, for this application, the focus will be on the LE movement. Focus on the movements at the pelvic girdle, hip, knee, and ankle. Select one of the following transitional movements, and fill in the answers in the space below.

    A. Supine to sitting
    B. Sitting to supine
    C. Sitting to standing
    D. Standing to sitting

Table 6-4 Muscles, Nerves, Spinal Root Level, and Actions of Muscles of the Ankle

Muscle	Nerve	Spinal Nerve root				Ankle Plantarflexion	Ankle Dorsiflexion	Ankle Inversion	Ankle Eversion
		L4	L5	S1	S2				
Gastrocnemius	Tibial nerve			x	x	x			
Soleus	Tibial nerve			x	x	x			
Plantaris	Tibial nerve		x	x		x			
Tibialis anterior	Deep peroneal nerve	x	x	x			x	x	
Extensor hallucis longus	Deep peroneal nerve	x	x	x			x	x	
Extensor digitorum longus	Deep peroneal nerve	x	x	x			x		x
Peroneus longus	Superficial peroneal nerve	x	x	x		x			x
Peroneus brevis	Superficial peroneal nerve	x	x	x		x			x
Peroneus tertius	Superficial peroneal nerve	x	x	x			x		x
Tibialis posterior	Tibial nerve		x	x		x		x	
Flexor digitorum longus	Tibial nerve		x	x		x		x	
Flexor hallucis longus	Tibial nerve		x	x	x	x		x	

Adapted from Lippert, L. S. (2006). *Clinical kinesiology for physical therapy assistants* (3rd ed.). Philadelphia, PA: F. A. Davis Company; Stone, R. J., & Stone, J. A. (2003). *Atlas of skeletal muscles* (4th ed.). New York, NY: McGraw Hill.

LE Movement Sequence
Transitional movement selected: _____

Joint Movement	Muscles Involved	Identify ROM Needed
1.		
2.		
3.		
4.		
5.		
6.		
7.		

2. **The Pelvic Girdle:** The pelvic girdle is very important due to its influence on the trunk and LE in sitting and standing. This activity will help you identify the different motions of the pelvic girdle. First, with a partner or on your own, identify the location of the ASIS, which is a bony landmark located on the pelvic bone on the front side of the body. The ASIS bony landmark provides a reference point to identify the motions of the pelvic girdle. Palpate the ASIS on each pelvic bone to identify if they are roughly symmetrical or if one ASIS is not a mirror image of the other ASIS on the contralateral (or other) side of the body. Standing upright, both ASIS landmarks should be level. Anterior tilt occurs if the ASIS landmarks are more anterior than the pubic symphysis. Posterior tilt occurs if the ASIS landmarks are more posterior than the pubic symphysis. In lateral tilt, one ASIS landmark is more superior than the contralateral, or opposite, side ASIS. The more superior ASIS landmark is the reference point. If the left ASIS is more inferior to the right ASIS, then the pelvic girdle is in left lateral tilt. Pelvic rotation is the final motion and occurs if one ASIS is more anterior or posterior as compared to the contralateral side. The reference point is the ASIS landmark that moves anteriorly as in frontal pelvic rotation or posteriorly as in backward pelvic rotation.

    A. While facing another student, place your thumbs over the ASIS landmarks. Spread your hands out to cover the sides of the hip with fingers abducted, as if you were going to catch a basketball. By moving your wrists in ulnar and radial deviation, try to palpate the movement of anterior and posterior pelvic tilt. Can you palpate the other pelvic girdle motions of pelvic tilt and pelvic rotation?

    B. Sit on the edge of a mat. Is your pelvic girdle in anterior or posterior pelvic tilt? Hopefully, the pelvic girdle is in anterior pelvic tilt. Being careful not to fall off the mat, try to make your pelvic girdle go into posterior pelvic tilt. Does it feel like you could easily slide off the mat? Why? Quite often, OT practitioners treat clients sitting on the edge of a mat. Anterior pelvic tilt is important to enable an active trunk that supports reaching and decreases the risk for falls.

3. **Lower Extremity PROM** In some settings, it may be necessary for the OTA to perform PROM on the LE as a preparatory treatment. With another student, either sitting or supine on a mat, practice moving each joint of the LE through its available ROM. Remember, in PROM, the therapist provides the force to create joint movement. The hand placement proximal to the joint supports and isolates the joint through stabilization. The hand placement distal to the joint provides the force needed to move the joint and create PROM. Try to move each joint through its available ROM. Each joint is listed below.

Table 6-5	**Lower Extremity Active Range of Motion Application**				
Position	Joint and Motion	Landmark	Stable Arm	Moving Arm	Recorded ROM
Supine	Hip flexion	Lateral aspect of greater trochanter	Parallel to the midaxilla line of the trunk	Parallel to the lateral aspect of the femur	
Supine	Hip extension				
Supine	Hip abduction	Over ASIS	Horizontal between ASIS	Parallel to the anterior midline of the femur	
Supine	Hip adduction				
Sitting	Hip internal rotation	Over midpoint of the patella	Perpendicular to the floor	Parallel to the anterior midline of the tibial midway between the two malleoli	
Sitting	Hip external rotation				
Sitting or supine	Knee flexion	Over the lateral epicondyle of the femur	Parallel to the lateral midline of the femur	Parallel to the lateral midline of the fibula	
Sitting or supine	Knee extension				
Sitting	Ankle plantar-flexion	Lateral aspect of the lateral malleolus	Parallel to the lateral midline of the fibula	Parallel to the lateral midline of the 5th metatarsal	
Sitting	Ankle dorsi-flexion				
Sitting	Ankle eversion	Over the anterior aspect of the ankle midway between malleoli	Parallel to the anterior midline of the lower leg	Parallel to the anterior midline of the 2nd metatarsal	
Sitting	Ankle inversion				

Adapted from Latella, D., & Meriano, C. (2003). *Occupational therapy manual for evaluation of range of motion and muscle strength*. Clifton Park, NY: Delmar Cengage Learning.

Joint Motions:
1. Hip flexion
2. Hip extension
3. Hip internal rotation
4. Hip external rotation
5. Hip abduction
6. Hip adduction
7. Knee flexion
8. Knee extension
9. Ankle plantarflexion
10. Ankle dorsiflexion
11. Ankle inversion
12. Ankle eversion

4.   **Lower Extremity AROM:** In some settings, it may be necessary for the OTA to measure the available joint ROM for the LE. For this application, measure the available AROM of the LE with a partner. Use Table 6-5 for this application.

5. **Lower Extremity Adaptive Equipment for Mobility:** OTA practitioners frequently need to educate and reinforce safety and proper use of adaptive equipment for safe mobility during engagement in occupations. Examples of adaptive equipment related to enhancing mobility include rolling walkers, standard walkers, wheelchairs, and various types of canes. Using a standard or rolling walker, answer the following questions:
   A. Describe the BOS without the adaptive equipment.
   B. Describe the BOS with the adaptive equipment.
   C. If the client is sitting down and tries to stand by pulling on the walker handholds, is this safe? What happens to the BOS? Is there a better alternative method to stand?
   D. When the client stands and holds the walker by the handholds as far to the front as possible, is this safe? Answer these questions:
      - Is the BOS larger or smaller?
      - Where is the center of gravity?
      - How could you make this safer for the client to stand with a walker?
   E. Is it safe for the client to stand and turn with a walker by only twisting the trunk, not changing foot placement, so that the front of the walker is more toward the side of the person during turning?
      - How is the BOS affected?
      - Where is the center of gravity?
      - How could you make this safer for the client to stand with a walker?

6. **Stride Length:** This application will help comprehend that while components of gait are similar for each person, each person has his or her own individualized characteristics. Anatomical characteristics, environmental adaptations, and contextual factors all influence gait and stride length. Individuals can have different leg lengths or body structure components that affect gait. A person walking downhill may have a greater stride length than when walking uphill. A person may also have a different stride length when walking on a level surface versus an unlevel surface.

   Knowing your stride length is useful in determining distances traveled for functional mobility. As stated previously, stride length is the distance traveled during the gait cycle or from one heel strike to the same heel strike on the ground. You can measure one stride length to find the distance traveled; however, it may be inaccurate due to the conscious effort to take a step. A more accurate method may be to walk a premeasured distance of 50 or 100 feet and count the number of strides for that distance. For this application, identify the following:
   A. What is the step length for your right leg? What is the step length for your left leg? Are they the same or different? Why?
   B. What is your number of stride lengths for 50 feet? Is it the same or different than a friend or classmate? Why?
   C. Identify five factors that influenced the stride length that was recorded.

7. **OTPF-2 Areas of Occupation:** The OTPF-2, specifically areas of occupation, was introduced in Chapter 1. Remember, areas of occupation include life activities in which a person engages (AOTA, 2008). This application will build on the use of the OTPF-2 by using Sarah's occupational profile. Identify areas of occupation that may apply to Sarah by using the occupational profile and Table 6-6. If you cannot identify an area of occupation from the occupational profile, identify what may be appropriate for Sarah considering her age and the information provided.

8. **OTPF-2 Activity Demands:** The OTPF-2, specifically activity demands, was introduced in Chapter 1. Remember, activity demands include what an activity requires for it to be doable (AOTA, 2008). This application will build on the use of the OTPF-2 by using Sarah's occupational profile. Identify an activity and its area of occupation in the first column of Table 6-7. Then, identify the activity demands for this activity that apply to Sarah to be able to complete that activity. Remember, some activities may need to be adapted in order for Sarah to complete the activity due to her impairments. Record your examples in Table 6-7.

Table 6-6	Occupational Therapy Practice Framework, 2nd Edition Domain Aspect: Areas of Occupation							
Areas of Occupation								
ADL	IADL	Rest and Sleep	Education	Work	Play	Leisure	Social Participation	
Upper & lower body dressing	Sweep floor	Sleep at night	Sunday school at church	Retired CNA	Golf league	Talk show	Volunteer at a long-term care facility	

Table 6-7	Occupational Therapy Practice Framework, 2nd Edition Activity Demands							
Activity and Areas of Occupation	Objects Used	Space Demands	Time Demands	Sequencing and Timing	Required Actions	Required Body Functions	Required Body Structures	
Toileting—self-care ability; area of occupation is ADL	Bedside commode, bed pan, grab bars, toilet paper	Lighting needs, area for a wheelchair, reaching for toilet paper	Typical time needed to complete toileting task	Needed items present, safe multistep processing, timeliness with toilet hygiene	Transfer to commode, lower pants, peri-hygiene, stand balance	Level of arousal, impulse control, sensory functions, urinary and bowel functions	Nerves, muscles, eyes, ears, sensory receptors	

9.   **OTPF-2 Consideration of Health Condition:** This application will build on the use of the OTPF-2 by using Sarah's occupational profile. The OTPF-2, specifically considerations of health conditions, was introduced in Chapter 1. Remember from Chapter 1, the ICF identifies three levels of human functioning to include **body part**, **whole person**, and **societal**. These levels coincide with levels of dysfunction labeled **impairment** (body part), **activity limitation** (individual level or whole person), and **participation restrictions** (societal). For this application, identify the impact of Sarah's health condition to the OTPF-2 domains. First, identify the level of human functioning and an example for Sarah. Second, identify the level of dysfunction and an example. Examples are provided to get you started. Fill in Table 6-8.

Table 6-8

Occupational Therapy Practice Framework, 2nd Edition Consideration of Health Condition

Health Condition	Domains	Domain Aspects	CVA		Foot Drop	
			Level of Human Functioning	Level of Dysfunction	Level of Human Functioning	Level of Dysfunction
Impact of health condition on OTPF-2 domains	Areas of Occupation	Activities of daily living	Toileting—whole person	Activity limitation		
		Instrumental ADL				
		Rest and sleep				
		Education				
		Work				
		Play				
		Leisure				
		Social participation				
		Values, beliefs, and spirituality				
	Client Factors	Body functions	Muscle tone—Body part	Impairment		
		Body structures				
	Performance Skills	Sensory perceptual				
		Motor and praxis				
		Emotional regulation				
		Cognitive				
		Communication and social				

(continued)

Table 6-8	*Occupational Therapy Practice Framework, 2nd Edition* **Consideration of Health Condition** *(continued)*					
Health Condition			**CVA**		**Foot Drop**	
	Domains	Domain Aspects	Level of Human Functioning	Level of Dysfunction	Level of Human Functioning	Level of Dysfunction
Impact of health condition on OTPF-2 domains	Performance Patterns	Habits				
		Routines				
		Roles				
		Rituals	*Unable to attend church—societal level*	*Participation restriction*		
	Context and Environment	Cultural				
		Personal				
		Physical				
		Social				
		Temporal				
		Virtual				
	Activity Demands	Objects used				
		Space demands				
		Social demands				
		Sequencing and timing				
		Required actions				
		Required body functions				
		Required body structures				

Adapted from American Occupational Therapy Association. (2008). Occupational therapy practice framework: Domain and process (2nd ed.). *American Journal of Occupational Therapy, 62,* 625-683.

REFERENCES

American Occupational Therapy Association. (2008). Occupational therapy practice framework: Domain and process (2nd ed.). *American Journal of Occupational Therapy, 62*, 625–683.

Cruz, T., & Dhaher, Y. (2007). *Compensatory gait movements post stroke: The influence of synergies.* Retrieved from http://web.x-cdtech.com/nacob/abstracts/233.pdf.

Foti, D., & Kanazawa, L. M. (2006). Activities of daily living. In H. M. Pendleton & W. Schultz-Krohn (Eds.), *Pedretti's occupational therapy: Practice skills for physical dysfunction* (6th ed., p. 150). St Louis, MO: Mosby Elsevier.

Greene, D. P., & Roberts, S. L. (2005). *Kinesiology: Movement in the context of activity* (2nd ed.). St. Louis, MO: Elsevier-Mosby.

Hayes, S. M. (2004). Gait awareness. In G. Gillen & A. Burkhardt (Eds.), *Stroke rehabiliation: A function-based approach* (2nd ed., pp. 312-337). St. Louis, MO: Mosby.

Jeka, J. (1997). Light contact as a balance aid. *Physical Therapy, 77*(5), 476–487.

Lippert, L. S. (2006). *Clinical kinesiology for physical therapy assistants* (3rd ed.). Philadelphia, PA: F. A. Davis Company.

Loudon, J., Swift, M., & Bell, S. (Eds.). (2008). *The clinical orthopedic assessment guide* (2nd ed.). Champaign, IL: Human Kinetics.

Merriam-Webster's collegiate dictionary (9th ed.). (1991). Springfield, MA: Merriam-Webster.

Moore, S., Schurr, K., Wales, A., Moseley, A., & Herbert, R. (1993). Observation and analysis of hemiplegic gait: Swing phase. *Australian Journal of Physiotherapy, 39*(4), 271-278.

Moseley, A., Wales, A., Herbert, R., Schurr, K., & Moore, S. (1993). Observation and analysis of hemiplegic gait: Stance phase. *Australian Journal of Physiotherapy, 39*(4), 259-267.

Neckel, N., Nichols, D., & Hidler, J. (2010). *Lower limb synergy patterns of stroke subjects while walking in a Lokomat Robotic Orthosis.* Retrieved from http//www.asweb.org/conference/2007/pdf/233.pdf.

Pritchett, J. W., & Porembski, M. A. (2010). *Foot drop.* Retrieved from http://emedicine.medscape.com/article/1234607-print.

Skinner, S. R., Antonelli, D., Perry, J., & Lester, K. (1985). Functional demands on the stance limb in walking. *Orthopedics, 8*, 355-361.

Thomas, C. L. (Ed.). (1997). *Taber's cyclopedic medical dictionary* (18th ed.). Philadelphia, PA: F. A. Davis.

Winstein, C. J., Gardner, E. R., McNeal, D. R., Barto, P. S., & Nicholson, D. E. (1989). Standing balance training: Effect on balance and locomotion in hemiparetic adults. *Archives of Physical Medicine and Rehabilitation, 70*, 755–762.

Yavuzer, G., & Süreyya, E. (2002). Effect of an arm sling on gait patterns in patients with hemiplegia. *Archives of Physical Medicine & Rehabilitation, 83*, 960–963.

chapter 7

Function and Movement of the Shoulder and Scapula

Carolyn L. Roller, OTR/L; Susan J. Sain, MS, OTR/L, FAOTA;
and Jeremy L. Keough, MSOT, OTR/L

OCCUPATIONAL PROFILE

The following occupational profile is provided to demonstrate how body functions and body structure are related to the shoulder complex and tie into occupational therapy (OT) intervention of shoulder impairments. Linda, the client in the following occupational profile, will be referred to throughout the chapter.

Linda is a 77-year-old grandmother who is participating in OT with a physician's referral to improve right, dominant shoulder function.

During the evaluation, the following data were gathered:

Subjective: Linda reports decreased function in her right shoulder for approximately 3 months with an increase in her signs and symptoms of right shoulder pain and stiffness over the past month. Her main complaints include an inability to properly care for her grandchildren. She also reports difficulty with grooming, toileting, bathing, and sleeping. Her occupational role includes caring for her two grandchildren since her daughter returned to part-time employment. Linda has a grandson who is 3 years old and a granddaughter who is 6 months old.

Linda states her biggest problem occurs when she is providing care for her grandchildren, especially when getting them in and out of their car seats. She also reports that it is difficult to change diapers on her 6-month-old granddaughter safely and without increased pain. The client denies any injury to her right shoulder. However, she states that she slipped while gardening about 6 months ago and caught herself with her right arm, breaking her fall. She stated that she had some "achy"-type pain in her whole arm occasionally, especially at night after this incident. She reported an inability to sleep on her right side, which has always been her most comfortable position. The client reports a past medical history of Type 2, insulin-dependent diabetes, hypertension, and high cholesterol. She reports that she does not have a pacemaker. Besides the insulin, she takes medication to control her blood pressure and cholesterol. She denies any other health problems and states that "she feels healthy and gets around quite well."

Objective: The client rates her pain on a 0 to 10 scale, 0 being no pain and 10 being "emergency room" pain. She rates her pain as a 3/10 at rest and an 8/10 at worst. She reports her worst pain with right shoulder movement during resistive functional activities. Examples of functional activities provided by Linda include lifting her granddaughter out of her car seat, attempting to shampoo her own hair, and unhooking her bra while undressing.

Keough, J. L., Sain, S. J., Roller C. L.
Kinesiology for the Occupational Therapy Assistant:
Essential Components of Function and Movement (pp. 175-216).

Active range of motion (AROM) is within functional limits in both upper extremities except the right, dominant shoulder. Formal measurements are described below:

- Glenohumeral (GH) joint flexion: Right: 75 degrees   Left: 170 degrees
- GH joint abduction: Right: 60 degrees   Left: 165 degrees
- GH joint external rotation: Right: 25 degrees   Left: 75 degrees
- GH joint internal rotation: Right: 35 degrees   Left: 70 degrees

The client reports pain at the end of AROM in the right shoulder during strength measurements. Grip strength is tested bilaterally with the right grip averaging 45 pounds and the left grip averaging 50 pounds. Linda denies any numbness or tingling in her upper extremities. There was no edema observed in the upper extremities at the time of the evaluation.

Goals were established by the occupational therapist in collaboration with Linda and are presented below:

Short-Term Goals:
1. Client will be instructed in and comply with a home exercise program.
2. Client will decrease pain from 3/10 to 0/10 at rest and will be able to sleep all night within 4 weeks by following ergonomic postural changes.
3. Client will decrease pain from 8/10 to 4/10 at worst during resistive functional activities within 4 weeks by using modified lifting techniques and adaptive equipment.
4. Client will increase AROM in all limited planes of right shoulder range of motion (ROM) by 10 degrees within 3 weeks.
5. Client will increase right grip strength by 5 pounds within 4 weeks.
6. Client will be able to perform toileting task using right hand independently and with fewer complaints of pain within 4 weeks.

Long-Term Goals:
1. Client will demonstrate compliance and independence in home exercise program at discharge.
2. Client will be independent with use of right upper extremity in self-care and occupational roles with only minimal complaints of discomfort within 3 months.
3. Client will demonstrate AROM and grip strength to within functional limits within 3 months.

BODY FUNCTIONS OF THE SHOULDER COMPLEX

Joint motions, as well as the strength characteristics, of the GH joint and scapula will be identified in the following sections as they relate to function. Scapulohumeral rhythm will also be defined and explained. Additionally, four common problems seen in OT treatment will be identified and discussed. Throughout this chapter, references will be made to the occupational profile of Linda.

The **shoulder complex** includes all of the body structures that provide motion at the GH joint and scapula. The shoulder complex includes in one part the activities of the scapula and clavicle, which can also be referred to as the shoulder girdle. Additionally, activities of the scapula and humerus are often referred to as the shoulder joint or GH joint. Overall, the shoulder complex consists of four joints that function in a coordinated and rhythmic manner. Changes in the position of the upper extremity involve movements of the clavicle, scapula, and humerus (Peat, 1986). This is accomplished by the sternoclavicular joint, acromioclavicular joint, GH joint, and the scapulothoracic gliding mechanism (Oatis, 2004).

The design of the shoulder complex is related to overall function of the upper extremity. For example, the shoulder complex controls placement of the hand in its occupational space in front of the body. The shoulder complex provides the upper extremity with a ROM that is greater than any other joint in the body. This ROM is more than what is required for most activities of daily living

(Peat, 1986). Linda, in the occupational profile, may not need to regain all of her right shoulder movement to resume care of her grandchildren, although that may be a treatment goal. She may be able to compensate with the other joints of her right arm and her left upper extremity to safely lift her grandchildren from the car seat. Even though she may not regain full ROM, she may have functional movement of a very mobile body part, the shoulder complex.

Motions of the Shoulder Girdle and Glenohumeral Joint

Movements of the shoulder complex rely on the motion of all components. Specifically, the humerus moves in synchronization with the scapula at the GH joint. The scapula moves while in contact with the clavicle at the acromioclavicular joint, while the clavicle attaches to the sternum at the sternoclavicular joint. Movement at all of these joints must occur for the arm to reach 180 degrees of GH joint flexion or abduction (Schenkman & Rugo De Cartaya, 1987). The ability to achieve full AROM of the upper extremity, however, depends more heavily on certain joints, namely the GH and scapulothoracic joints.

Motions of the scapula are identified as scapular elevation, scapular depression, scapular adduction or retraction, scapular abduction or protraction, scapular upward rotation, and scapular downward rotation. Scapular elevation is achieved when the client elevates his or her shoulder complex as in shrugging the shoulders. Scapular depression is achieved when the client attempts to depress the shoulder complex as in reaching toward the ground. Scapular adduction, also called retraction, is when the client moves his or her scapula closer to the vertebrae. This can be achieved by sticking the chest out and pulling the shoulder complex toward the rear of the person. The opposite is scapular abduction, also referred to as protraction. Scapular abduction is achieved when the client moves the shoulder complex toward the front of the person as when reaching forward, resulting in an increase in distance between the scapula and vertebrae. Scapular upward rotation is achieved with either GH joint flexion or GH joint abduction. This occurs when the inferior angle of the scapula moves upward and away from the spinal column. Downward rotation occurs when the arm returns to the neutral or anatomical position. Of importance, scapular upward rotation is important and necessary to achieve full GH joint AROM. Each scapular motion is labeled in Figures 7-1 to 7-6.

Motions of the GH joint are identified as GH joint flexion, extension, abduction, adduction, internal rotation, external rotation, horizontal adduction, and horizontal abduction. GH joint flexion is achieved when the client raises his or her arm overhead in front of the body, such as

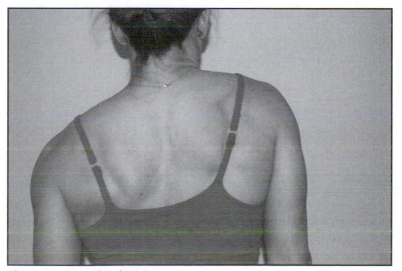

Figure 7-1. Scapular elevation.

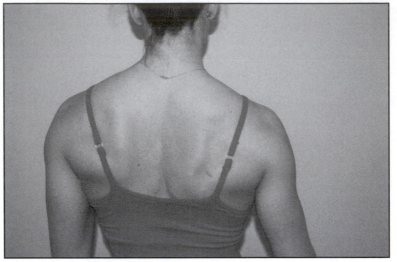

Figure 7-2. Scapular depression.

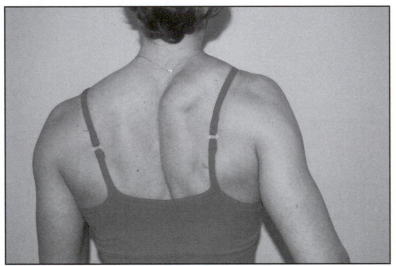

Figure 7-3. Scapular retraction (also called adduction).

placing an item in a cupboard above the head. GH joint extension, sometimes called hyperexten-sion, is when the client moves his or her arm straight back from the neutral or anatomical position at the side of the body. This movement could be used to place an object in the back seat of the car with the right arm while seated in the driver's seat. GH joint abduction occurs when the client moves his or her arm away from the body out to the side away from the anatomical position. This movement may be seen functionally when the client reaches up and out to the side to turn on a light switch. GH joint adduction is the movement of the client's arm returning to the side of the body from GH joint abduction. GH joint internal rotation is achieved when the greater tubercle of the humerus rotates toward the midline in front of the body. Functionally, during this motion, the client would be reaching behind the small of his or her back as though he or she was tucking in a shirt or placing the palm of the hand on his or her stomach. GH joint external rotation is seen

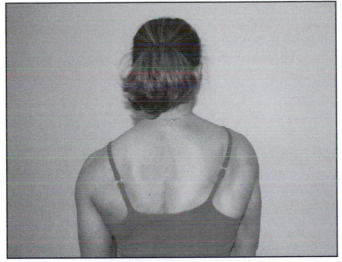

Figure 7-4. Scapular protraction (also called abduction).

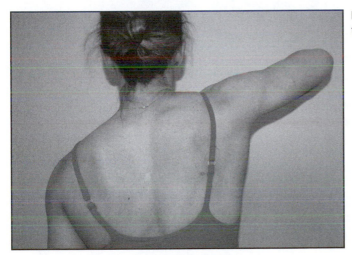

Figure 7-5. Scapular upward rotation.

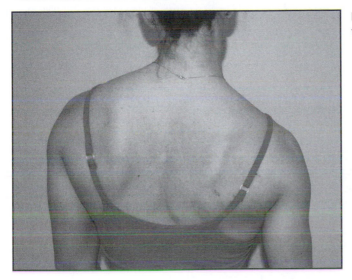

Figure 7-6. Scapular downward rotation.

when the client rotates the greater tubercle of the humerus away from the midline. This movement can be seen when a client is reaching with his or her left arm for the shoulder belt prior to driving the car or placing the palm of the hand on the back of the head. GH joint horizontal adduction is shown when the client moves the arm in a horizontal or transverse plane toward and across the chest, such as reaching across the body to bathe the left shoulder with the right hand. Finally, GH joint horizontal abduction is achieved when the person moves the arm in a horizontal or transverse plane away from the chest. Each motion is identified in Figures 7-7 to 7-14.

Scapulohumeral Rhythm

Understanding the concept of scapulohumeral rhythm may be enhanced by multiple definitions. According to Lippert (2000), **scapulohumeral rhythm** describes the movement relationship between the scapula in the shoulder girdle and the GH joint. This movement can be described as a synchronization of combined movements that occur between the scapula and humerus

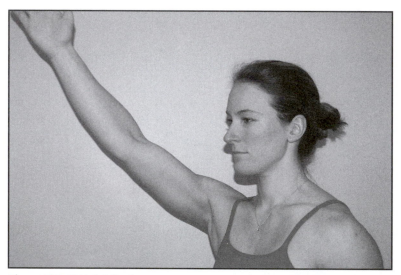

Figure 7-7. GH joint flexion.

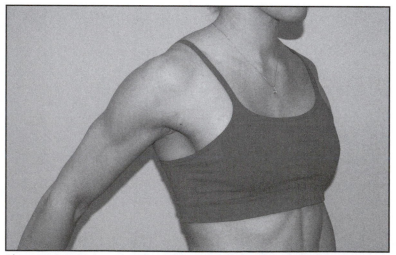

Figure 7-8. GH joint extension (also called hyperextension).

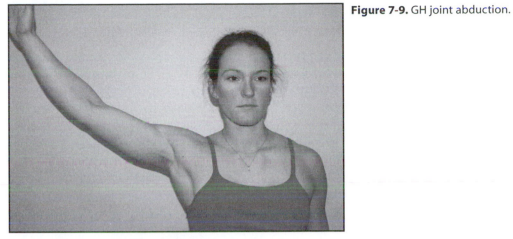

Figure 7-9. GH joint abduction.

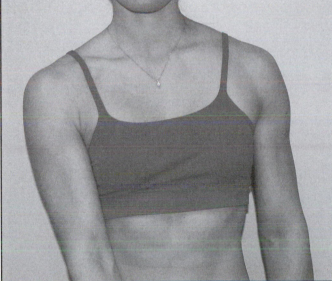

Figure 7-10. GH joint adduction.

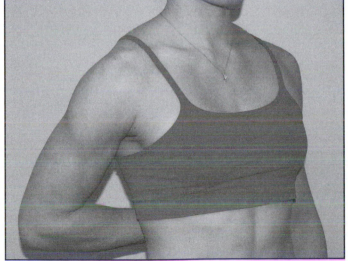

Figure 7-11. GH joint internal rotation.

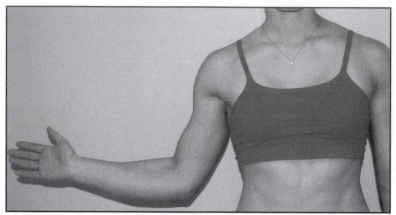

Figure 7-12. GH joint external rotation.

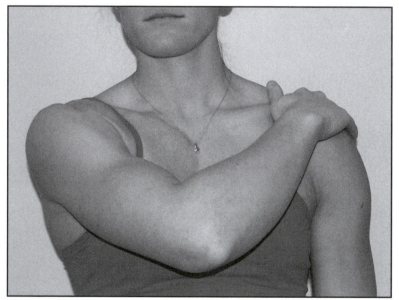

Figure 7-13. GH joint horizontal adduction.

during GH joint flexion or abduction (Dutton, 2004). Scapulohumeral rhythm can also be defined as motions of the clavicle, scapula, and humerus all working together to achieve full elevation of the arm (Hunter et al., 2002). Due to the importance of scapulohumeral rhythm, its definition is provided in Gold Box 7-1.

The first 30 degrees of GH joint flexion or abduction is called the "setting phase" of scapulohumeral rhythm. During this phase, scapulothoracic movement is very small and inconsistent (Schenkman & Rugo De Cartaya, 1987). During the second phase, the scapula abducts and upwardly rotates 1 degree of motion for every 2 degrees of GH joint flexion or abduction. The second phase occurs between 30 and 90 degrees of GH joint flexion or abduction (Glinn, 2008). This 2:1 ratio is the measurement of scapulohumeral rhythm. After 90 degrees of GH joint movement, 60 degrees of motion occurs at the GH joint, with the remaining 30 degrees consisting of scapular movement. In this final phase of scapulohumeral rhythm, this 2:1 ratio is not consistent

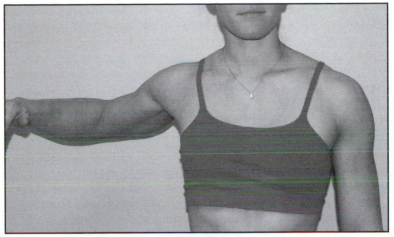

Figure 7-14. GH joint horizontal abduction.

Gold Box 7-1

Scapulohumeral rhythm: The motion of the clavicle, scapula, and humerus working together to achieve full elevation of the arm. This movement relationship exists between the scapula in the shoulder girdle and the GH joint.

Dutton (2004); Hunter et al. (2002)

---

throughout the ROM. Early movement as in the first phase involves more GH joint motion, while end-range movement involves more scapular movement (Dutton, 2004).

Scapulohumeral rhythm serves two purposes. First, scapular upward rotation allows the GH joint muscles to maintain the length-tension relationship. This allows the muscles to sustain their force through a larger portion of the available ROM and effectively limits active insufficiency. Second, simultaneous movement of the humerus and scapula during GH joint flexion or abduction prevents impingement between the greater tubercle of the humerus and the acromion process (Hunter et al., 2002).

Strength Characteristics of the Shoulder Girdle and Glenohumeral Joint

Most muscles of the shoulder complex perform a variety of movements. Additionally, most muscles work together to either strengthen a movement or provide stability. **Synergists** are muscles that work together to increase the strength of a desired movement as they work in unison. If stability is the goal rather than increased strength, then muscles will work in unison to counter each other, thus stabilizing a joint. **Antagonists** are muscles that work against each other to equal or cancel out the movement and therefore gain stability. When muscles work against each other to provide stability, this is also called a co-contraction.

Synergists are muscles whose fibers (line of force) lie approximately in the same direction. Muscles that act as synergists to one another provide a stronger action on the joint, resulting in stronger functional movement for the client. A force couple, as seen in upward and downward rotation, is a special type of synergy. The muscles in the **force couple** still act together to provide a stronger functional movement; however, they do so in a different manner. To be classified as a force couple, two basic requirements must be met. First, the resulting movement must be rotary in nature. Second, the line of force and the pull or angle of muscle fibers of all muscles involved must be in opposing directions. One muscle's line of force might be vertical, another lateral, and still another medial. A common example given for a force couple is the motion used to turn a steering wheel when the power steering goes out. One hand pushes or turns the steering wheel upward while the other hand pushes or turns the steering wheel in a downward direction. The forces are in opposite directions but work together to strengthen the rotary movement of the steering wheel.

Table 7-1 can be used to readily identify muscles that act as synergists for scapular motions. Synergists can be found by selecting a movement and then looking in the column beneath it for the muscles marked with an X. To discuss specific movements required during selected daily activities, refer back to the client Linda. Looking at the table, we see that scapular protraction, which Linda uses when she reaches forward to get her grandchild out of the car seat, is performed by the serratus anterior and pectoralis minor muscles working as synergists. In a similar manner, this table can also be used to find antagonists for each movement. Retraction is the motion that is opposite to, or antagonist to, protraction. Therefore, the muscles that cause retraction are antagonists to the muscles that cause protraction. Using the table as a reference, one sees that the middle trapezius and rhomboid muscles cause scapular retraction; thus, they are antagonists to the serratus anterior and pectoralis minor for the motion of scapular protraction.

Some muscles of the shoulder girdle are so large that the muscle fibers in different portions of the muscle are oriented in different directions, meaning that their line of pull will be different. In this case, the different portions of the same muscle may work as synergists to each other or as antagonists, depending on the motion desired at a given joint. The trapezius and deltoid muscles both fit this description and are both divided into three parts. The trapezius muscle is divided into upper, middle, and lower sections while the deltoid muscle is divided into anterior, middle, and posterior sections. Again, refer to the table to note that the upper portion of the trapezius functions as a synergist with the lower portion of the trapezius for scapular upward rotation. The upper portion of the trapezius also functions as an antagonist to the lower portion of the trapezius for the movement of scapular depression.

To determine motions necessary at the shoulder complex to complete specific daily activities, refer again to Linda in the occupational profile. The inter-relatedness of joint actions, muscular control, and innervations can be seen in reference to an activity important to Linda. One of Linda's activities of daily living (ADL), shampooing her hair, requires her to use many movements to include scapular elevation and upward rotation, GH joint flexion and abduction, and GH joint external rotation. Examples of motions, muscles, nerves, and innervations that may be needed to shampoo hair are provided in Table 7-2.

An instrumental activity of daily living (IADL) for Linda, caring for her grandchildren, includes diapering and getting the children into and out of car seats. For these actions, Linda uses scapular protraction and GH joint internal rotation in reaching forward and holding the child, GH joint extension and scapular retraction in lifting the child toward herself, and GH joint horizontal abduction and adduction in reaching for and placing a diaper on the baby. Scapular depression and downward rotation accompany GH joint extension. As you can see, all of the motions of the shoulder girdle listed earlier in this chapter are necessary for our client to engage in her chosen occupations. Typically, in order for most people to accomplish their daily chosen activities, they will need to be able to perform all the motions of the shoulder girdle. The ability to perform these motions will require an intricate and detailed coordination of muscle, nerve, and joint motion.

Table 7-1 Motions of the Scapula

Muscle	Nerve	Nerve Root						Depression	Elevation	Protraction	Retraction	Upward Rotation*	Downward Rotation*
		C3	C4	C5	C6	C7	C8						
Trapezius (upper)	Spinal accessory	x	x						x			x	
Trapezius (middle)	Spinal accessory	x	x								x		
Trapezius (lower)	Spinal accessory	x	x					x				x	
Levator scapulae	Dorsal scapular	x	x						x				x
Rhomboids	Dorsal scapular			x							x		x
Serratus anterior	Long thoracic			x	x	x				x		x	
Pectoralis minor	pectoral				x	x	x	x		x			x

Adapted from Kendall, F. P., McCreary, E. K., Provance, P. G., Rodgers, M. M., & Romani, W. A. (2005). *Muscle testing and function with posture and pain* (5th ed.). Baltimore, MD: Lippincott, Williams & Wilkins.

*Indicates force couple.

Table 7-2	Shampooing Hair: Movements, Muscles, and Nerve Innervation	
Muscle	**Nerve**	**Nerve Roots**
Scapular Elevation		
Trapezius (upper)	Spinal accessory	C3, C4
Levator scapulae	Dorsal scapular	C3, C4
Scapular Upward Rotation		
Trapezius (upper)	Spinal accessory	C3, C4
Trapezius (lower)	Spinal accessory	C3, C4
Serratus anterior	Long thoracic	C5, C6, C7
GH Joint Flexion		
Deltoid (anterior)	Axillary	C5, C6
Biceps brachii	Musculocutaneous	C5, C6
Pectoralis major (clavicle)	Medial pectoral	C8, T1
Coracobrachialis	Musculocutaneous	C5, C6
GH Abduction		
Deltoid	Axillary	C5, C6
Supraspinatus	Suprascapular	C5, C6
GH External Rotation		
Deltoid (posterior)	Axillary	C5, C6
Infraspinatus	Suprascapular	C5, C6
Teres minor	Axillary	C5, C6

Common Problems With the Shoulder Girdle and Glenohumeral Joint

There are many injuries and diseases that can affect the scapula and GH joint, requiring OT intervention. Four of the most common shoulder injuries and diseases seen in OT will be presented in the following section. While reading about these injuries and diseases, consider Linda in the occupational profile. Think about Linda's signs and symptoms and the functional tasks that are limited. Appendix C will provide further information on Linda's treatment plan and the outcome of her interventions.

Primary Adhesive Capsulitis: "Frozen Shoulder"

Most clients report a history of progressive shoulder stiffness with **primary adhesive capsulitis** or **"frozen shoulder."** The stiffness is usually preceded by diffuse pain with no prior obvious shoulder problem, which may last from 2 weeks to several months. At times, there may have been a period of immobilization or minor trauma to the extremity. According to Hunter and colleagues (2002), female clients over the age of 40 appear to be more commonly affected with adhesive capsulitis. Clients with insulin-dependent diabetes, degenerative disk disease of the cervical spine, and those with a history of stroke involving shoulder hemiplegia are also more likely to experience adhesive capsulitis (Boyle-Walker, Gabard, Bietsch, Masek-Van Arsdale, & Robinson, 1997).

There are three clinical stages in primary adhesive capsulitis. The first stage is called the *painful stage*. The client often complains of diffuse pain that is progressive and worse at night. The first stage can last from 2 to 9 months. As the client uses his or her extremity less, he or she begins to lose ROM. This leads to the second phase, which is called the stiffening phase. The client loses more ROM and complains of an inability to use the affected extremity in ADL. Dull, achy pain continues and becomes worse with AROM. The second stage can last from 4 to 12 months. The final clinical stage is called the thawing stage and occurs as the client begins to regain lost ROM. The client reports less pain with movement and gradually returns to independence in ADL tasks over a time period of 6 to 9 months (Dutton, 2004).

Shoulder Hemiplegia and Subluxation After Stroke

Hemiplegia is the paralysis of one side of the body after a cerebrovascular accident (CVA) or stroke. A stroke can be caused when a clot reduces or blocks blood flow through an artery supplying blood to the brain. When the brain is without blood or oxygen for even a short period of time, damage occurs (WebMD, 2009). **Shoulder subluxation** is a partial dislocation of the humerus at the GH joint and is seen in many individuals after a stroke (Ohio Health, 1995). When the shoulder complex is affected by weakness or paralysis after a stroke, subluxation of the GH joint can occur. In particular, the shoulder is vulnerable to stretch, especially when the arm is hanging unsupported by the side of the body and there is less stability at the GH joint (Ryerson & Levit, 1987).

GH joint integrity and rhythm are important for typical and pain-free shoulder movement. Even after recovery from stroke is achieved, pain and stiffness can lead to limitations in movement and function (Vliet, Sheidan, Kerwin, & Fenton, 1995). Another example of pain-limiting movement is in the previous condition of adhesive capsulitis.

Rehabilitation of clients after stroke is very complex; however, an overview of treatment applications will be focused on the subject of this impairment, subluxation. It is important to protect the affected arm from injury and to keep the affected extremity in a supported position early in the treatment of clients with shoulder hemiplegia after stroke. Pillows can be used in bed or a lap board can be used in the wheelchair to support the arm while positioned to help keep the shoulder joint intact and prevent shoulder subluxation. According to Zorowitz, Hughes, Idank, Idai, and Johnston (1996), the client should be educated in movement techniques to maximize functional recovery with AROM and active assist range of motion (AAROM). Additionally, OT techniques may also include neuromuscular re-education, modalities, shoulder cuffs or adaptive therapeutic equipment, taping protocols, and forced use/constraint-induced movement programs. Ideally, the therapist will focus on functional tasks to achieve rehabilitation of the affected upper extremity.

Erb's Palsy or Upper Obstetric Brachial Plexus Palsy

Erb's palsy is often seen in newborns after a difficult delivery. The difficult birth can cause an injury to the baby's brachial plexus, which is an interconnected group of nerves passing through the shoulder. The brachial plexus includes the nerves that control movement and sensation to the arm, hand, and fingers. Erb's palsy is characterized by weakness or paralysis of the arm by affecting nerve roots C5, C6, and C7. Typically, the paralyzed limb is positioned in internal rotation, elbow extension, forearm pronation, and wrist and finger flexion. Approximately one to two babies per 1,000 births are affected with this impairment.

Erb's palsy can result from several causes connected to a difficult delivery. Breech birth and larger-than-average baby weight, which is greater than 8 pounds 13 ounces, presents an increased risk. During breech birth, which is feet first, the baby's arms are usually raised, and excess pressure can cause a stretching injury to the brachial plexus. In births where the baby is larger than average, a condition called shoulder dystocia occurs more frequently. In **shoulder dystocia**, the infant's head is delivered normally, but one shoulder becomes stuck under a portion of the mother's pelvic bones. The doctor's use of manipulations such as forceps or a vacuum extractor to free the baby can then increase the risk of a brachial plexus injury. Women who are short, have gestational diabetes, have pelvic abnormalities, or have experienced prolonged labor are more at risk for a birth involving shoulder dystocia. A cesarean birth may be scheduled for mothers at greater risk of shoulder dystocia (Brain and Spinal Cord.org, 2009).

Most cases of Erb's palsy are due to stretching of the brachial plexus and will heal within 6 to 12 months. Sometimes, total recovery is not possible due to scar tissue that forms around healthy nerves after the stretching injury. Only 10% of brachial plexus birth injuries result in permanent paralysis or impairment. Erb's palsy is almost always apparent immediately because it is caused by an injury at birth. The extent of the injury may not be known for months to years due to the slow rate of nerve healing. Signs and symptoms that parents may notice are limited spontaneous arm movement of the baby's affected side and decreased grip or fisting in the affected hand. Infants with Erb's palsy may lack a Moro reflex on the injured side. The Moro reflex, which is present in healthy newborns, occurs when the infant is startled. A healthy infant, when startled, will throw out the arms to the side with the palms up and the thumbs flexed. Figure 7-15 illustrates a baby with a Moro reflex.

OT treatment for infants with Erb's palsy may include gentle massage and passive range of motion (PROM) to improve circulation and prevent joint contractures while the injured nerves are healing. Neoprene serpentine splinting, which promotes supination, or splinting to bring the affected hand to midline near the chin may also be incorporated.

Rotator Cuff Tendonitis and Shoulder Impingement

The **rotator cuff** is a tendon connecting four muscles, which covers the head of the humerus. The muscles are the supraspinatus, the infraspinatus, the teres minor, and the subscapularis. Gold Box 7-2 provides an easy acronym to memorize these muscles. The rotator cuff muscles work together to lift and rotate the humerus and maintain the head of the humerus in the glenoid fossa. **Rotator cuff tendonitis** and **shoulder impingement** are one of the most common causes of pain in the shoulders for adults. Impingement happens when there is pressure on the surface of the rotator cuff from the acromion process as the arm is lifted.

Impingement can cause local swelling and soreness in the front of the shoulder. Pain and stiffness may occur when raising the arm and sometimes when the arm is lowered from an elevated position. As the condition progresses, there may also be pain at night and difficulty sleeping. Over time, strength and movement may continue to be lost, and functional movements requiring

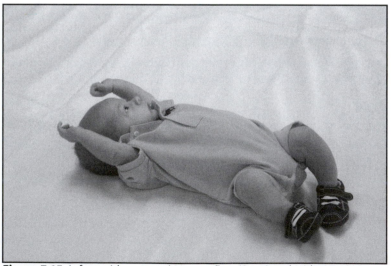

Figure 7-15. Infant with a normal Moro reflex. (Reprinted with permission of Robb Seahorn.)

placement of the arm behind the back may also become difficult and painful. Figure 7-16 illustrates a picture of shoulder impingement.

A history of forward-head posture with rounded shoulders, clinically called thoracic kyphosis, is especially seen in clients 45 years and older with shoulder impingement. Clients may also report a history of overuse of the upper extremities. Other signs and symptoms may include pain after activity, pain at night, and a "catching" sensation in the shoulder with overhead activities. Clients may report arm fatigue during and after functional activities as well. The symptom of night pain, which often involves sleeplessness, is usually the main reason an individual seeks medical attention (Glinn, 2008).

Risk factors that can lead to shoulder impingement are categorized as structural or functional. Structural risk factors include degenerative spurring of the acromion process, inflammation of the bursa, calcification or thickening of the rotator cuff tendon, or tears of the rotator cuff.

Gold Box 7-2

Rotator Cuff Muscles: Use the Acronym SITS

S = Supraspinatus
I = Infraspinatus
T = Teres minor
S = Subscapularis

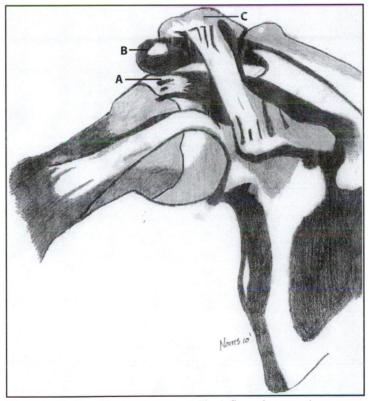

Figure 7-16. Shoulder impingement. The inflamed supraspinatus tendon (A) becomes impinged between the humeral head and the swollen bursa (B) and acromion process (C). (Reprinted with permission of Kevin Norris.)

Additionally, there are three types of acromion shapes (Figure 7-17). Type 1 is flat, type 2 is curved, and type 3 is hooked. Individuals with a type 2- or type 3-shaped acromion process are also at greater structural risk for shoulder impingement.

Unfortunately, the majority of individuals have either type 2 or type 3 acromion process shapes, which are more often associated with impingement. The hook or curved shape can lead to degeneration and eventual tearing of the rotator cuff (Weiss & Falkenstein, 2005). Functional risk factors include abnormal scapular and GH joint positioning during functional use from thoracic kyphosis, depression of the humeral head in the glenoid fossa due to rotator cuff weakness or tear, and tightness of the posterior capsule.

Over time, these conditions can lead to decreased blood flow, inflammation, and rotator tendon tears or rupture (American Academy of Orthopaedic Surgeons, 2007). Supraspinatus tendonitis accounts for 80% to 90% of rotator cuff tendonitis, possibly because of this tendon's location at the GH joint. There is constant pressure on the supraspinatus tendon from the humeral head that impinges against the coracoacromial arch during normal joint movements (Weiss & Falkenstein, 2005).

OT treatment may focus on decreasing pain and inflammation, which will promote the healing process and assist in regaining normal GH joint motion required for typical shoulder function. Treatment approaches may also include education on positioning of the shoulder to decrease pain and inflammation, activity modification, and protective positions for the shoulder during sleeping, sitting, and walking. Ideally, rotator cuff tears can be prevented as well as subsequent surgical intervention (Burke, Higgins, McClinton, Saunders, & Valdata, 2006).

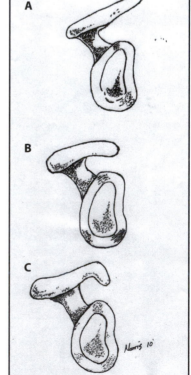

Figure 7-17. Acromion types (A) Type 1, flat; (B) type 2, curved; (C) type 3, hooked. (Reprinted with permission of Kevin Norris.)

BODY STRUCTURES OF THE SHOULDER COMPLEX

Muscle Actions

A significant number of muscles controls movement at the shoulder complex. The movements of the shoulder complex will be discussed in terms of their kinetic functional roles. These functional roles include **scapular pivoters, humeral positioners, humeral propellers,** and **shoulder protectors** (Glinn, 2008). The functional roles are identified in Gold Box 7-3. An overview of the shoulder complex muscles and their functional roles are presented in Table 7-3.

Gold Box 7-3

Kinetic Functional Roles of the Shoulder Complex

Scapular pivoters: Muscles that are involved with motion at the scapulothoracic joint.

Humeral positioners: Muscles that position the humerus in space during or after actions of the scapular pivoters.

Humeral propellers: Muscles that propel the humerus.

Shoulder protectors: Muscles that act as a force couple with the humeral positioners to keep the structures of the shoulder complex safe. These include the rotator cuff muscles.

Glinn (2008)

The **scapular pivoters** include the trapezius, serratus anterior, levator scapulae, and the rhomboid major and minor muscles. Together, these muscles are involved with movement at the scapulothoracic joint. The trapezius muscle is divided into upper, middle, and lower portions because of its different actions.

The upper portion of the trapezius is a prime mover in scapular elevation and upward rotation. The middle trapezius muscle is effective at scapular retraction. The lower portion of the trapezius depresses and upwardly rotates the scapula (Lippert, 2000). One of the main functions of the trapezius is to provide shoulder girdle elevation on the fixed cervical spine. For the trapezius to perform its job well, the cervical spine must be stabilized by anterior neck flexors, which will prevent forward head posture if stable and strong. The trapezius muscle is used strenuously when using the hands to hold a heavy object overhead or when an individual is moving a heavy wheelbarrow, for example (Floyd & Thompson, 2001).

The serratus anterior muscle is a prime mover in scapular protraction. It forms a force couple with the trapezius muscle in rotating the scapula upward. Again, a force couple is defined as muscles pulling in different directions to provide the same motion. According to Weiss and Falkenstein (2005), another function of the serratus anterior muscle is to hold the vertebral border of the scapula against the ribs, preventing **"winging of the scapula."** Winging of the scapula occurs when the inferior angle of the scapula sticks out from the body. Figure 7-18 illustrates winging of the scapula.

The action of the serratus anterior muscle is commonly seen in functional movements used to throw a baseball, tackle in football, or shoot a gun while hunting (Floyd & Thompson, 2001). According to Lippert (2000), an individual could not raise his or her arm overhead without the action of the serratus anterior.

The levator scapula muscle elevates the scapula and allows us to shrug our shoulders. It is also a prime mover in downward rotation. The rhomboid muscles retract and elevate the scapula. Along with the levator scapula, they assist in downward rotation of the scapula as well. The proper

Table 7-3	Functional Roles of Shoulder Complex Muscles			
Scapular Pivoters	Humeral Positioners	Humeral Propellers	Shoulder Protectors (Rotator Cuff)	Muscles of the Shoulder Complex
Trapezius Serratus anterior Levator scapulae Rhomboids	Deltoid, anterior fibers Deltoid, middle fibers Deltoid, posterior fibers	Latissimus dorsi Pectoralis major Teres major	Supraspinatus Infraspinatus Teres minor Subscapularis	Biceps brachii Coracobrachialis Triceps brachii (long head only) subclavius Pectoralis minor

Adapted from Dutton, M. (2004). *Orthopaedic examination, evaluation, and intervention.* New York, NY: McGraw Hill.

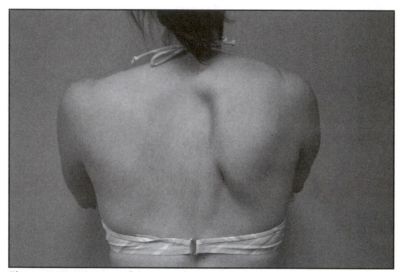

Figure 7-18. Winging of the scapula.

function of these scapular pivoters is important to normal movement of the entire shoulder complex and functional tasks involving the upper extremity (Van Dyck, 2000).

Humeral positioners are muscles that position the humerus in space during or after actions of the scapular pivoters. The humeral positioner muscles include the anterior, middle, and posterior deltoid. The different sections of the deltoid are separated by their different origins and functions. All sections have a common insertion, the deltoid tuberosity of the lateral humerus. The *anterior* fibers of the deltoid muscle originate on the clavicle and perform actions of shoulder GH joint abduction, flexion, horizontal adduction, and internal rotation. The *middle* fibers of the deltoid originate on the acromion process of the scapula and perform shoulder GH abduction. The *posterior* fibers originate on the spine of the scapula. The posterior deltoid abducts, extends, horizontally abducts, and externally rotates the GH joint.

The deltoid muscle is commonly used in lifting movements with the arms at the side. Floyd and Thompson (2001) identify that the trapezius muscle stabilizes the scapula as the deltoid pulls on the humerus. Any movement of the humerus on the scapula will involve all or a portion of the deltoid muscle.

Humeral propellers are muscles that propel the humerus and include the latissimus dorsi, pectoralis major, and teres minor. These muscles have been shown to have a positive impact on pitching speed and the propulsive phase of the swim stroke in athletes (Dutton, 2004). The latissimus dorsi muscle functions include GH extension, adduction, and internal rotation. It also assists with scapular depression, retraction, and downward rotation. If the arms are stabilized, the latissimus dorsi will elevate the pelvis. This is an example of reversal of muscle function described in earlier chapters of this text. Examples of this reversal action could be seen in walking with crutches or while performing a sitting push-up.

The pectoralis major and teres major muscles are other muscles that serve as humeral propellers. The pectoralis major has different lines of pull depending on its attachments. It is a large chest muscle originating on the clavicle and sternum and inserts on the lateral lip of the bicipital groove of the humerus. The clavicular portion of the pectoralis major has a vertical line of pull and assists in GH joint flexion during the first part or to approximately 90 degrees. The sternal portion of the pectoralis major, named due to its origin on the sternum, assists in GH joint extension from 180 degrees to approximately 90 degrees. Both the clavicular and sternal portions provide GH joint adduction, internal rotation, and horizontal adduction (Glinn, 2008).

Even though the pectoralis major muscle does not insert on the scapula, it acts on the scapulothoracic joint through its insertion on the humerus (Dutton, 2004). The pectoralis major muscle works closely with the anterior deltoid muscle while performing push-ups, pull-ups, and during tennis serves. The teres major muscle is the last of the humeral propeller muscles discussed. It assists the latissimus dorsi and the pectoralis major muscles in adduction, internal rotation, and extension of the humerus along with one of the rotator cuff muscles, the subscapularis. According to Floyd and Thompson (2001), it is commonly called the latissimus dorsi's "little helper."

The **shoulder protectors** act as a force couple with the humeral positioners (the anterior, middle, and posterior deltoid) to keep the structures of the shoulder complex safe. Another role is to "fine tune" the humeral head position during arm elevation. This allows for a greater surface area of the head of the humerus to remain in contact with the smaller glenoid fossa. The shoulder protectors also serve as decelerators to prevent subluxation and/or dislocation during repetitive motions such as pitching or in heavy lifting. The shoulder protectors are known as the rotator cuff muscles and consist of the supraspinatus, infraspinatus, teres minor, and subscapularis muscles. These four muscles have different origins on the scapula, and they all insert on the humerus as displayed in Figure 7-19. The rotator cuff acts as a dynamic unit, playing an important role in movements of the GH joint (Peat, 1986).

The muscles of the rotator cuff assist in rotation of the GH joint. They also stabilize the humeral head in the glenoid cavity during functional tasks of the upper extremities, especially when the arms are abducted to 45 degrees and externally rotated (Dutton, 2004).

The supraspinatus is the most superior muscle of the rotator cuff group. It acts in GH joint abduction along with the middle deltoid as well as in GH joint extension. This muscle stabilizes the humeral head in the glenoid fossa, mainly inferiorly. The "empty can" exercise can be used to show supraspinatus action, according to Floyd and Thompson (2001). During "empty can" exercises, the client is asked to position his or her arm at approximately 90 degrees of GH joint flexion with the elbow extended as the person moves into full GH joint internal rotation, as in emptying a can. Figure 7-20 shows a client performing an "empty can" exercise.

The infraspinatus and the teres minor muscles act together to provide external rotation, horizontal abduction, and extension of the GH joint. These two muscles also work with the other rotator cuff muscles to stabilize the humeral head in the glenoid fossa. The infraspinatus muscle is important in maintaining posterior stability of the GH joint with the help of the teres minor muscle. The infraspinatus is the strongest external rotator of the shoulder complex and is the second most commonly injured of the rotator cuff group (Floyd & Thompson, 2001).

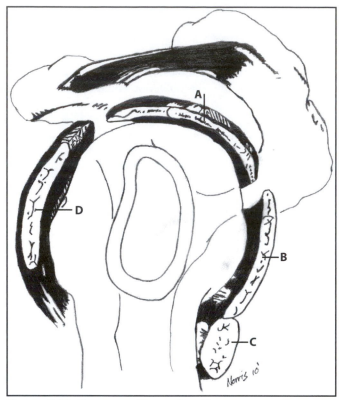

Figure 7-19. Rotator cuff muscles. The rotator cuff muscles from top clockwise: (A) supraspinatus, (B) infraspinatus, (C) teres minor, and (D) subscapularis. (Reprinted with permission of Kevin Norris.)

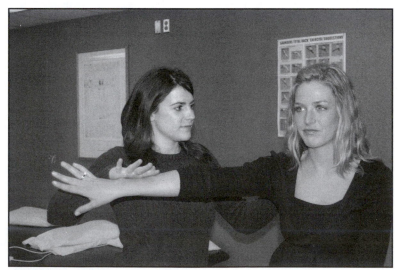

Figure 7-20. Client in empty can exercise.

The subscapularis muscle is the largest muscle of the rotator cuff muscles. It has the prefix "sub" because it lies under or on the anterior surface of the scapula. It lies between the scapula and ribcage; therefore, it is so deep that it cannot be palpated. It acts to internally rotate, adduct, and extend the GH joint in unison with the latissimus dorsi and teres major muscles. Oatis (2004) states that it has the most anterior attachment of the four rotator cuff muscles, which allows it to stabilize the head of the humerus in front and below. It is rare for the subscapularis to receive an isolated tear. Occasionally, partial ruptures have been reported, associated only with anterior dislocation of the GH joint (Weiss & Falkenstein, 2005).

There are additional muscles that play a lesser role in functional movement of the shoulder complex. They will be briefly discussed here along with their motions at the scapula and/or GH joint.

The biceps brachii muscle is better known as an elbow flexor and a forearm supinator; however, due to the origin of its two heads on the scapula, it does act as a weak flexor of the shoulder joint. It also assists in anterior stabilization of the humeral head of the glenoid fossa (Floyd & Thompson, 2001). It has been called the "fifth" tendon of the rotator cuff group (Weiss & Falkenstein, 2005).

The coracobrachialis muscle is not a strong muscle, but it assists in flexion and adduction of the GH joint. It is most functional in moving the arm across the chest during horizontal adduction of the shoulder (Dutton, 2004).

The subclavius muscle pulls the clavicle toward the sternum or assists in depressing the clavicle and the shoulder girdle. Its significant function is protecting and stabilizing the sternoclavicular joint during upper extremity movements (Floyd & Thompson, 2001).

The pectoralis minor muscle produces scapular downward rotation and is used with the serratus anterior muscle in scapular abduction or protraction. This is seen in movements like performing push-ups. The above muscles work together in most movements requiring pushing with the hands.

The long head of the triceps brachii muscle originates on the glenoid fossa of the scapula and inserts on the olecranon process of the ulna. Its main action is to extend the elbow; however, the long head is also an important GH joint extensor (Lippert, 2000). The long head of the triceps brachii also aids in shoulder adduction. It is always used in any pushing movement of the upper extremity (Floyd & Thompson, 2001). The sternocleidomastoid muscle is a strong flexor of the neck. It is mentioned here because of its origin on the shoulder girdle, specifically on the sternum and clavicle (Lippert, 2000).

In summarizing the motions and muscles of the shoulder and scapula, it is important to remember that the incredible movement and consequent function available in the shoulder complex cannot be achieved by independent muscles and joints. As each structure works together to provide mobility and stability to the shoulder and scapula, each muscle group relies on the other to provide functional motion in the upper extremities. For example, the rotator cuff muscles cannot work together to move and protect the shoulder if the scapular pivoters, such as the rhomboids, are not stabilizing and rotating the scapula.

To demonstrate how integrated the shoulder complex movements are during functional roles, let's return to Linda. One of the problems that Linda reported was pain in her right shoulder while unhooking her bra with a back closure. For Linda, this functional task requires the following movements from the shoulder complex: scapular elevation, depression, retraction, and downward rotation and GH joint horizontal adduction, abduction, extension, and internal rotation. Performing just this one task during undressing requires 13 muscles of the shoulder complex working together to stabilize and move the structures to complete this functional role.

Muscles, Nerves, and Spinal Cord Levels

The majority of the muscles in the shoulder complex are innervated by nerve roots C3 through C6 with C7, C8, and T1 playing a lesser role. All of the nerve branches, except the long thoracic nerve and the spinal accessory nerve, are considered part of the brachial plexus. The long thoracic nerve and the spinal accessory nerve originate prior to the formation of the plexus, from the nerve roots themselves (Gench, Hinson, & Harvey, 1999). The fact that most of the innervations in shoulder girdle movement emerge from the brachial plexus indicates a certain protection for these motions. Injury or damage to one nerve or nerve root will most likely only weaken a given movement, not render it completely unusable.

In general, the muscles that act on the scapula originate on the trunk and insert on the scapula. Muscles that act at the GH joint also originate on the trunk, as well as on the scapula, but insert on the humerus. The muscles needed for each movement and the innervation required for these movements will be discussed in relation to Linda's daily activities. Given that upward rotation of the scapula must accompany GH flexion or abduction, strengthening these muscles, and therefore the associated movements, would have a positive impact on Linda's ability to raise her arms above her shoulders, thus allowing her to complete her daily activity of shampooing hair.

Again, the muscles for these movements, and their respective innervations, can be found in Table 7-2. One sees that the upper and lower sections of the trapezius muscle, in addition to the serratus anterior, act together to cause the movement of scapular upward rotation. Other information found on the table indicates that the spinal accessory nerve, from roots C3 and C4, innervates the trapezius muscle and the long thoracic nerve, roots C5, C6, and C7, innervates the serratus anterior muscle. In other words, all of the nerve roots from C3 through, and including, C7 contribute to scapular upward rotation.

What other scapular movements might Linda need to use to shampoo her hair? Think of how you perform this activity. The actual movements may vary from person to person. Identify the movements you use and then determine, by referencing Tables 7-1 and 7-2, which muscles you are using.

In addition to scapular movements, GH movements must be used to raise the arms above shoulder level for shampooing hair. Table 7-4 can be used in the same manner as Table 7-1 to determine synergists or antagonists for a given GH joint movement. Information on innervation and normative ranges of motion is also included. The normative ROM for GH flexion is between 150 and 180 degrees, depending on the source. This amount of motion, however, is not necessary to perform most daily activities. A more functional ROM for GH flexion is 100 to 110 degrees.

Another use of these tables is to determine what effects certain nerve damage might have on the client's movements. Considering the movement of scapular protraction in Table 7-1, injury to the spinal accessory or dorsal scapular nerves would have no effect, nor would damage to nerve roots C3 or C4. On the other hand, injury to the long thoracic nerve would cause weakened protraction just as injury to any nerve root C5 through C8 would also weaken this movement. Consider the movements you identified above, in relation to performing your own ADL tasks. Consult the tables to determine the innervations needed for these motions. Consider what would happen if you had an injury to nerve root C5.

Reviewing the tables will give a clear picture of the muscles that Linda uses and necessary innervations for successful completion of this one ADL. Would Linda be able to wash her own hair if she sustained an injury to nerve roots C5 and C6? Defend your answer. Select a daily activity that is important to you. Determine the scapular and GH motions necessary to complete this activity. Create a table similar to the one created for Linda. What do you learn about yourself and your movement needs for this activity from analyzing this table?

Table 7-4 Motions of the Glenohumeral Joint

Muscle	Nerve	Nerve Root C5	C6	C7	C8	T1	Flexion 0 to 180 degrees	Extension 0 to 50 degrees	Abduction 0 to 180 degrees	Adduction 180 to 0 degrees	Internal Rotation 0 to 90 degrees	External Rotation 0 to 90 degrees	Horizontal Abduction 0 to 45 degrees	Horizontal Adduction 0 to 135 degrees
Deltoid (anterior)	Axillary	x	x				x		x		x			x
Deltoid (middle)	Axillary	x	x						x					
Deltoid (posterior)	Axillary	x	x					x	x			x	x	
Coracobrachialis	Musculo-cutaneous	x	x				x							
Biceps brachii	Musculo-cutaneous	x	x				x							
Pectoralis major (clavicular)	Medial Pectoral				x	x	x			x				x
Pectoralis major (sternal)	Lateral Pectoral	x	x	x				x						x
Latissimus dorsi	Thoracodorsal		x	x	x			x		x	x			
Teres major	Lower sub-scapular	x	x					x		x	x			
Triceps brachii	Radial		x	x	x	x		x						
Rotator Cuff Muscles														
Supraspinatus	Suprascapular	x	x						x					
Infraspinatus	Suprascapular	x	x									x	x	
Teres Minor	Axillary	x	x									x	x	
Subscapularis	Subscapular	x	x								x			

Adapted from Kendall, F. P., McCreary, E. K., Provance, P. G., Rodgers, M. M., & Romani, W. A. (2005). *Muscle testing and function with posture and pain* (5th ed.). Baltimore, MD: Lippincott, Williams & Wilkins.

Tendons and Ligaments

The shoulder complex and its associated joints allow more ROM than any other joint in the body, but in so doing lose much of their stability. The skeletal structure allows movement in all planes but these bony structures do not provide needed stability. In the GH joint, the relatively lateral position of the glenoid fossa, along with its small size and shallow depth, allow the potential for the head of the humerus to easily slip out of the glenoid fossa. Additionally, the looseness of the joint capsule, necessary to allow full movement, provides little stability. Were it not for other structures, such as tendons and ligaments, this joint would not be able to sustain the weight of the arm or the resistance needed during daily activities. Generally speaking, tendons, via contraction of the attached muscles, cause joint movement, while ligaments provide stability for the skeletal system. However, in addition to providing movement, the tendons around the GH joint provide stability as well. One of the primary functions of the rotator cuff muscles is to hold the head of the humerus in the glenoid fossa, in other words, to provide joint stability. The tendons of these muscles combine with a variety of ligaments to strengthen and stabilize this joint. Additional stability is provided by the glenoid labrum, which deepens the shallow glenoid fossa, especially inferiorly.

Stability is not provided by the skeletal structure of the other joints of the shoulder complex either. Laterally, at the acromioclavicular joint, the relatively flat acromion process could slide over the clavicle. Medially, at the sternoclavicular joint, the clavicle and sternum present with flat surfaces that could glide past one another. The sternoclavicular joint needs added support as it is the only structural or bony attachment of the scapula, clavicle, and upper extremity to the axial skeleton. Along with ligaments, the sternoclavicular joint has a thick articular disk that aids in stability and, perhaps more importantly, absorbs forces from falling or leaning on the upper extremity.

The strength and stability of these joints is provided by ligaments. The ligaments of all of the joints of the shoulder complex are named for their locations. Each ligament performs a unique function in counteracting dislocation in a certain direction. Together, they allow the GH joint to move safely in any plane, or in a combination of planes, allowing us to perform any activity of our choosing. Trauma or stress to the GH joint can occur from any direction and is more common than one would initially think. Falling and catching yourself with your hand, performing closed-chain actions with the upper extremity, such as pull-ups or push-ups, carrying heavy objects, or even carrying a heavy backpack or purse over one shoulder can lead to trauma of the GH joint. Refer to Table 7-5 for a listing of shoulder complex ligaments and their respective functions.

APPLICATIONS

The following activities will help you apply knowledge of the shoulder girdle and GH joint in real-life applications. Activities can be completed individually or in small groups to enhance learning.

1. **The Shoulder Girdle/Scapula:** The shoulder girdle is another term to describe the motion of the scapula. The shoulder joint is more accurately referred to as the GH joint. Scapular motion and GH joint motion combine to allow for stability and mobility of the arm and ultimately placement of the arm in numerous positions in space. Limitations in scapular motion may affect GH joint motion, and likewise limitations in GH joint motion may affect scapular motion. As such, ROM of the GH joint cannot be fully appreciated without first considering the influence of the scapula on movement. With a partner, complete the following activities to increase your familiarity with aspects and movements of the scapula.

    A.   Palpate the scapula and identify the bony landmarks of the scapula.

        ▪   Identify the inferior angle and superior angle, and trace your fingers along the vertebral border and axillary border.

Table 7-5	Ligaments and Their Functions	
Joint	Ligament	Function
Glenohumeral	Coracohumeral	Major structure to prevent downward or upward displacement; limits lateral rotation and extension of humeral head; supports weight of upper extremity
	Superior glenohumeral	Prevents downward displacement of humeral head; limits lateral rotation; provides anterior stability
	Middle glenohumeral	Provides anterior stability; limits lateral rotation of humeral head
	Inferior glenohumeral	Prevents anterior displacement; limits lateral rotation; supports GH abduction
Sternoclavicular	Costoclavicular	Major stabilizing structure, especially in GH elevation or scapular protraction; supports weight of upper extremity
	Anterior sternoclavicular	Limits excessive retraction; supports weight of upper extremity
	Posterior sternoclavicular	Limits excessive protraction; supports weight of upper extremity
	Interclavicular	Provides stability on superior aspect of joint; supports weight of upper extremity; protects brachial plexus via limiting clavicular depression
Acromioclavicular	Supracromioclavicular	Strengthens upper portion of joint; prevents clavicle over-riding acromion process; controls anterior-posterior joint stability
	Coracoclavicular	Major stabilizer; maintains clavicle in contact with acromion process; prevents dislocation here; limits upward rotation of scapula
	Coracoacromial	With acromion and coracoid process forms protective arch over GH joint; prevents superior displacement

Adapted from Peat, M. (1986). Functional anatomy of the shoulder complex. *Physical Therapy, 66*(12), 1855-1865.; Schenkman, M., & Rugo De Cartaya, V. (1987). Kinesiology of the shoulder complex. *Journal of Orthopaedic and Sports Physical Therapy, 8*(9), 438-450.; Levangie, P., & Norkin, C. (2005). *Joint structure and function: A comprehensive analysis* (4th ed.). Philadelphia, PA: F. A. Davis.

- Also trace your fingers along the spine of the scapula ending at the acromion process.
- Follow the acromion process around to the top of the GH joint all the way to the acromioclavicular joint. Then, follow the clavicle to the sternum, and palpate the sternoclavicular joint. Of importance, the acromion process is a reference point for a goniometer in measuring multiple GH joint motions. Additionally, the sternoclavicular and acromioclavicular joints minimally influence the movement of the GH joint. It may be easier to palpate these joints if the client moves his or her GH joint at the same time.

    B.   Observe the position of the scapula on the back of your partner. Are both scapulas relatively mirrored on the left and right sides of the body? If not, what seems different?

- Look at the vertebral border of the scapula. Is it equally distant from the spinal column?
- Look at the height of both shoulders at rest. Are they equal, or is one shoulder slightly higher than the other? Developed shoulder musculature as in the pitching arm of a pitcher or the dominant arm of a client may present slightly depressed as compared to the other arm.

    C.   Lastly, refer to the movements and pictures of the scapula earlier in this chapter. As your partner moves his or her scapula, palpate it. Palpate the scapular movements of retraction, protraction, elevation, depression, upward rotation, and downward rotation. You are not trying to move the scapula, but feeling the scapula move under your hand. Scapular mobilization refers to a therapeutic treatment technique whereby the therapist assists with the movement of the scapula. Due to the complexity of scapular mobilization, additional training may be necessary to incorporate this treatment technique into OT practice.

    D.   Identify the position of the scapula during the following functional movements:

- Brushing the hair on the back of your head: _____.
- Bringing your arm back to throw a ball: _____.
- Standing, reaching down to scratch your knee: _____.
- Doing a push-up when arms are extended: _____.
- Reaching up to touch the ceiling: _____.

    E.   Identify the position of the GH joint during the following functional movements:

- Brushing the hair on the back of your head: _____.
- Bringing your arm back to throw a ball: _____.
- Standing, reaching down to scratch your knee: _____.
- Doing a push-up when arms are extended: _____.
- Reaching up to touch the ceiling: _____.

2.   **ROM Chart:** Proceed through each joint motion with your partner, and record the available ROM in Table 7-6.

3.   **ROM of the GH Joint:** Motions of the GH joint and ROM norms are identified in Table 7-7. ROM norms can vary depending on the reference source. One norm is provided for

Table 7-6	**Range of Motion Application Table**		
	Motions	**Available ROM (degrees)**	**ROM of your partner**
Glenohumeral Joint	Flexion	0 to 180	
	Extension (also called hyperextension)	0 to 50	
	Abduction	0 to 180	
	Adduction	180 to 0	
	Internal rotation	0 to 90	
	External rotation	0 to 90	
	Horizontal abduction	0 to 45	
	Horizontal adduction	0 to 135	

Table 7-7	Range of Motion of the Shoulder—Glenohumeral Joint	
Glenohumeral Joint/ Shoulder Motion	**Range of Motion (degrees)**	**Associated Shoulder Girdle Motions****
Flexion	0 to 180	Abduction, upward rotation, slight elevation
Extension (also referred to as hyperextension)	0 to 50	Depression, adduction
Abduction	0 to 180	Elevation and upward rotation
Adduction	180 to 0	Depression, downward rotation, and adduction
Internal rotation	0 to 90	Abduction
External rotation	0 to 90	Adduction
Horizontal abduction	0 to 45*	Abduction
Horizontal adduction	0 to 135*	Abduction

Modified from The Guides to the Evaluation of Permanent Impairment, 6th ed.

*Identified from Latella, D., & Meriano, C. (2003). *Occupational therapy manual for the evaluation of range of motion and muscle strength.* Clifton Park, NY: Delmar Carnage Learning.

**Identified from Killingsworth, A., & Pedretti, L. (2006). Joint range of motion. In: H. M. Pendleton & W. Schultz-Krohn (Eds.), *Pedretti's occupational therapy: Practice skills for physical dysfunction*, (6th ed., pp. 437-468). St. Louis, MO: Mosby Elsevier.

Gold Box 7-4

Referenced Works for Range of Motion

Sections Referenced (a to e)	Reference
Goniometric landmark, end feel, and start and end positions	Latella & Meriano (2003)
Muscles responsible	Hislop & Montgomery (2002)
Available range of motion	American Medical Association (2008)

---

each motion within this text to increase ease of applications. Additionally, while multiple muscles may influence a particular motion, only the main muscles responsible for a joint motion are included. References for the following information can be found in Gold Box 7-4. With your partner, practice using a goniometer to measure each motion available at the GH joint.

A. **GH Joint Flexion**
   a. Goniometric landmark: Lateral surface of the acromion process
      Moving arm: Midline of the humerus
      Stable arm: Mid axilla/thorax.
   b. Available ROM: 0 to 180 degrees
   c. End feel: Firm
   d. Muscles responsible: Anterior deltoid
   e. Start and end position: Figure 7-21 displays the start position. The arm is positioned at the side of the body with the arm in the functional position. Raise the arm up straight to the front with the thumb up, while maintaining elbow extension. Figure 7-22 displays the end position. The arm is raised to full length reaching up.

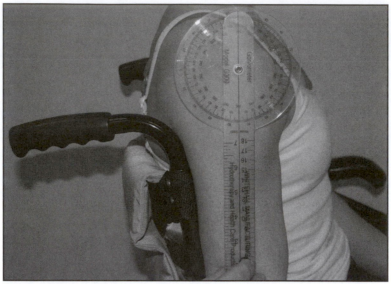

Figure 7-21. Start position for GH joint flexion ROM testing.

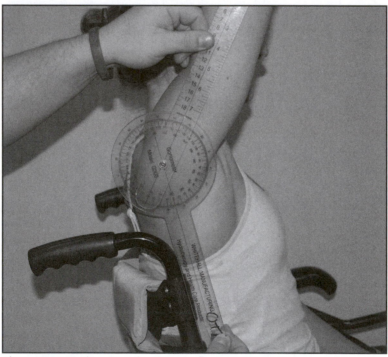

Figure 7-22. End position for GH joint flexion ROM testing.

B.   **GH Joint Extension (also called hyperextension in some texts)**
    a.   Goniometric landmark: Lateral surface of the acromion process
                      Moving arm: Midline of the humerus
                      Stable arm: Mid axilla/thorax.
    b.   Available ROM: 0 to 50 degrees (also called hyperextension in some texts)
    c.   End feel: Firm
    d.   Muscles responsible: Latissimus dorsi, posterior deltoid, and teres major

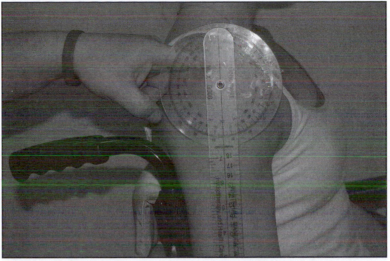

Figure 7-23. Start position for GH joint extension ROM testing

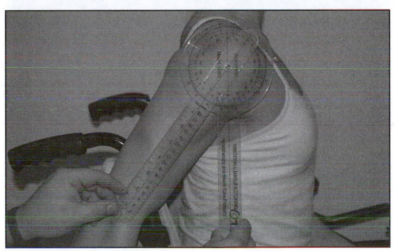

Figure 7-24. End position for GH joint extension ROM testing.

    e.   Start and end position: Figure 7-23 displays the start position. During GH joint extension, the arm returns to the side of the body after GH joint flexion to return the hand to the side of the body. With GH joint extension, the start position is the hand at the side of the body and the arm moves posteriorly to the furthest position available. Figure 7-24 displays the end position.

C.   **GH Joint Abduction**

    a.   Goniometric landmark: Anterior surface of the acromion process

                Stable arm: Parallel to the spine

                Moving arm: Medial aspect of the humerus

    b.   Available ROM: 0 to 180 degrees

    c.   End feel: Firm

    d.   Muscles responsible: Middle deltoid and supraspinatus

    e.   Start and end position: Figure 7-25 displays the start position. The arm is by the side of the body in the anatomical position. The client raises his or her arm to the side at the shoulder with shoulder abduction maintain-

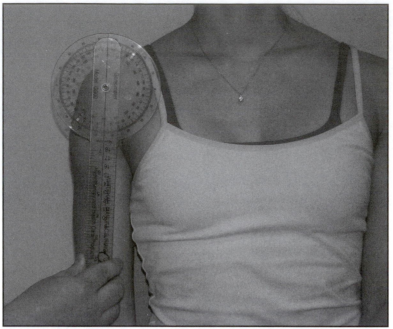

Figure 7-25. Start position for GH joint abduction ROM testing.

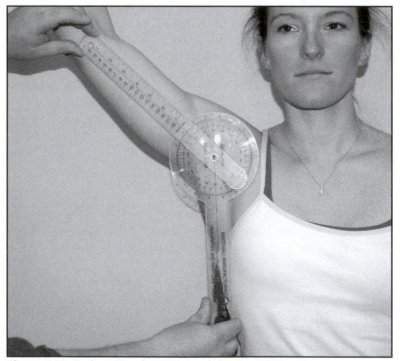

Figure 7-26. End position for GH joint abduction ROM testing.

ing the position of all other joints of the arm. The arm is raised to the full height. The end position is pictured in Figure 7-26. Remember the thumb has to remain facing up when raising the arm.

D.   **GH Joint Adduction**

   a.   Goniometric landmark: Anterior surface of the acromion process

                          Stable arm: Parallel to the spine

                                  Moving arm: Medial aspect of the humerus

- b.   Available ROM: 180 to 0 degrees
- c.   End feel: Soft
- d.   Muscles responsible: Pectoralis major, teres major, latissimus dorsi
- e.   Start and end position: Figure 7-27 displays the start position. The client's arm is raised above his or her head at full GH joint abduction, elbow and wrist extended. The client returns the arm to the side of the body, ending in the anatomical position. Figure 7-28 displays the end position.

E.   **GH Joint Internal Rotation**

- a.   Goniometric landmark: Middle of the olecranon process

                             Stable arm: Maintains parallel to the fore arm at the start position.

                             Moving arm: Parallel to the midline of the ulna

- b.   Available ROM: 0 to 90 degrees
- c.   End feel: Firm
- d.   Muscles responsible: Subscapularis
- e.   Start and end position: Figure 7-29 displays the start position. The client's GH joint is adducted with the upper arm positioned by the side of the body. The client's elbow is bent at 90 degrees to the front with the forearm at neutral, wrist extended. The client keeps the elbow positioned at the side of the body and rotates the hand and forearm in an arc around to the front side of the body. Figure 7-30 displays the end position.

F.   **GH Joint External Rotation**

- a.   Goniometric landmark: Middle of the olecranon process

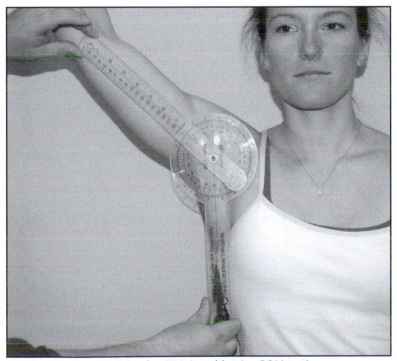

Figure 7-27. Start position for GH joint adduction ROM testing.

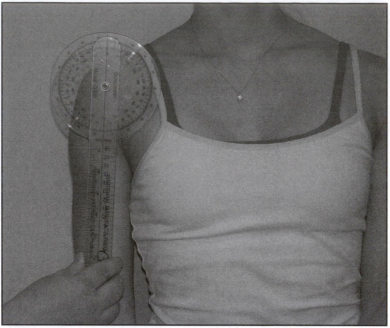

Figure 7-28. End position for GH joint adduction ROM testing.

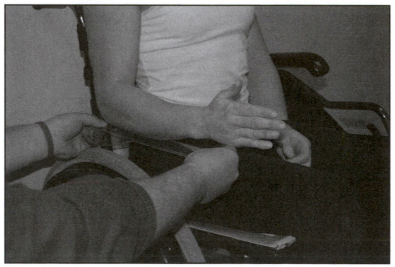

Figure 7-29. Start position for GH joint internal rotation ROM testing.

Stable arm: Parallel to the forearm at the start position.

Moving arm: Parallel to the midline of the ulna

b. Available ROM: 0 to 90 degrees
c. End feel: Firm
d. Muscles responsible: Infraspinatus, teres minor
e. Start and end position: Figure 7-31 displays the start position. The client's GH joint is adducted with the upper arm positioned by the side of the body. The client's elbow is bent at 90 degrees to the front

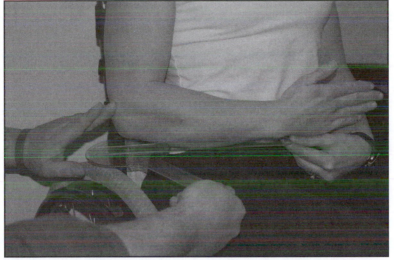

Figure 7-30. End position for GH joint internal rotation ROM testing.

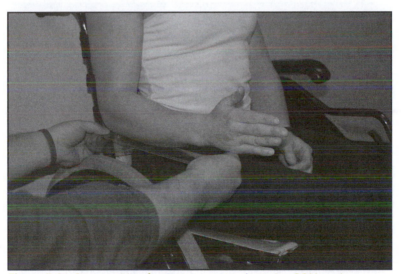

Figure 7-31. Start position for GH joint external rotation ROM testing.

with the forearm at neutral, wrist extended. The client keeps the elbow positioned at the side of the body and rotates the hand and forearm in an arc away from the midline of the body. Figure 7-32 displays the end position.

G.   **GH Joint Horizontal Adduction**

    a.   Goniometric landmark: Superior aspect of the acromion process

                Stable arm: Remains parallel to the humerus position prior to motion.

                Moving arm: Remains parallel to the humerus position during motion.

    b.   Available ROM: 0 to 135 degrees

    c.   End feel: Firm/Soft

    d.   Muscles responsible: Pectoralis Major

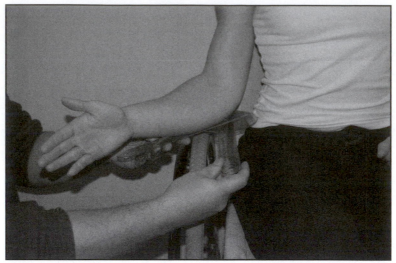

Figure 7-32. End position for GH joint external rotation ROM testing.

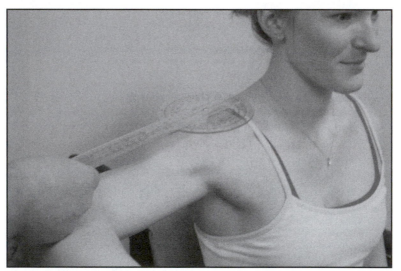

Figure 7-33. Start position for GH joint horizontal adduction ROM testing.

      e.   Start and end position: Figure 7-33 displays the start position. The GH joint is positioned at 90 degrees shoulder abduction, and elbow can be flexed at 90 degrees or extended. Thumb is facing up. The client moves the arm horizontally above the ground with the arm moving across the front of the body. Figure 7-34 displays the end position.

H.   **GH Joint Horizontal Abduction**

      a.   Goniometric landmark: Superior aspect of the acromion process

                          Stable arm: Remains parallel to the humerus position prior to motion.

                          Moving arm: Remains parallel to the humerus position during motion.

      b.   Available ROM: 0 to 45 degrees

      c.   End feel: Firm

      d.   Muscles responsible: Posterior deltoid

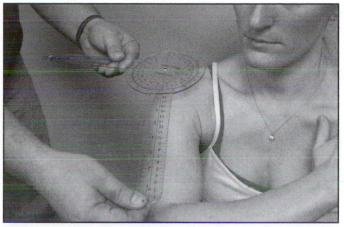

Figure 7-34. End position for GH joint horizontal adduction ROM testing.

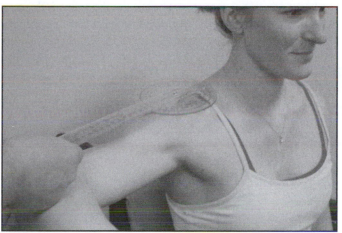

Figure 7-35. Start position for GH joint horizontal abduction ROM testing.

  e. Start and end position: Figure 7-35 displays the start position. The GH joint is positioned at 90 degrees shoulder abduction, and elbow can be flexed at 90 degrees or extended. Thumb is facing up. The client moves the arm horizontally above the ground with the elbow moving posteriorly. Figure 7-36 displays the end position.

4. **Manual Muscle Testing (MMT):** Complete gross MMT for motions of the GH joint using Table 7-8.

5. **MMT of the GH Joint:** With your partner, practice the standardized procedure for identifying gross MMT for each GH joint motion.

  A. **GH Joint Flexion and Extension:** Testing procedure: Figure 7-37 displays the start position for GH joint flexion. The client moves his or her arm halfway into GH joint flexion or to about 90 degrees of flexion. The therapist stabilizes just proximal to the GH joint to avoid compensation. Resistance is applied just distal to the GH joint, half the distance to the elbow. The client is asked to maintain his or her arm position as resistance is provided on the humerus in the opposite direction to GH joint flexion. Figure 7-38 displays the testing position.

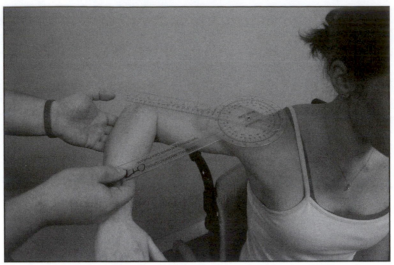

Figure 7-36. End position for GH joint horizontal abduction ROM testing.

Table 7-8	Manual Muscle Testing Application Table		
	Motions	**Palpate Muscle Group/Muscles**	**Gross MMT Score**
Glenohumeral Joint	Flexion		
	Extension		
	Hyperextension		
	Abduction		
	Adduction		
	Internal rotation		
	External rotation		
	Horizontal abduction		
	Horizontal adduction		

GH joint extension is tested similarly. The arm is positioned at the side of the body. The client moves his or her GH joint posteriorly to about 25 degrees. Some books identify this motion as hyperextension. The therapist stabilizes just proximal to the GH joint to avoid compensation. Resistance is applied just distal to the GH joint, half the distance to the elbow. The client is asked to maintain his or her arm position while resistance is provided on the humerus in the opposite direction to GH joint extension.

B. **GH Joint Abduction and Adduction:** Testing procedure: Figure 7-39 displays the start position for GH joint abduction. The arm is positioned at 90 degrees shoulder abduction. The therapist stabilizes just proximal to the GH joint to avoid compensation. Resistance is applied just distal to the GH joint, half the distance to the elbow. The client is asked to maintain this position as resistance

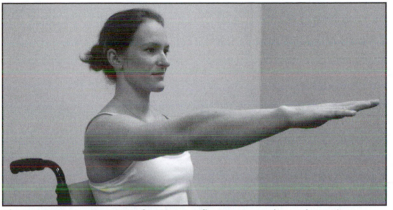

Figure 7-37. Start position for GH joint flexion manual muscle testing.

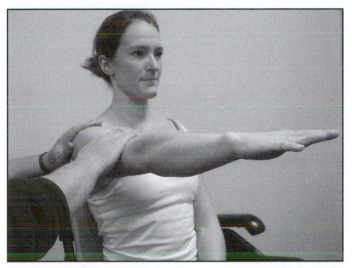

Figure 7-38. Test position for GH joint flexion manual muscle testing.

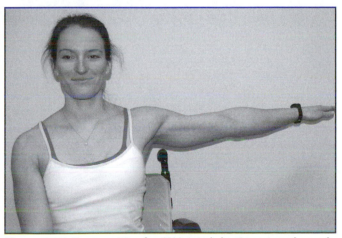

Figure 7-39. Start position for GH joint abduction manual muscle testing.

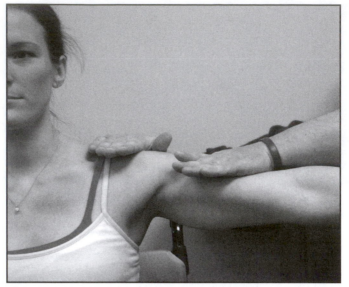

Figure 7-40. Test position for GH joint abduction manual muscle testing.

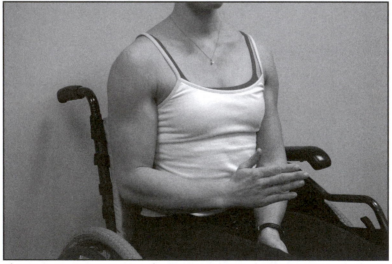

Figure 7-41. Start position for GH joint internal rotation manual muscle testing.

is provided on the humerus in the opposite direction to GH joint abduction. Figure 7-40 displays the testing position.

GH joint adduction is tested similarly. The arm is positioned at 90 degrees shoulder abduction. The client is asked to maintain his or her arm position while resistance is provided on the humerus in the opposite direction to GH joint adduction.

C. **GH Joint Internal Rotation and External Rotation:** Testing Procedure: Figure 7-41 displays the start position for GH joint internal rotation. The arm is positioned at the side of the body with the elbow bent at 90 degrees to the front with the thumb facing up. The forearm is positioned at 45 degrees internal rotation. The therapist stabilizes the arm at the elbow against the body to avoid com-

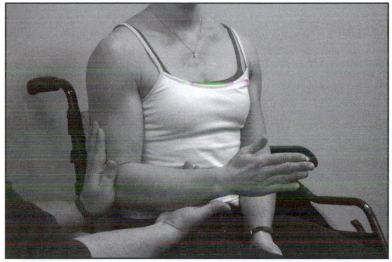

Figure 7-42. Test position for GH joint internal rotation manual muscle testing.

pensation. Resistance is applied just distal to the elbow. The client is asked to maintain his or her position of the arm while resistance is provided on the side of the forearm in the opposite direction to GH joint internal rotation. Figure 7-42 displays the testing position.

GH joint external rotation is tested similarly, except the arm is positioned in 45 degrees of external rotation. Again, the client is asked to maintain his or her arm position as resistance is provided on the humerus in the opposite direction to GH joint external rotation.

D.   **GH Joint Horizontal Adduction and Horizontal Abduction:** Testing procedure: Figure 7-43 displays the start position for GH joint horizontal adduction. The arm is positioned at 90 degrees shoulder abduction and 90 degrees elbow flexion with the palm facing the ground. The arm is then positioned about 70 degrees GH joint horizontal adduction. The therapist stabilizes the arm distal to the GH joint to avoid compensation. Resistance is applied just distal to the shoulder, against the humerus, halfway to the elbow. The client is asked to maintain the arm position as resistance is provided on the side of the humerus in the opposite direction to GH joint horizontal adduction. Figure 7-44 displays the testing position.

GH joint horizontal abduction is tested similarly. The arm is positioned at about 20 degrees GH joint horizontal abduction. Again, the client is asked to maintain his or her arm position as resistance is provided on the humerus in the opposite direction to GH joint horizontal abduction.

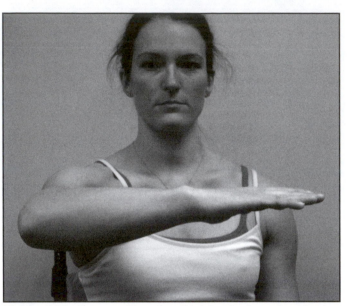

Figure 7-43. Start position for GH joint horizontal adduction manual muscle testing.

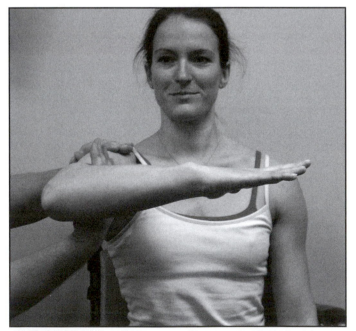

Figure 7-44. Test position for GH joint horizontal adduction manual muscle testing.

REFERENCES

American Academy of Orthopaedic Surgeons. (2007). *Shoulder impingement*. Retrieved from http//orthoinfo.aaos.org/topic.cfm?topic=a00032.

American Medical Association. (2008). *Guides to the evaluation of permanent impairment* (6th ed.). Chicago, IL: Author.

Boyle-Walker, K. L., Gabard, D. L., Bietsch, E., Masek-Van Arsdale, D. M., & Robinson, B. L. (1997). A profile of patients with adhesive capsulitis. *Journal of Hand Therapy, 10*(3), 222–227.

Brain and Spinal Cord.org. (2009). *Erb's palsy*. Retrieved from http://www.brainandspinalcord.org/cerebralpalsy/types/erbs-palsy.html.

Burke, S. L., Higgins, J. P., McClinton, M. A., Saunders, R., & Valdata, L. (2006). *Hand and upper extremity rehabilitation: A practical guide* (3rd ed.). St. Louis, MO: Elsevier-Mosby.

Dutton, M. (2004). *Orthopaedic examination, evaluation and intervention*. New York, NY: McGraw-Hill.

Floyd, R. T., & Thompson, C. W. (2001). *Manual of structural kinesiology* (14th ed.). New York, NY: McGraw-Hill.

Gench, B., Hinson, M., & Harvey, P. (1999). *Anatomical kinesiology* (2nd ed.). Dubuque, IA: Eddie Bowers Publishing.

Glinn, J. E., Jr. (2008). Shoulder biomechanics. *Physical Therapy's Clinical Educator*, 49–53.

Hislop, H. J., & Montgomery, J. (2002). Daniel's and Worthingham's muscle testing: Techniques of manual examinations (7th ed.). Philadelphia, PA: Saunders.

Hunter, J. M., Macklin, E. J., Callahan, H. D., Skirven, T. M., Schneider, L. H., & Osterman, A. E. (2002). *Rehabilitation of the hand and upper extremity* (5th ed.). St. Louis, MO: Mosby.

Latella, D., & Meriano, C. (2003). *Occupational therapy manual for the evaluation of range of motion and muscle strength*. Clifton Park, NY: Delmar Carnage Learning.

Lippert, L. S. (2000). *Clinical kinesiology for physical therapist assistants* (3rd ed.). Philadelphia, PA: F. A. Davis.

Oatis, C. A. (2004). Kinesiology: *The mechanics and pathomechanics of human movement*. Philadelphia, PA: Lippincott, Williams & Wilkins.

Ohio Health. (1995). Shoulder subluxation. Retrieved from www.ohiohealth.com.

Peat, M. (1986). Functional anatomy of the shoulder complex. *Physical Therapy, 66*(12), 1855–1865.

Ryerson, S., & Levit, K. (1987). The shoulder in hemiplegia. In R. Donatelli (Ed.), *Physical therapy of the shoulder* (pp. 105–129). New York, NY: Churchill Livingston.

Schenkman, M., & Rugo De Cartaya, V. (1987). Kinesiology of the shoulder complex. *Journal of Orthopaedic and Sports Physical Therapy, 8*(9), 438–450.

Van Dyck, W. R. (2000). The trunk-upper extremity connection: Understanding the origins of scapula control. *AOTA's Physical Disabilities SI Section Quarterly, 23*(2), 1–4.

Vliet, P., Sheidan, M., Kerwin, D., & Fenton, P. (1995). The influence of functional goals on the kinematics of reaching following stroke. *Neurology Report, 9*(1), 111–116.

WebMD. (2009). Shoulder and hemiplegia. Retrieved from http://emedicine.medscape.com/article/328793-overview.

Weiss, S., & Falkenstein, N. (2005). *Hand rehabilitation: A quick reference guide and review*. St. Louis, MO: Elsevier Mosby.

Zorowitz, R., Hughes, M., Idank, D., Idai, T., & Johnston, M. (1996). Shoulder pain and subluxation after stroke: Correlation or coincidence. *The American Journal of Occupational Therapy, 50*(3), 194–201.

chapter 8

Function and Movement of the Elbow Complex

Carolyn L. Roller, OTR/L

OCCUPATIONAL PROFILE

The following occupational profile is provided to demonstrate how body functions and body structures are related to the elbow complex. Through the client, David, this profile will show how occupational therapy (OT) intervention can affect elbow complex impairment. References to David will be made throughout this chapter.

David is a 47-year-old carpenter working in construction and receiving OT with a physician's referral to improve right dominant elbow function with less pain.

During the OT evaluation, the following data were gathered:

Subjective: David states that he has experienced pain in his right lateral elbow for about 8 months. The pain has worsened over the past month, negatively affecting his function. He reports that he was referred to OT and placed on a 10-pound weightlifting restriction at work using the right upper extremity after seeing the doctor last week. David reports his signs and symptoms have included pain in the right elbow, which is exacerbated when gripping with the elbow extended and palm facing down. He states that his grip has weakened, causing him to drop items at times while working. David has been using his carpentry skills at home, remodeling his kitchen on the weekends for the past 6 months. He says that he has been unable to work on his remodeling project over the past month due to right elbow pain and weakness. He has not been able to enjoy his favorite leisure activity of fishing and has not been able to play catch with his son, who is a star pitcher for the high school baseball team.

David denies any history of past medical problems. He reports taking over-the-counter medicine for his elbow pain occasionally.

Objective: David rates the pain in his right elbow as 2/10 at rest and 7/10 at worst during active range of motion (AROM). He reports his worst pain is with resistive gripping, such as using a hammer at work, casting a fishing line and reeling it in, or throwing the baseball back to his son during practice. He states, "It hurts my arm when I start the truck or shift it into gear, and I even have pain when I brush my teeth!"

AROM is within normal limits in the bilateral upper extremities; however, the client reports pain in the lateral epicondyle at the end range of motion (ROM) of elbow extension, full wrist extension, and full forearm pronation.

Upper extremity strength was tested using manual muscle testing (MMT), dynamometer, and pinch meter. MMT was 5/5 in the bilateral upper extremities, except wrist extensors in the

Keough, J. L., Sain, S. J., Roller, C. L.
*Kinesiology for the Occupational Therapy Assistant:
Essential Components of Function and Movement* (pp. 217-246).

right upper extremity, which were 4/5 with complaints of pain. A dynamometer was used to evaluate grip strength in standard and stressed positions. The standard position is performed with arm at the side, elbow at 90 degrees of flexion, and forearm in neutral. The stressed position is performed with the elbow fully extended and the forearm pronated. Grip strength was recorded as follows:

Standard position:
- Average male 45 to 50 years old Right: 110 lbs   Left: 100 lbs
- Grip   Right: 90 lbs   Left: 120 lbs

Stressed position:
- Grip   Right: 75 lbs   Left: 135 lbs

Note: The client reports pain with grip on the right more so in the stressed position.

- Pinch (key or lateral)   Right: 28 lbs   Left: 29 lbs
  - Average   Right: 27 lbs   Left: 25 lbs
- Pinch (palmar or three jaw chuck)   Right: 20 lbs   Left: 26 lbs
  - Average   Right: 24 lbs   Left: 24 lbs

Note: The client reports pain with right palmar pinch only.

David denies any numbness or tingling in his upper extremities. There was mild localized edema observed just distal to the right lateral epicondyle, and thickness was palpated in this area. The client was extremely tender to deep palpation over the insertion of the extensor carpi radialis brevis (ECRB) tendon at the right lateral epicondyle at the time of the OT evaluation.

Goals were established by the occupational therapist in collaboration with David and are presented below:

Short-Term Goals:
1. Client will be instructed in and comply with a home exercise program within 1 week.
2. Client will present with decreased pain from 7/10 to 3/10 at worst during resistive functional tasks within 4 weeks by using modified lifting techniques, adapting tool handles, using cold modalities, and performing stretches.
3. Client will increase right grip strength by 5 pounds with report of no greater pain within 4 weeks.
4. Client will be able to drive his truck and brush his teeth with no complaints of pain in the right elbow within 3 weeks.
5. Client will be able to work with a 20-pound lifting restriction and fewer complaints of pain in the right elbow within 6 weeks.

Long-Term Goals:
1. Client will demonstrate compliance and independence in a home exercise program at discharge.
2. Client will be independent in self-care and occupational roles using the right upper extremity with no complaints of pain and the utilization of ergonomic considerations within 12 weeks.
3. Client will demonstrate MMT and grip pinch strength within functional limits in the right upper extremity within 12 weeks.
4. Client will demonstrate independence and pain-free use of his right upper extremity during the leisure activity of fishing at discharge.

The outcome of David's OT intervention along with treatment techniques and goals achieved can be found in Appendix C.

BODY FUNCTIONS OF THE ELBOW COMPLEX

Joint motions and strength characteristics of the elbow and radioulnar joint as they relate to function will be described in the following section. Also, three common problems seen in the elbow complex and treated in OT will be defined and discussed. References will be made to David's occupational profile throughout this chapter.

The **elbow complex** consists of the body structures that provide motion at the elbow and the forearm. There are also body structures in the forearm that provide motion at the wrist and the hand; however, these will be discussed in Chapter 9 of this text. According to Floyd and Thompson (2001), the elbow consists of two inter-related joints, the humeroulnar joint and the humeroradial joint. The forearm consists of the proximal radioulnar joint. The primary role of the elbow complex is positioning and stabilizing the hand for functional activities, just like the shoulder complex. The elbow complex is made to be strong and stable. Unfortunately, this stability does not allow much room for compensatory adjustments. This makes the elbow complex prone to repetitive stress injuries (Dutton, 2004). A definition of repetitive stress injuries is provided in Gold Box 8-1. David demonstrates one of the many overuse injuries seen in the elbow. Fortunately for David and many clients like him, he can return to his prior level of function with the assistance of OT interventions.

Gold Box 8-1

Repetitive stress injuries (RSIs) are also known as repetitive motion injuries, repetitive strain injuries, or cumulative trauma disorders. RSIs are defined as a group of signs and symptoms that commonly affect the joints and the soft tissues of the arms, hands, knees, and back. RSIs are seen in individuals who perform tasks that are often repetitive and resistive. The signs and symptoms may include pain, fatigue, tingling, numbness, and decreased function.

Hertfelder & Gwin (1989)

Motions of the Elbow Complex

Movements of the elbow complex include motion at the elbow and forearm of the upper extremity. According to Weiss and Falkenstein (2005), the arc of motion needed to perform most activities of daily living (ADL) is lower than typical available motion. Elbow ROM required to perform the majority of ADL tasks is between 30 and 130 degrees of flexion and extension. Forearm supination and pronation used is also 50 degrees each for a total arc of motion of 100 degrees. The ROM chart shown later in this chapter provides ROM norms for each of these movements. The movement of elbow flexion and extension involves the humeral articulations. The motion of forearm pronation and supination involves the proximal radioulnar joint.

In particular, motions of the elbow are described as elbow flexion and elbow extension. Elbow flexion occurs when David bends his elbow bringing the hand to the mouth, such as in the activity of self-feeding. Elbow extension occurs when David straightens his elbow, such as reaching down to take the hand of a small child, for example.

The motions of the forearm or proximal radioulnar joint are called forearm supination and forearm pronation. Forearm supination happens when David moves his hand from the palm-down position to the palm-up position. Carrying a full bowl of soup in the palm of the hand is an example of forearm supination. Forearm pronation is the opposite motion as when David moves his hand from palm-up to palm-down, as in reaching out to pick up a cellular phone from the table. When the movement of forearm rotation occurs, the radius moves around the ulna. The ulna does not rotate, as it is fixed by its bony shape at the proximal end at the olecranon process. Figure 8-1 illustrates elbow flexion, while Figure 8-2 illustrates elbow extension. Figure 8-3 illustrates forearm supination, while Figure 8-4 illustrates forearm pronation.

The carrying angle of the elbow provides for improved functional ROM with elbow joint motion. The **carrying angle** of the elbow is described as the angle formed by the long axis of the humerus and forearm. This angle is evident when the arm is in the anatomical position and the forearm and humerus do not display a continuous straight line. When the elbow is fully extended,

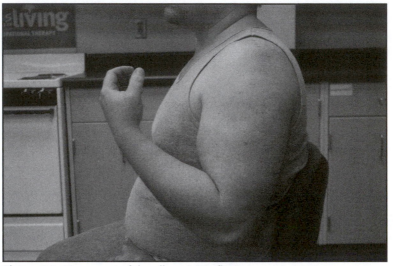

Figure 8-1. Movement of the elbow joint: flexion.

Figure 8-2. Movement of the elbow joint: extension.

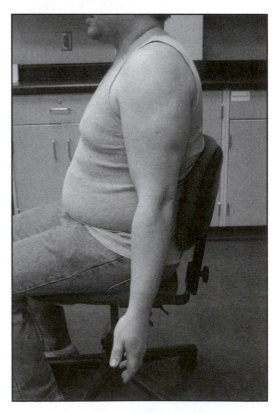

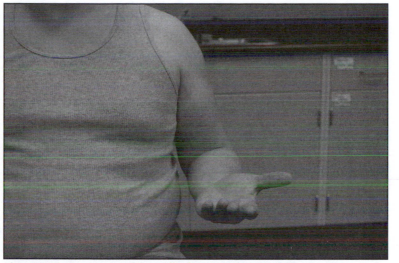

Figure 8-3. Movement of the radioulnar joint: supination.

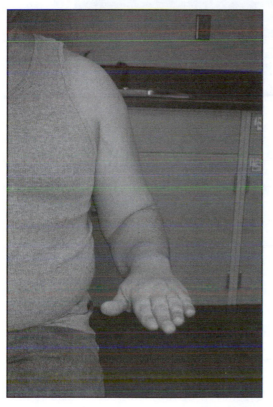

Figure 8-4. Movement of the radioulnar joint: pronation.

the carrying angle is typically greater in women than men. The carrying angle in women is typically about 10 to 15 degrees, while the carrying angle for men is about 5 degrees. When the elbow is flexed, the carrying angle serves to create improved function as the carrying angle assists in bringing the hand to the mouth (Dutton, 2004). Figure 8-5 and Figure 8-6 provide examples of the carrying angle.

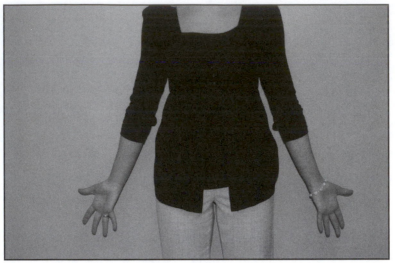

Figure 8-5. Elbow carrying angle, anatomic position.

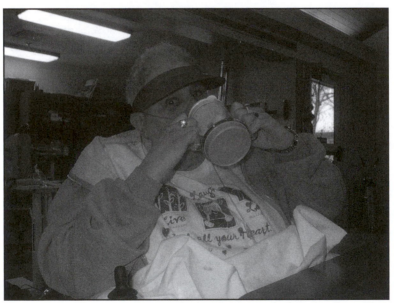

Figure 8-6. Elbow carrying angle, hand to mouth functional position. (Reprinted with permission of Jeremy Keough.)

Strength Characteristics of the Elbow Complex

The structure of the elbow, as compared to the shoulder, shows increased stability and decreased mobility. The elbow is a strong and stable joint. The tightly fitting bony articulations of the elbow joint and proximal radioulnar joint restrict extreme motion in elbow extension. It is essential for the elbow joint to be strong, as it needs to withstand forces of one to three times the weight of the body (Oatis, 2004). Upper extremity weight-bearing activities, such as crutch walking or wheelchair propulsion, can increase forces to the elbow up to one time the body's weight. Forceful, repetitive upper extremity activity as seen in overhead throwing has shown to be up to three times the body's weight in force to the elbow joint (Hertling & Kessler, 2006). Additionally, forces may be increased if the individual has weakness in the scapula stabilizers or the rotator cuff muscles of the shoulder complex.

The muscles of the elbow complex provide some joint stability, but their main role is ROM (Oatis, 2004). The four elbow flexors are the biceps, brachialis, brachioradialis, and to a lesser degree the pronator teres. The elbow flexors are synergists as they work together to bend the elbow. The elbow flexor muscles are strongest at the midrange of elbow flexion or at about 90 degrees. Additionally, the biceps muscle is a stronger flexor muscle when combined with forearm supination. The biceps supinates the forearm along with the supinator muscle. The brachialis muscle is a true elbow flexor, having no effect on forearm rotation. The brachioradialis muscle helps flex the elbow; however, it only aids resisted forearm pronation and supination as the forearm moves to neutral. The pronator teres contributes to elbow flexion only against resistance. The pronator teres assists the pronator quadratus during forearm pronation as well (Dutton, 2004).

The elbow flexors are stronger than their antagonists, the elbow extensors. The muscles that extend the elbow include the triceps and the anconeus muscle. These muscles act as synergists and are the only muscles that work together to straighten the elbow. They have no effect on forearm rotation due to their attachment on the ulna, which does not rotate during forearm pronation or supination. Like the elbow flexors, the elbow extensors are the most powerful at midrange (Hunter et al., 2002). You may notice that most activities that require upper body strength are performed with the elbow at least slightly flexed, if not flexed at 90 degrees. Functionally, pushing a door open, rising from a chair, or walking with crutches recruit the extensor muscles of the elbow.

Force couples are muscles that work together in opposite directions to produce a stronger functional movement and stabilize the joint. Force couples of the elbow complex are elicited during activities that require elbow stabilization. The three force couples of the elbow include the triceps/biceps, brachioradialis, and pronator teres/supinator, along with the extrinsic wrist flexors/extensors.

David's occupational profile will be used to help determine the movement and strength required to complete certain daily activities using the elbow complex. David is unable to participate in his favorite leisure activity of fishing. A portion of this activity consists of casting and reeling the fishing rod, which causes pain in his right dominant elbow. As a result, he has stopped performing an occupational role in which he enjoys participating. Refer to Table 8-1 to identify how the joints, muscles, and nerves enable David to participate in fishing.

As you can see, one of David's instrumental activities of daily living (IADL) occupations is casting and reeling the fishing rod. This requires elbow flexion, extension, and forearm pronation. The muscles listed in Table 8-1 work with other muscles in the upper extremity and trunk to enable participation in the fishing activity. According to Dutton (2004), the main function of the elbow complex is to help the shoulder position the hand for ADL and IADL. In order for David to return to independent and pain-free use of his right arm, improved coordination of the muscles and joint motion at the elbow complex is required.

Common Problems of the Elbow Complex

Many injuries and diseases affect the elbow and forearm of clients seen in OT. Therapists work with clients who have a variety of functional impairments. The elbow complex is especially susceptible to overuse injuries, dislocations, fractures, and tears. Consider David's occupational profile while reading the following three common elbow injuries and diseases seen in OT. Think about David's signs and symptoms and functional limitations, and see if you can identify his injury. As in the previous chapter, you can find David's epilogue in Appendix C. The epilogue will provide additional information about David's outcomes during and after OT intervention.

Table 8-1	Movements, Muscles, and Innervation of the Elbow Complex Using a Fishing Rod	
Elbow Flexion		
Biceps brachii	Musculocutaneous	C5, C6
Brachialis	Musculocutaneous	C5, C6
Brachioradialis	Radial	C5, C6
Elbow Extension		
Triceps	Radial	C6, C7, C8
Anconeus	Radial	C6, C7, C8
Forearm Pronation		
Pronator teres	Median	C7, C8
Pronator quadratus	Anterior interosseous radial	C7, C8, T1

Ulnar Nerve Entrapment (Cubital Tunnel Syndrome)

There are a variety of nerve injuries that occur in and around the elbow. Ulnar nerve injury is the most common nerve injury after carpal tunnel syndrome in the upper extremity. The ulnar nerve is the most superficial nerve in the upper extremity as it passes through the cubital tunnel on the medial side of the elbow joint (Dutton, 2004).

Causes of cubital tunnel syndrome include pressure at the medial side of the elbow over the nerve, frequent positioning of the elbow in extreme flexion, and repetitive motion. These activities may cause inflammation and swelling, which in turn limit normal ulnar nerve gliding. The elbow in full flexion can cause pressure on the ulnar nerve at the medial epicondyle and the cubital tunnel retinaculum where the flexor carpi ulnaris inserts (Hertling & Kessler, 2006).

Signs and symptoms of cubital tunnel syndrome may include activity-related tingling and numbness in the ring and small fingers of the hand, which may worsen at night. The above signs and symptoms are often accompanied by pain in the medial elbow and can progress to include decreased sensation in the ulnar nerve distribution of the hand. Loss of grip, coordination, and muscle atrophy in the involved hand are seen frequently as well (Hunter et al., 2002).

Conservative treatment is very successful if initiated before symptoms progress to include sensory loss in the ulnar nerve distribution and intrinsic weakness of the hand. OT treatment may include education about the diagnosis, ergonomic considerations, and restrictions. Clients are instructed to rest the affected extremity, avoid repetitive elbow movement, avoid postures that place the elbow in full flexion, and protect the medial elbow from pressure or being bumped (Cannon, 2003).

The occupational therapy assistant (OTA) will instruct the client in a home exercise program that may include nerve gliding exercises and a padded sleeve for protection for use during the day. Towel splinting at night is very effective during early conservative OT treatment. In this treatment technique, the client uses a towel wrapped around the elbow to prevent full elbow flexion during sleep. When the elbow is not allowed to bend past 90 degrees of flexion during rest, there is less pressure on the ulnar nerve, allowing it to heal. This treatment technique is very effective in decreasing numbness and tingling in the client's small and ring fingers (Cannon, 2003).

If conservative treatment fails, the client may require surgical intervention. The surgery is called ulnar nerve transposition. The surgeon releases the ulnar nerve in the cubital tunnel and moves the nerve to the medial side of the medial epicondyle, securing it with a flap of fascia or muscle. The client would then be seen postsurgically in OT for rehabilitation (Weiss & Falkenstein, 2005).

Distal Biceps Tendon Rupture

In a distal biceps tendon rupture, the distal portion of the biceps tendon, which attaches at the radial tuberosity, completely tears or ruptures. This sudden injury is most often seen in muscular male clients between the ages of 35 and 60 years. The client usually reports that he was moving a heavy object when his elbow forcibly straightened against the heavy-load. This caused increased stress on the biceps muscle and tearing of the tendon from the bone. In most cases, the tear is complete. A distal biceps tear is rarely associated with other medical conditions; however, smokers are more likely to experience the injury due to decreased tendon nutrition caused from the nicotine in the cigarettes (American Academy of Orthopaedic Surgeons, 2009a).

The signs and symptoms of a distal biceps tendon rupture or tear may include the following:

- A "pop" is heard at the elbow at the time of the injury when the tendon ruptures.
- Pain in the elbow that subsides about 1 to 2 weeks after injury.
- Visible swelling and bruising at the elbow and forearm.
- Weakness with elbow flexion and forearm supination.
- A bulging in the upper arm where the biceps muscle has recoiled.

It is recommended that a distal biceps tendon tear is surgically repaired, especially in an active individual. Without repair, there is a 30% loss of elbow flexion and a 40% loss of supination strength. After surgical repair, the injured extremity is protected for 6 to 8 weeks. During this protective phase, the client is seen in OT. The client is referred to therapy approximately 2 weeks postoperatively after the cast is removed. The OT practitioner will fit the client with a hinged elbow brace locked between 90 and 70 degrees of flexion. The client is then instructed in AROM to the shoulder, wrist, and hand as part of a home exercise program. The client is also instructed in scar and edema management techniques to promote healing and to improve ROM. Only passive range of motion (PROM) is allowed for elbow flexion and forearm supination. The client is also limited to 40 degrees of elbow extension to protect the repair. At 6 weeks after surgery, the client is allowed to perform AROM out of the brace, but the hinged brace continues to be worn unlocked for protection until 8 weeks postoperatively. The OTA will begin instructing the client in light resistive exercises, as well as in light functional tasks, at 8 weeks after repair.

The individual with a distal biceps tendon repair has to restrict functional activities somewhat until the tendon is fully healed, which takes 3 to 6 months. Most individuals can return to full ROM and heavy activities, including jobs requiring manual labor, at the end of 6 months (Hertling & Kessler, 2006).

Lateral Epicondylitis (Tennis Elbow)

Lateral epicondylitis or tennis elbow commonly presents with inflammation and pain in the elbow caused from overuse. As the term *tennis elbow* explains, playing racquet sports can cause this condition, as well as other recreational and work-related activities that require repetitive use of the forearm muscles. Carpenters, cooks, painters, and butchers develop tennis elbow more often than other occupations. Individuals between the ages of 30 and 50 years also get tennis elbow more frequently. Men develop the condition more often than women and more frequently in their dominant elbow (American Academy of Orthopaedic Surgeons, 2009b).

The symptoms include pinpoint pain at the lateral epicondyle of the elbow, that slowly worsens over weeks and months. There is usually no specific injury related to the beginning of symptoms. Individuals will also complain of a weak grip and report more pain with activities that require sustained gripping, such as holding a tool or shaking hands. More pain is also reported in lifting an object with the forearm in pronation (DeSmet & Fabry, 1997).

Inflammation and pain are caused by microscopic tears in the ECRB tendon where it attaches at the lateral epicondyle. Because the ECRB muscle stabilizes the wrist in extension when the elbow is extended, the increased risk of weakening from overuse occurs, causing small tears. When treated conservatively, tennis elbow resolves in approximately 90% of clients (Hertling & Kessler, 2006). OT conservative treatment may consist of the following:

- Client education, rest
- Ergonomic considerations
- Bracing
- Use of cold and heat
- Stretching
- Scar mobilization
- Strengthening

The OT goals of conservative treatment in tennis elbow are to decrease pain and inflammation, prevent recurrence of signs and symptoms, and increase functional use of the injured arm. Client education of the diagnosis and the rehab process can increase compliance. The client is taught to rest the injured upper extremity as much as possible and to use cold to decrease inflammation and pain. The client is shown how to adapt tools by making the handles larger and pacing him- or herself throughout the workday with rest breaks. Clients are educated to lift with the weight closer to their center of gravity and with their palms up to lessen the strain on the forearm extensor muscles (Dutton, 2004). The above adaptations are a few examples of ergonomic considerations. A definition of ergonomics is provided in Gold Box 8-2.

Gold Box 8-2

Ergonomics: This is the study of the interaction between human capabilities and the demands of their occupational roles. Occupational therapy and ergonomics are both concerned with an individual's adaptation to his or her physical environment.

Hertfelder & Gwin (1989)

Bracing the wrist in neutral for a time can decrease the tension and avoid additional microtearing on the ECRB tendon when extending the wrist and fingers. This is because the ECRB muscle originates on the lateral epicondyle of the humerus and inserts in the hand and fingers. Observe or palpate approximately 1 inch distal to your lateral epicondyle, and wiggle your fingers. You can feel or see the movement where the extensor tendon originates at the lateral epicondyle.

The OTA would teach the client to perform a home exercise program of passive stretching by bending the wrist into flexion with the elbow extended. This stretch elongates the tendons at the lateral epicondyle to avoid additional microtearing and promotes blood flow and healing. A friction massage over the origin of the tendon at the lateral elbow will decrease scar tissue and increase blood flow as well. To perform a friction massage, the client would use two to three fingers and massage perpendicular to the muscle fibers on dry skin with moderate pressure for about 1 minute three times a day or as tolerated. Figures 8-7 and 8-8 illustrate examples of passive stretching and friction massage.

When the client's pain and inflammation have decreased, the treatment would include gradual forearm strengthening. Progression would continue in a home exercise program as long as signs and symptoms are lessened. Clients tend to do well with conservative treatment due to the fact they now understand what has caused their pain and dysfunction. The epilogue on the occupational profile of David will follow his treatment and progress during OT. The epilogue will provide the reader with additional information on the lateral epicondylitis or tennis elbow.

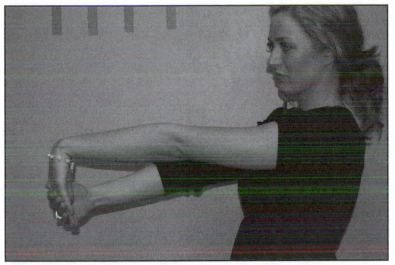

Figure 8-7. Tennis elbow stretch.

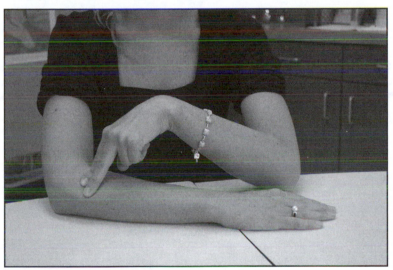

Figure 8-8. Friction massage exercise for tennis elbow.

BODY STRUCTURES OF THE ELBOW COMPLEX

Muscles, tendons, ligaments, nerves, and spinal cord levels of the elbow complex will be identified and discussed as they relate to function in this section. The ability to place the hand in space in order to perform personal care and daily activities is important to our independence and self-esteem. The motions of feeding and toileting, for example, are performed by the elbow and radioulnar joints and their supporting neuromuscular system (Hunter et al., 2002). Of course, these activities are made possible by all of the upper extremity structures working together; however, the elbow complex is of vital importance to the performance of these functional activities.

Table 8-2	Muscle Function and Occupational Roles	
Muscle	**Function**	**Examples of Occupational Roles**
Biceps brachii Brachialis Brachioradialis	Elbow flexion	• Phone to ear • Brush teeth • Put objects to mouth • Shave • Button shirt
Triceps brachii Anconeus	Elbow extension	• Reach for object on table • Rise from chair • Put arm in sleeve • Don/doff socks • Tie shoes
Pronator teres Pronator quadratus	Forearm pronation	• Use keyboard or mouse • Write • Cut food • Pour from cup • Wipe table
Biceps brachii Supinator	Forearm supination	• Carry a bowl in palm • Turn page of a book • Wash face • Pericare • Clasp a chain at back of neck

Adapted from Latella, D., & Meriano, C. (2003). *Occupational therapy manual for the evaluation of range of motion and muscle strength.* Clifton Park, NY: Delmar Carnage Learning.; Weiss, S., & Falkenstein, N. (2005). *Hand rehabilitation: A quick reference guide and review.* St. Louis, MO: Elsevier Mosby.

Muscle Actions

The muscles of the elbow complex are divided by function into flexors, extensors, pronators, and supinators. Certain muscles perform more than one action just as other muscles can work differently in combination with each other. An overview of the elbow complex muscles and their functional roles can be found in Table 8-2.

The flexors of the elbow complex are the biceps brachii, brachialis, and the brachioradialis muscles. The biceps brachii is considered a multiarticular muscle. It serves as a weak shoulder flexor, but flexes the elbow and supinates the forearm (Floyd & Thompson, 2001). The biceps muscle is a stronger elbow flexor with the radioulnar joint supinated. When the forearm is in pronation, the effectiveness of the biceps muscle lessens as an elbow flexor. To show this, perform a chin-up holding the bar with the forearms in supination. Now, try the same chin-up grasping the bar with the forearms in pronation. Your arms do not have as much strength to pull up your body weight in the second position.

The brachialis muscle is the primary elbow flexor and is strong whether the forearm is in supination or pronation. This is due to its insertion on the ulna, which is stationary during forearm rotation (Lippert, 2000). The brachialis muscle lies deeper in relation to the biceps muscle and contracts whenever the elbow flexes, gaining the nickname the "workhorse" of elbow flexion (Oatis, 2004).

The brachioradialis muscle is the third elbow flexor. It is the strongest when flexing the elbow with the forearm in neutral due to its more lateral and distal attachment at the styloid process of the radius. The brachioradialis also provides stabilization of the elbow joint during rapid elbow flexion, such as pounding a nail into a block of wood with a hammer.

The extensor muscles of the elbow complex are the triceps brachii and the anconeus. The triceps muscle makes up all the muscle mass on the posterior side of the arm and receives its name from three heads. Because it inserts on the olecranon process of the ulna, it is very effective at extending the elbow. It has no role in forearm rotation because it has no attachment to the rotating radius. The triceps muscle is assisted by a very small muscle called the anconeus. The main role of the anconeus is to pull on the annular ligament when it contracts, which keeps the ligament from being pinched in the olecranon fossa with elbow extension. The functional action of the elbow extensors can be seen when using the hand to push open a door, bearing weight on the arm while moving in bed, or rising from a sofa or a chair.

The muscles that cause pronation at the radioulnar joint or place the palm facing down are the pronator teres and the pronator quadratus muscles. The pronator teres is primarily a pronator but assists with elbow flexion due to its origin at the medial epicondyle of the humerus, especially when a heavy object is held in the hand. The pronator teres is recruited only with resisted pronation. Elbow position does not affect the action of the pronator teres. The pronator quadratus muscle is the only muscle working when pronation is unresisted. It is a deep, small, and flat muscle that cannot be palpated, but connects the distal portion of the ulna to the radius with a horizontal pull (Lippert, 2000). The pronator muscles hold the forearm in a palm-down position during functional tasks, such as typing or cleaning table tops.

Supination or the palm facing up is accomplished by the biceps brachii and the supinator muscles. The biceps brachii muscle was discussed with the elbow flexors; however, it is important to mention it here again as it is the primary supinator of the radioulnar joint. In forearm supination, the biceps is active even if there is no weight in the hand. The supinator muscle is a secondary forearm supinator. It acts alone with unresisted supination, but the biceps is activated with resistance (Hunter et al., 2002). The two muscles combine in a force couple action to move the radius around a stable ulna, bringing the hand from a palm-down position to a palm-up position.

The muscle actions of the elbow complex cannot be separated, even though we try to do so for learning purposes. As in the entire body, rarely is there one muscle that works alone to stabilize or move a joint. To summarize the muscle actions of the elbow and forearm, let's return to David in the occupational profile. Because leisure activities are so important to maintain a balance in our lives, we can look at the meaning of fishing to David. He had stated in the occupational profile that he had been unable to fish due to pain and weakness in his right dominant elbow. Performing an activity analysis of casting and reeling the rod during fishing, think about what movements and muscle actions would be required at the elbow and forearm. You will find that you will use every movement and muscle in the elbow complex along with the joints and muscles of the entire upper extremity to participate in this leisure activity.

Muscles, Nerves, and Spinal Cord Levels

Nerve roots C5, C6, C7, and C8 supply the joints and muscles of the elbow complex. The muscles that flex the elbow and supinate the forearm are innervated by the C5 and C6 nerve roots and the musculocutaneous and radial nerves, respectively. The muscles that extend the elbow receive their innervation from nerve roots C6, C7, and C8 and only from the radial nerve branch. The forearm pronators are supplied by nerve roots C7, C8, and T1. The pronator teres muscle is innervated by the median nerve branch, and the pronator quadratus muscle is innervated by the anterior interosseous branch of the radial nerve (Weiss & Falkenstein, 2005). All of the muscles of the elbow complex are innervated by the terminal nerves of the brachial plexus. Table 8-3 displays the muscles, movements, and innervations of the elbow complex.

The muscles needed for each movement and the nerve innervations required for these movements will be discussed again in relationship to David's favorite leisure activity of fishing. Table 8-1 names the movements, muscles, and nerve innervations necessary to cast and reel a fishing rod. Think about the following questions:

Table 8-3 Motions of the Elbow Complex

Muscle	Nerve	Nerve root					Elbow Flexion 0 to 140 degrees	Elbow Extension 140 to 0 degrees	Forearm Pronation 0 to 80 degrees	Forearm Supination 0 to 80 degrees
		C5	C6	C7	C8	T1				
Biceps brachii	Musculocutaneous	x	x				x			x
Brachialis	Musculocutaneous	x	x				x			
Brachioradialis	Radial	x	x				x			
Triceps	Radial		x	x	x			x		
Anconeus	Radial		x	x	x			x		
Pronator teres	Median			x	x				x	
Pronator quadratus	Anterior interosseous (radial)			x	x	x			x	
Supinator	Posterior interosseous (radial)		x							x

Adapted from Dutton, M. (2004). *Orthopaedic exam, evaluation and intervention*. New York, NY: McGraw-Hill.; Latella, D., & Meriano, C. (2003). *Occupational therapy manual for the evaluation of range of motion and muscle strength*. Clifton Park, NY: Delmar Carnage Learning.; Oatis, C. A. (2004). *Kinesiology: The mechanics and pathomechanics of human movement*. Philadelphia, PA: Lippincott, Williams & Wilkins.; Floyd, R. T., & Thompson, C. W. (2001). *Manual of structural kinesiology* (14th ed.). New York, NY: McGraw-Hill.

    A.   Which muscles required for casting and reeling a fishing rod are innervated by the radial nerve?

    B.   If David's radial nerve was damaged, where would he have weakness, and which elbow movements would be limited?

    C.   If he had a neck injury that affected the nerve roots C5, C6, and C7, which muscles of the elbow complex would be affected?

Elbow flexion and extension are prevalent movements in the activity of fishing. Strengthening the biceps and triceps muscles, after decreasing David's pain and inflammation, may prevent a recurrence of his tennis elbow. For David to continue his occupational roles in the future and prevent injury as he ages, a structured muscle-strengthening program will be required. He can also preserve his well-being with participation in his chosen leisure activity, fishing.

The elbow complex also serves as protection for the nerve branches that innervate structures more distally. Function of the distal forearm, wrist, and hand can be affected negatively if a peripheral nerve is damaged at the elbow. The radial nerve innervates distal muscles as well as the elbow extensors. If the radial nerve is damaged in the humeral area of the upper extremity, not only will the triceps muscle be weakened, but the wrist, finger, and thumb extensors will be affected. Referring to one of the common problems of the elbow complex discussed earlier in this chapter, cubital tunnel syndrome is seen when the ulnar nerve becomes compressed or irritated at the medial elbow. Even though the ulnar nerve does not innervate the muscles of the elbow complex, it is impairment at the elbow that affects the distal muscles.

Tendons and Ligaments

The tendons of a muscle are strong and show the ability to elongate during muscle stretch and contraction. The tendons, however, have a decreased blood supply compared to the muscle, which increases risk of injury and slows healing after injury or surgical repair. When a muscle or tendon tears, it is usually where the tendon inserts or originates at the bone or where the tendon and muscle join, called the musculotendinous junction. One of the problems of the elbow complex discussed earlier in this chapter, for example, is the distal biceps tendon rupture. The distal tendon of the biceps muscle tears in most cases at the insertion, which is the radial tuberosity. In the case of David's diagnosis, tennis elbow, microscopic tears occurred at the musculotendinous junction where the ECRB attaches at the lateral epicondyle of the humerus. Figure 8-9 provides a view of the musculotendinous junction at the lateral epicondyle.

In comparison to the shoulder complex, the elbow complex relies on its collateral ligaments for stabilization of mediolateral movement. The ligaments of the elbow also contribute to the limits of elbow extension and prevent subluxation in this more rigid joint (Oatis, 2004). Remember that the shoulder depends on its muscles to stabilize the joints for the most part. Because the ligaments of the elbow complex are so vital for its stability, they will be named and discussed in this section. Table 8-4 identifies the elbow complex ligaments and their functions.

The lateral collateral ligament (LCL) complex attaches proximally at the lateral epicondyle and distally on the annular ligament and on the ulna (Lippert, 2000). This ligament provides stability against excessive varus deviation anywhere in the full range of elbow flexion and extension. *Varus* is defined as being angled inward or when a distal segment of a joint is adducted. The LCL stabilizes the ulnohumeral and radiohumeral joints when using the elbow resistively, especially when the forearm is supinated (Oatis, 2004).

The medial collateral ligament (MCL) complex is larger than the LCL and attaches proximally at the medial epicondyle of the humerus and distally to the medial sides of the olecranon and coronoid processes of the ulna (Lippert, 2000). The elbow's normal alignment is valgus, as seen in the anatomic position, where the forearm (the joint distal segment) is abducted or angled outward (Oatis, 2004). This predisposes the elbow joint to valgus stress. The MCL complex protects the stability of the elbow joint against excessive valgus stress especially with the elbow flexed between 60 and 90 degrees (Hunter et al., 2002).

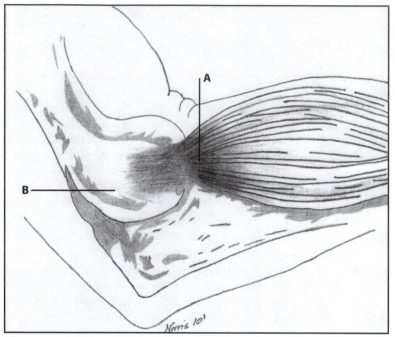

Figure 8-9. (A) The musculotendinous junction at the (B) lateral epicondyle. (Reprinted with permission of Kevin Norris.)

Table 8-4	**Elbow Complex Ligaments and Their Functions**	
Joint	**Ligament**	**Function**
Elbow	Lateral collateral	Maintain the ulnohumeral and radio-humeral joints when the elbow is loaded in supination
	Annular	• Prevents subluxation of the radial head. • Restrains the radial head and maintains the relationship with the ulna and humerus.
Radioulnar	Medial collateral	Most important to provide stability against valgus stress, especially in the range of 20 to 130 degrees of extension and flexion.
	Annular	See above.
	Interosseous membrane	Supports radius and ulna keeping them from separating.

Adapted from Dutton, M. (2004). *Orthopaedic exam, evaluation and intervention.* New York, NY: McGraw-Hill.; Lippert, L. S. (2000). *Clinical kinesiology for physical therapist assistants* (3rd ed.). Philadelphia, PA: F. A. Davis.

The annular ligament is a strong, broad band that surrounds the radial head, like a sling binding it to the ulna (Hunter et al., 2002). The annular ligament is effective in preventing subluxation of the head of the radius and provides protection against dislocation of the proximal radioulnar joint. An injury that is seen involving the annular ligament is known as "pulled elbow" or "nursemaids' elbow." It is seen mainly in children less than 6 years of age and is caused from a traction

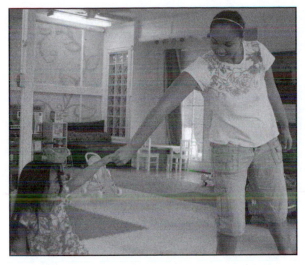

Figure 8-10. Child pulling away from mother, which demonstrates mechanics of "nursemaids' elbow." (Reprinted with permission of Joy Jonah.)

force pulling the forearm distally from the elbow. This may occur by swinging or lifting a young child by the hands (Oatis, 2004). It is believed that the weight of the child's body applies traction, pulling the radial head through the underdeveloped, looser annular ligament causing dislocation. The lateral aspect of the radial head is narrower in a child and can slip through the annular ligament more easily when the elbow is extended and the forearm pronated (Weiss & Falkenstein, 2005). Figure 8-10 shows the mechanics of "nursemaids' elbow."

The interosseous membrane (IM) is located between the ulna and the radius and helps to keep the two bones from separating through the length of the forearm (Lippert, 2000). It also plays a role in distributing loads applied during weight bearing on the hand. When an individual falls on an outstretched hand, the radius takes the load initially. The orientation of the fibers of the IM allows the ulna to receive a portion of the load, lessening the chance of distal radius fractures (Oatis, 2004). As in all the joint movements of the body, the elbow complex relies on the coordination of muscles, the nerves that innervate them, and the supporting soft tissue structures of the tendon and ligament for functional movement. All of these structures work in harmony to allow clients, such as David, to participate in their preferred occupational roles that may include carpenter, father, or fisherman.

APPLICATIONS

Elbow and Radioulnar Joint Range of Motion

The following activities will help you apply knowledge of the elbow and radioulnar joints in real-life applications. Activities can be completed individually or in a small group to enhance learning.

1. **The Elbow and Radioulnar Joints:** The elbow joint is the articulation of the humerus with the radius and the ulna and is called a uniaxial joint because it allows for only extension and flexion. The radioulnar joint involves the proximal articulation between the ulna and the radius. This is a pivot joint because the radius moves around the ulna but it is still considered a uniaxial joint because it only allows supination and pronation of the forearm. Complete the following activities to increase your familiarity with the aspects and movements of the elbow and radioulnar joints.

A. Locate and palpate the following landmarks of the humerus, radius, and ulna on a partner or human skeleton:

- Lateral and medial epicondyles
- Radial tuberosity
- Radial head
- Olecranon process
- Coronoid process
- Capitulum
- Trochlea

B Now, locate and palpate the following bony landmarks on a skeleton or partner:

- Lateral epicondyle
- Medial epicondyle
- Olecranon fossa
- Olecranon process

C Identify all motions of the elbow and forearm during the following functional activities:

- Drying the hair on the back of your head: _____.
- Bringing your arm back to throw a ball: _____.
- Turning the key in the ignition of your car: _____.
- Doing a chin-up with your palms facing you: _____.
- Reaching up to unscrew a light bulb: _____.

2. **ROM of the Elbow and Radioulnar Joints:**
Motions of the elbow and radioulnar joints and ROM norms are identified in Table 8-5. ROM norms can vary depending on the reference source. One norm is provided for each motion within this text to increase ease of applications. Additionally, while multiple muscles may influence a particular motion, only the main muscles responsible for a joint motion are included. References for the following information can be found in Gold Box 8-3. With your partner, practice using a goniometer to measure each motion available at the elbow and radioulnar joints. Use Table 8-5 to record your and your partner's ROM for the joints of the elbow complex.

Table 8-5	**Range of Motion Application Table**			
	Motions	Available ROM	Your ROM	Partner's ROM
Elbow and Radioulnar Joints	Flexion	0 to 140 degrees		
	Extension	140 to 0 degrees		
	Forearm Supination	0 to 80 degrees		
	Forearm Pronation	0 to 80 degrees		

Gold Box 8-3	
Sections Referenced (a to e)	Referenced Works for Range of Motion
Goniometric landmark, end feel, and start and end positions	Latella & Meriano (2003)
Muscles responsible	Hislop & Montgomery (2002)
Available range of motion	American Medical Association (2008)

A. **Elbow Joint Flexion ROM Testing**
  a. Goniometric landmark: Lateral epicondyle of the humerus
      Moving arm: Midline of the radius
      Stable arm: Midline of the humerus
  b. Available ROM: 0 to 140 degrees
  c. End feel: Soft
  d. Muscles responsible: Biceps brachii, brachialis, brachioradialis
  e. Start and end position: Figure 8-11 displays the start position. The arm is positioned at the side of the body with the arm fully extended and in the anatomical position. Bend the arm at the elbow into maximum flexion with the palm up. Figure 8-12 displays the end position of ROM testing.

B **Elbow Joint Extension ROM Testing**
  a. Goniometric landmark: Lateral epicondyle of the humerus
      Moving arm: Midline of the radius
      Stable arm: Midline of the humerus
  b. Available ROM: 140 to 0 degrees
  c. End feel: Firm
  d. Muscles responsible: Triceps and anconeus
  e. Start and End Position: Figure 8-13 displays the start position for goniometric testing of elbow joint extension. During elbow extension, the arm returns to the side of the body after elbow flexion to return to the anatomical position. Figure 8-14 displays the end position.

C. **Forearm Supination ROM Testing**
  a. Goniometric landmark: Volar surface of the distal forearm, 1 cm proximal to the pisiform

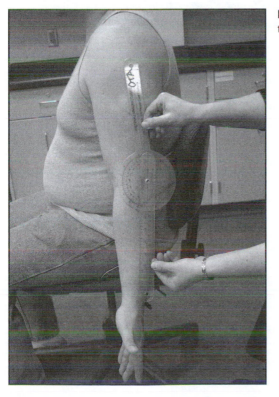

Figure 8-11. Start position for elbow flexion ROM testing.

Figure 8-12. End position for elbow flexion ROM testing.

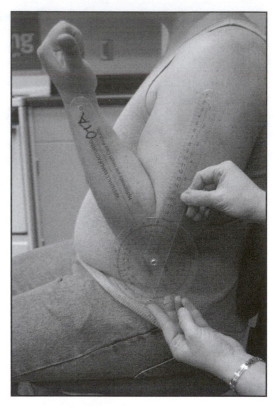

Figure 8-13. Start position for elbow extension ROM testing.

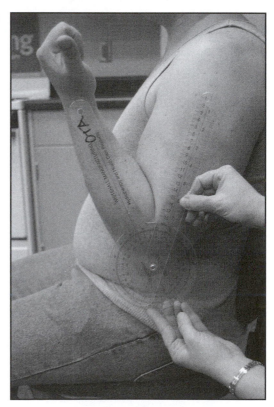

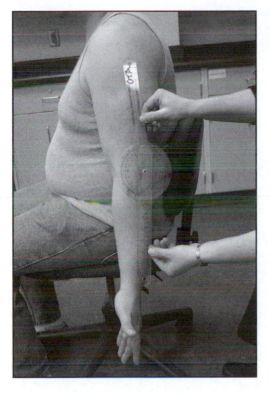

Figure 8-14. End position for elbow extension ROM testing.

          Stable arm: Perpendicular to the floor
          Moving arm: Across the volar aspect of the distal forearm

    b.   Available ROM: 0 to 80 degrees
    c.   End feel: Firm
    d.   Muscles responsible: Biceps brachii, brachioradialis, and supinator
    e.   Start and end position: Figure 8-15 displays the start position for goniometric testing of forearm supination. The arm is at the side of the body with the humerus adducted, the elbow flexed to 90 degrees, and the forearm in neutral. The client moves his or her forearm into full supination or palm up, without moving the shoulder. The end position is pictured in Figure 8-16.

  D.   **Forearm Supination ROM Testing (Alternate Method)**

Note: This method requires holding a pencil in the fingers and may be difficult for clients with a limitation in finger flexion.

    a.   Goniometric landmark: Head of third metacarpal
          Stable arm: Perpendicular to the floor
          Moving arm: Parallel to the pencil
    b.   Available ROM: 0 to 80 degrees
    c.   End feel: Firm
    d.   Muscles responsible: Biceps brachii, brachioradialis, and supinator
    e.   Start and end position: Figure 8-17 displays the start position. The client holds a pencil in the fist of the arm being tested. The arm is at the side of the body with the humerus adducted, the elbow flexed to 90 degrees, and the forearm in neutral. The client moves his or her forearm into full supination, or palm up, without moving the shoulder. Figure 8-18 displays the end position.

Figure 8-15. Start position for forearm supination ROM testing.

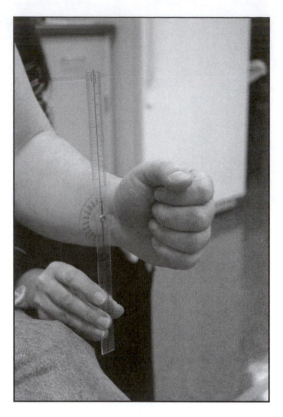

Figure 8-16. End position for forearm supination ROM testing.

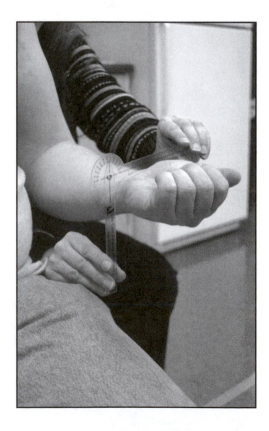

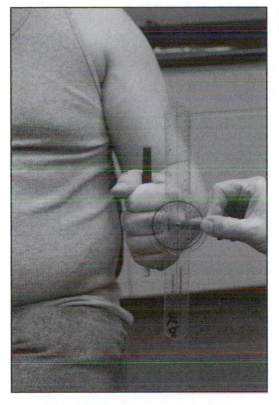

Figure 8-17. Start position for alternate forearm supination ROM testing.

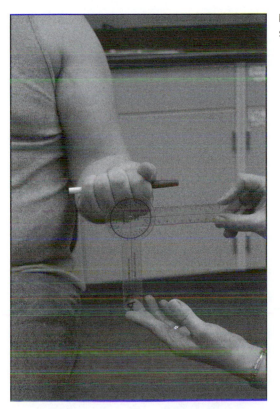

Figure 8-18. End position for alternate forearm supination ROM testing.

E. **Forearm Pronation ROM Testing**
   a. Goniometric landmark: Ulnar styloid process

   Stable arm: Perpendicular to the floor
   Moving arm: Dorsal surface of the distal forearm

   b. Available ROM: 0 to 80 degrees
   c. End feel: Hard
   d. Muscles responsible: Pronator teres, pronator quadratus, and brachioradialis
   e. Start and end position: Figure 8-19 displays the start position. The arm is at the side of the body with the humerus adducted, the elbow flexed to 90 degrees, and the forearm in neutral. The client moves his or her forearm into full pronation, or palm down, without moving the shoulder. Figure 8-20 displays the end position.

F. **Forearm Pronation ROM Testing (Alternate Method)**
   Note: This method requires holding a pencil in the fingers and may be difficult for clients with a limitation in finger flexion.
   a. Goniometric landmark: Head of third metacarpal

   Stable arm: Perpendicular to the floor
   Moving arm: Parallel to the pencil

   b. Available ROM: 0 to 80 degrees
   c. End feel: Hard
   d. Muscles responsible: Pronator teres, pronator quadratus, and brachioradialis
   e. Start and end position: Figure 8-21 displays the start position. The arm is at the side of the body with the humerus adducted, the elbow flexed

Figure 8-19. Start position for forearm pronation ROM testing.

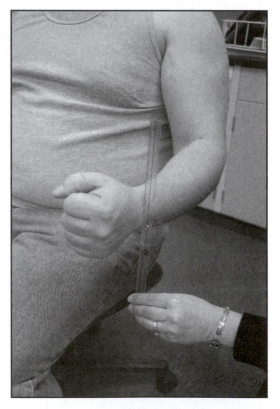

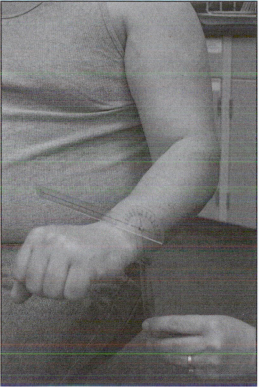

Figure 8-20. End position for forearm pronation ROM testing.

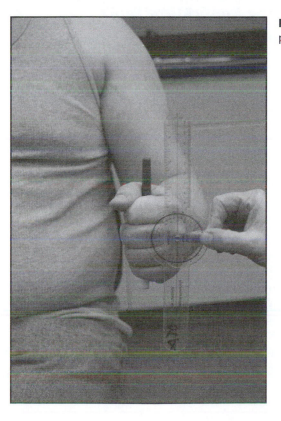

Figure 8-21. Start position for alternate forearm pronation ROM testing.

Figure 8-22. End position for alternate forearm pronation ROM testing.

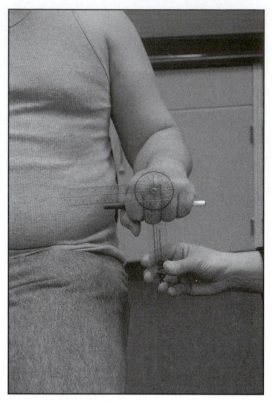

Table 8-6	Manual Muscle Testing Application Table		
	Motions	Palpate Muscle Group/ Muscles	Gross MMT Score
Elbow and Radioulnar Joints	Elbow Flexion		
	Elbow Extension		
	Forearm Supination		
	Forearm Pronation		

to 90 degrees, and the forearm in neutral. The client moves his or her forearm into full pronation or palm down, without moving the shoulder. Figure 8-22 displays the end position.

3. **MMT of the Elbow Complex:** Complete gross MMT for Motions of the elbow and radioulnar joints using Table 8-6. With your partner, practice the standardized procedure for identifying gross MMT for each elbow and radioulnar joint motion.

    A. **Elbow Joint Flexion and Extension:** Testing procedure: Figure 8-23 displays the start position for elbow joint flexion. The client moves his or her arm halfway into elbow flexion or to about 90 degrees. The therapist stabilizes the humerus over the biceps muscle to avoid compensation. Resistance is applied to the distal/volar forearm in the direction of elbow extension. The client is asked to move

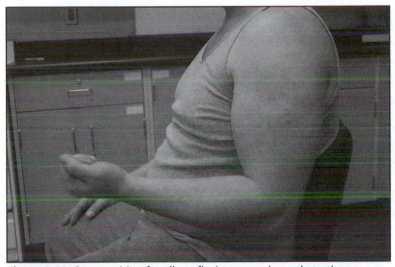

Figure 8-23. Start position for elbow flexion manual muscle testing.

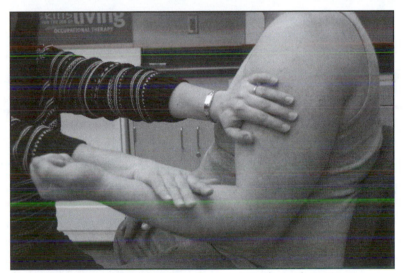

Figure 8-24. Test position for elbow flexion manual muscle testing.

his or her arm in the direction of elbow flexion. Figure 8-24 displays the testing position.

Figure 8-25 displays the start position for testing elbow joint extension. The client moves his or her shoulder to about 120 degrees of flexion with the elbow at 90 degrees of flexion. The therapist stabilizes the humerus over the triceps muscle to avoid compensation. Resistance is applied on the ulnar portion of the distal forearm in the direction of elbow flexion. The client is asked to move his or her arm in the direction of elbow extension. Figure 8-26 displays the testing position.

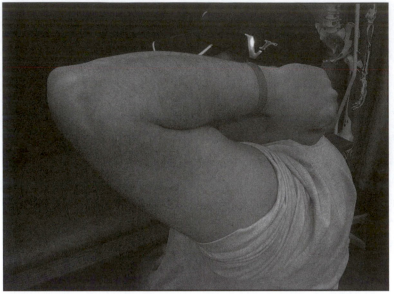

Figure 8-25. Start position for elbow extension manual muscle testing.

Figure 8-26. Test position for elbow extension manual muscle testing.

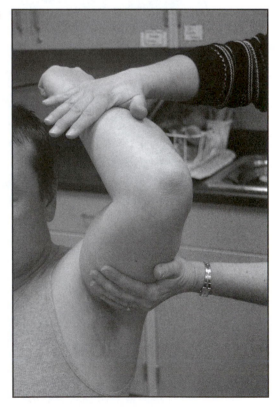

B. **Radioulnar Joint Supination and Pronation:** Testing procedure: Figure 8-27 displays the start position for radioulnar joint supination and pronation. The arm is at the side of the body with the humerus adducted, the elbow flexed to 90 degrees, and the forearm in neutral. The therapist stabilizes the arm at the elbow to avoid compensation. To test radioulnar joint or forearm supination, resistance is applied at the distal forearm in the direction of pronation. The client is asked to move his or her forearm in the direction of supination. Figure 8-28 displays the testing position.

To test radioulnar joint or forearm pronation, resistance is applied at the distal forearm in the direction of supination. The client is asked to move his or her forearm in the direction of pronation. Figure 8-29 displays the testing position.

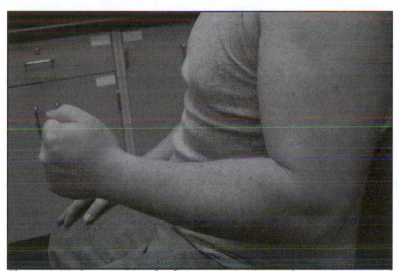

Figure 8-27. Start position for forearm supination and pronation manual muscle testing.

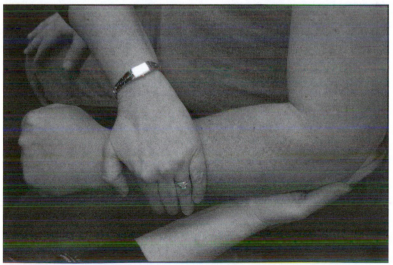

Figure 8-28. Test position for forearm supination manual muscle testing.

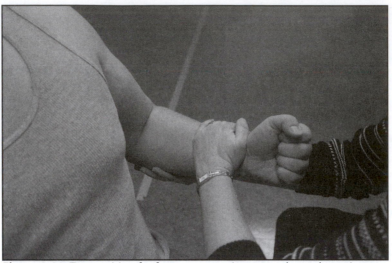

Figure 8-29. Test position for forearm pronation manual muscle testing.

REFERENCES

American Academy of Orthopaedic Surgeons. (2009a). Biceps tendon tear at the elbow. Retrieved from http://orthoinfo.aaos.org/topic.cfm?topic=A00376.

American Academy of Orthopaedic Surgeons. (2009b). Tennis elbow (Lateral epicondylitis). Retrieved from http://orthoinfo.aaos.org/topic.cfm?topic=A00068.

American Medical Association. (2008). *Guides to the evaluation of permanent impairment* (6th ed.). Chicago: Author.

Cannon, N. M. (2003). *Diagnosis and treatment manual for physicians and therapists: Upper extremity rehabilitation* (4th ed.). Indianapolis, IN: The Hand Rehabilitation Center of Indiana.

DeSmet, L., & Fabry, G. (1997). Grip force reduction in patients with tennis elbow: Influence of elbow position. *The Journal of Hand Therapy, 10*(3), 229–231.

Dutton, M. (2004). *Orthopaedic exam, evaluation and intervention.* New York, NY: McGraw-Hill.

Floyd, R. T., & Thompson, C. W. (2001). *Manual of structural kinesiology* (14th ed.). New York, NY: McGraw-Hill.

Hertfelder, S., & Gwin, C. (1989). *Work in progress: Occupational therapy in work programs.* Rockville, MD: American Occupational Therapy Association.

Hertling, D., & Kessler, R. (2006). *Management of common musculoskeletal disorders: Physical therapy principles and methods.* Philadelphia, PA: Lippincott, Williams & Wilkins.

Hislop, H. J., & Montgomery, J. (2002). *Daniel's and Worthingham's muscle testing: Techniques of manual examinations* (7th ed.). Philadelphia, PA: Saunders.

Hunter, J. M., Maklin, E. J., Callahan, H. D., Skirven, T. M., Schneider, L. H., & Osterman, A. E. (2002). *Rehabilitation of the hand and upper extremity* (5th ed.). St Louis, MO: Mosby.

Latella, D., & Meriano, C. (2003). *Occupational therapy manual for the evaluation of range of motion and muscle strength.* Clifton Park, NY: Delmar Carnage Learning.

Lippert, L. S. (2000). *Clinical kinesiology for physical therapist assistants* (3rd ed.). Philadelphia, PA: F. A. Davis.

Oatis, C. A. (2004). *Kinesiology: The mechanics and pathomechanics of human movement.* Philadelphia, PA: Lippincott, Williams & Wilkins.

Weiss, S., & Falkenstein, N. (2005). *Hand rehabilitation: A quick reference guide and review.* St. Louis, MO: Elsevier Mosby.

chapter 9

Function and Movement of the Hand

Carolyn L. Roller, OTR/L

OCCUPATIONAL PROFILE

The following occupational profile is provided to demonstrate occupational therapy (OT) intervention as related to the body functions and structures of the wrist and hand. Laura, the client in this profile, will show how a wrist and hand injury can negatively affect function. References to Laura will be addressed throughout this chapter. Laura is a 53-year-old teacher receiving OT with a physician's referral to increase range of motion (ROM) and decrease edema in her left dominant wrist and hand.

During the OT evaluation, the following data were gathered:

Subjective: Laura states that 6 weeks ago, she attended a roller skating field trip with her fourth-grade class. While skating, she fell, landing on her left outstretched hand. Laura reports that she noticed immediate pain and swelling in her left wrist and hand. She went to the hospital where x-rays were taken and a cast was applied to her left arm. Laura states she was last seen by her doctor 3 days ago at which time her cast was removed. She was given a wrist brace and was referred to OT.

Today, Laura complains of stiffness in her left wrist and hand, swelling in her left hand, and pain when she tries to use her arm. She states she cannot drive, write, brush her teeth, feed herself, dry her hair, push a cart in the grocery store, or type on the computer using her left hand. Laura reports, "I need to be able to drive, write, and type to return to my teaching position. The cast is off, and the doctor says the bone is healed, but my wrist is stiff, and my hand is so swollen that I can't make a fist. It hurts when I try to hold the steering wheel while using the turn signal. I don't feel safe driving."

Laura reports a past medical history of high cholesterol and high blood pressure, which are controlled with medication. She denies any other health problems and states she lost her husband to cancer 4 years ago. She currently lives alone but has two grown children and four grandchildren who live in the area and have been helpful since her injury. She reports that she has been very active, participating in yoga and walking frequently prior to her injury. Laura states that she loves to knit but has not been able to perform that leisure activity since her injury.

Objective: Laura rates the pain in her left wrist and hand as 0/10 at rest and 5/10 at worst. She states the worst pain is at end ROM with forearm supination, finger flexion, and wrist flexion and extension. She also reports pain as a 5/10 with inadvertent use of her injured wrist and hand.

Keough, J. L., Sain, S. J., Roller, C. L.
Kinesiology for the Occupational Therapy Assistant:
Essential Components of Function and Movement (pp. 247-320).

Active range of motion (AROM) is within normal limits in both upper extremities with the exception of her left forearm, wrist, and hand. Formal AROM measurements are taken with a goniometer where limitations were noted. The joints of the right forearm, wrist, and hand are measured for comparison purposes. AROM is recorded as follows:

Forearm:	**Right**	**Left**
Supination	0 to 90 degrees	0 to 35 degrees
Pronation	0 to 90 degrees	0 to 60 degrees

Wrist:	**Right**	**Left**
Extension	0 to 78 degrees	0 to 15 degrees
Flexion	0 to 93 degrees	0 to 30 degrees
Radial deviation	0 to 24 degrees	0 to 11 degrees
Ulnar deviation	0 to 36 degrees	0 to 16 degrees

Thumb:	**Right**	**Left**
Metacarpophalangeal (MCP) flexion	0 to 52 degrees	0 to 20 degrees
Interphalangeal (IP) flexion	0 to 90 degrees	0 to 15 degrees

Fingers:

	MCP Joints		**PIP Joints**		**DIP Joints**	
	Right	Left	Right	Left	Right	Left
Index (IF)	0 to 81 degrees	0 to 44 degrees	0 to 98 degrees	0 to 80 degrees	0 to 70 degrees	0 to 45 degrees
Long (LF)	0 to 79 degrees	0 to 43 degrees	0 to 108 degrees	0 to 81 degrees	0 to 72 degrees	0 to 35 degrees
Ring (RF)	0 to 78 degrees	0 to 49 degrees	0 to 109 degrees	0 to 78 degrees	0 to 68 degrees	0 to 33 degrees
Small (SF)	0 to 75 degrees	0 to 35 degrees	0 to 102 degrees	0 to 79 degrees	0 to 74 degrees	0 to 39 degrees

MCP = metacarpophalangeal; PIP = proximal interphalangeal; DIP = distal interphalangeal; Measurements are recorded as extension/flexion.

*Note: The fingers are often referred to as digits one through five beginning with the thumb and ending with the small or little finger. In this chapter, the digits will be referred to as thumb, index, long or middle, ring, and small fingers.

Laura is unable to make a full fist due to a lack of finger flexion. The linear edge of the goniometer is used to measure the gap from each finger pad to the distal palmar crease and is recorded as follows:

IF: 3.5 cm   RF: 3.0 cm

LF: 3.0 cm   SF: 2.5 cm

Edema is observed to be moderate in the left hand and fingers with pitting edema noted over the dorsum of the hand. Mild edema is noted in the wrist and distal forearm. Whole hand edema was evaluated using the volumeter with measurements as follows:

Right: 445 mL   Left: 520 mL

Laura complains of unresolved tingling and numbness in her left thumb, index, and long fingers, which began when her cast was applied after her injury. Visual examination reveals discoloration of the entire left hand as compared to her uninvolved hand, especially in the thumb and fingers. Manual examination reveals that the fingertips of the left hand feel cold as compared to the fingertips of the right hand. Palpation reveals tenderness over the medial and lateral sides of the PIP and DIP joints of all fingers and over the radial wrist.

Sensory screening is performed, revealing intact two-point discrimination in the left fingertips. Light touch sensation is evaluated using the Semmes-Weinstein monofilaments. Findings include normal light sensation (2.83 g) present on the volar surface of the fingertips of the right hand and the small finger and ulnar portion of the ring finger of the left hand. The left thumb, index finger, long finger, and radial aspect of the ring finger reveal diminished protective light touch sensation (4.31 g). Grip and pinch strength are not tested at this time due to pain and limitations in finger ROM.

Goals were established by the occupational therapist in collaboration with Laura and are presented as follows:

Short-Term Goals:

1. Client will be instructed in and comply with a home exercise program within 1 week.
2. Client will tolerate a formal evaluation of left grip and pinch strength when able and appropriate or within 4 weeks.
3. Client will demonstrate the ability to grade students' papers using the left dominant hand and adaptive writing implements within 3 weeks.
4. Client will demonstrate self-feeding with the left hand and adaptive utensils within 2 weeks.
5. Client will demonstrate decreased edema by 30 mL using edema control techniques within 3 weeks.
6. Client will demonstrate an increase in AROM in all limited joints by 5 degrees in each joint in 4 weeks.

Long-Term Goals:

1. Client will demonstrate compliance and independence in a home exercise program at discharge.
2. Client will be independent in self-care tasks and occupational roles using the left dominant hand and adaptive equipment within 3 months.
3. Client will demonstrate AROM to within functional limits in left forearm, wrist, and thumb and demonstrate a straight fist in left hand within 3 months.
4. Client will demonstrate a decrease in edema by 50 mL in the left hand volumetrically in 3 months.
5. Client will demonstrate functional ROM in the left dominant hand by knitting a scarf in 3 months.

The outcome of Laura's OT intervention along with treatment techniques and goals achieved can be found by reading Appendix C.

BODY FUNCTIONS OF THE WRIST AND HAND

In this part of the chapter, joint motions and strength characteristics of the wrist and hand as they relate to function will be described. Three problems of the wrist and hand commonly treated in OT will be identified and discussed. Throughout this chapter, references will be made to Laura and her functional problems, goals, and treatment.

Motions of the Wrist

The wrist joint is also known as the radiocarpal joint and is classified as a biaxial, or condyloid, joint (Lippert, 2000). The wrist joint allows flexion, extension, radial deviation, and ulnar deviation. Because it is a biaxial joint, the wrist also combines these four movements to produce circumduction, which is a circular movement of the hand on the forearm (Oatis, 2004).

The amount of wrist motion can vary significantly among clients and even in the same client when comparing the right to the left wrist (Rybski, 2004). Wrist ROM can vary due to ligament tightness or laxity, muscle mass, and articulating surface lubrication (Weiss & Falkenstein, 2005). Normal and functional wrist motions vary significantly according to different references. A table listing wrist ROM for this text and the references cited can be found later in this chapter. Normal wrist ROM can best be determined by comparison of the involved wrist to the uninvolved wrist of the client.

Studies show that individuals can perform independent functional activities with less than normal wrist ROM (Oatis, 2004). According to Weiss and Falkenstein (2005), functional wrist ROM for performing most activities of daily living is 40 degrees of wrist flexion and extension and 40 degrees of composite radial and ulnar deviation. For example, using a fork or holding a newspaper only requires 35 degrees of wrist extension, whereas weight bearing while using a cane may require 40 degrees of wrist extension (Oatis, 2004). These functional examples demonstrate less-than-normal wrist extension.

Wrist flexion occurs when the client bends his or her wrist down as if trying to touch the fingers to the volar aspect of the distal forearm. A daily self-care task that uses wrist flexion is toileting. Wrist extension (occasionally called dorsiflexion) occurs when the client bends his or her wrist back, such as holding a cell phone to the ear. Weight-bearing activities, such as pushing up from a chair or using a walker, are additional examples of functional activities that require wrist extension.

The side-to-side wrist motions are called radial and ulnar deviation. Wrist radial deviation is seen when the client moves his or her wrist toward the thumb side of the hand. Wrist ulnar deviation is the opposite of radial deviation and occurs when the client moves his or her wrist toward the small finger side of the hand. These movements most likely occur when the client casts a fishing rod or uses a hammer.

The combination of all four wrist motions together is called circumduction and occurs when a client washes his or her hands or beats an egg with a fork. Figures 9-1 through 9-4 demonstrate wrist flexion, extension, radial deviation, and ulnar deviation.

Motions of the Hand

Think of your hands as tools used to perform activities of daily living. The hand is used in simple, everyday activities such as eating and in complex tasks such as creating an intricate piece of

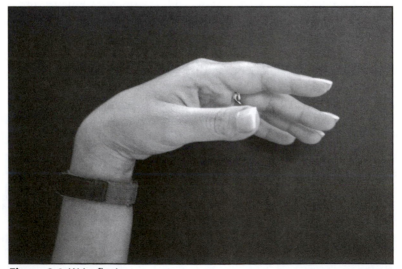

Figure 9-1. Wrist flexion.

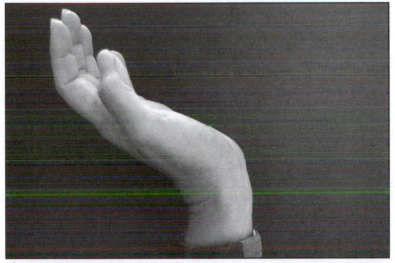

Figure 9-2. Wrist extension.

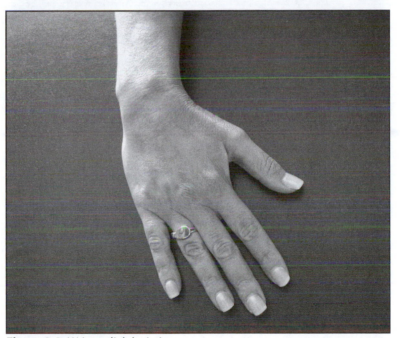

Figure 9-3. Wrist radial deviation.

sculpture. The hand is used as a means of expression, to identify where the body is in space using touch, and unfortunately as a weapon. The hands are extremely versatile and coordinated. The main purpose of the other joints of the upper extremity is to place the hand in various positions to complete the vast array of tasks we perform on a daily basis.

The thumb is named the first joint or digit of the hand and has three joints: the carpometacarpal (CMC) joint, the MCP joint, and the interphalangeal (IP) joint (Lippert, 2000). The CMC joint of the thumb is a saddle joint, providing mobility in all directions (Hertling & Kessler, 2006). The thumb CMC joint is formed by the trapezium bone proximally and the first metacarpal bone distally. The trapezium is rotated anteriorly out of the plane of the hand, which facilitates opposition of the thumb (Oatis, 2004). Figure 9-5 illustrates a hand in a relaxed position and the way the thumb is positioned out of the plane of the hand.

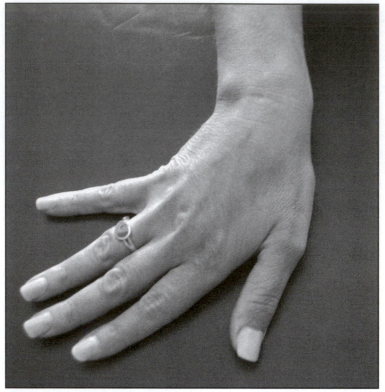

Figure 9-4. Wrist ulnar deviation.

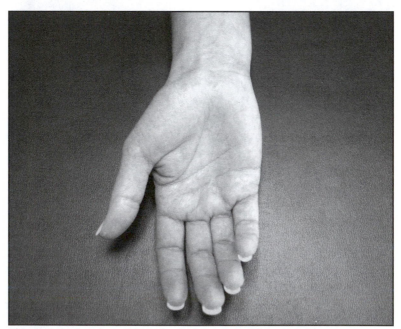

Figure 9-5. Thumb positioned out of the plane of the hand.

Because the MCP and IP joints of the thumb are similar to the MCP and PIP/DIP of the fingers, they will be discussed later in this section with the joints of the fingers.

Motions of the thumb include flexion, radial abduction (also called extension), palmar abduction, adduction, and opposition. When the forearm is supinated and the palm is facing up, thumb flexion and radial abduction (extension) is the side-to-side movement across the palm and out. A functional example of thumb radial abduction (extension) and flexion would be turning the page of a book using the left hand. Figure 9-6 demonstrates thumb radial abduction (extension) while Figure 9-7 demonstrates thumb flexion.

Again, with the forearm supinated and the palm facing up, the movement of the thumb in palmar abduction and adduction can be displayed. This time, the thumb moves up toward the ceiling for palmar abduction and returns to touch the second digit or index finger for adduction. Functionally, palmar abduction can be seen when a client prepares to pick up a glass of water as

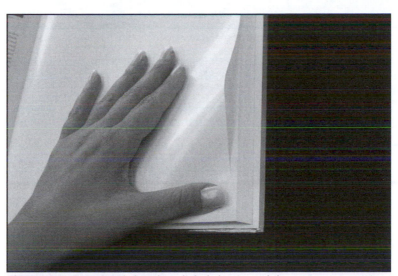

Figure 9-6. Functional thumb radial abduction while turning a page in a book.

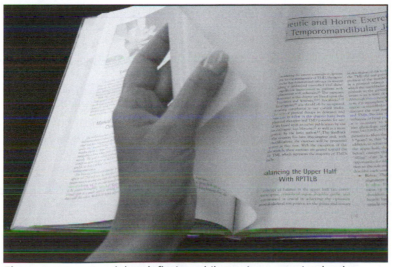

Figure 9-7. Functional thumb flexion while turning a page in a book.

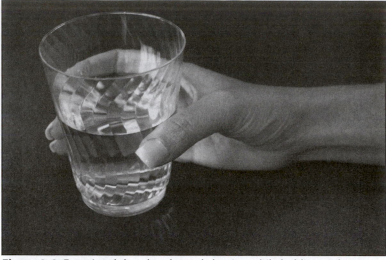

Figure 9-8. Functional thumb palmar abduction while holding a glass.

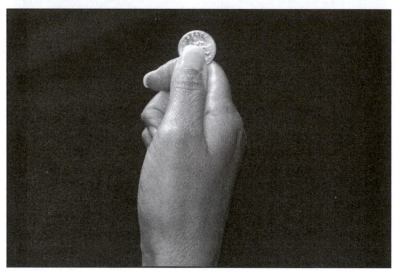

Figure 9-9. Functional thumb adduction while holding a coin.

illustrated in Figure 9-8. Adduction is seen when a client uses a lateral pinch to hold a coin as illustrated in Figure 9-9.

Thumb opposition is a combination of thumb flexion and abduction. This combined movement positions the pad of the thumb to oppose or touch the pad of a finger. The ability to oppose the thumb is what separates humans from other animals. A functional task that requires opposition is writing. Figure 9-10 illustrates opposition to the fifth digit while Figure 9-11 illustrates functional opposition during writing.

The MCP joint of the thumb is a hinged uniaxial joint, allowing only flexion and extension. Thumb MCP movement combines with the CMC joint and IP joint of the thumb to provide full opposition and reposition. Reposition is the movement of the thumb as it returns from opposition. The MCP joints of the fingers are biaxial condyloid joints and are commonly called the "knuckles" when a fist is made (Lippert, 2000). The movements allowed at the MCP joints are flexion, extension, hyperextension, abduction, and adduction. MCP joint abduction occurs when the second, fourth, and fifth digits move away from the middle finger or third digit, which is used as a

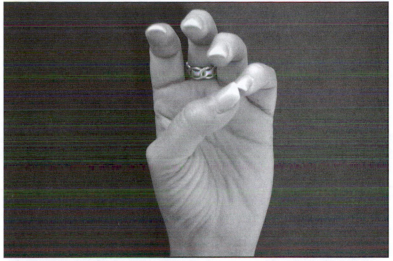

Figure 9-10. Opposition to the fifth digit.

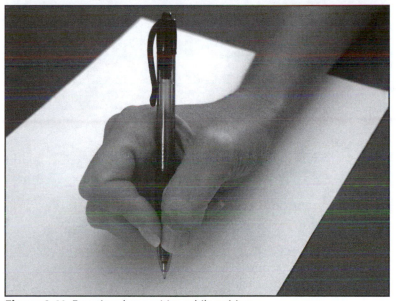

Figure 9-11. Functional opposition while writing.

reference point for abduction and adduction of the other three digits. Adduction is the return from abduction of the second, fourth, and fifth digits. Only the third digit or middle finger abducts in either direction and does not adduct.

The IP joint of the thumb and the PIP/DIP joints of the fingers are uniaxial hinge joints that allow only flexion and extension (Hertling & Kessler, 2006). The finger PIP joints are created by the articulations between the proximal and middle phalanges, and the DIP joints are created by the articulations between the middle and distal phalanges. The joints of the fingers and the thumb move together to open and close the hand for functional gripping. Figures 9-12 through 9-15 illustrate full finger flexion, extension, abduction, and adduction, respectively.

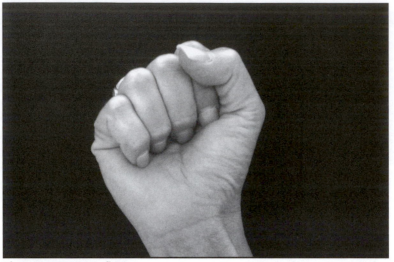

Figure 9-12. Finger flexion.

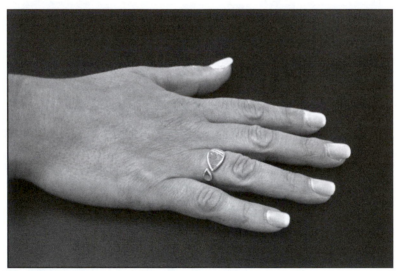

Figure 9-13. Finger extension.

Strength Characteristics of the Wrist and Hand

Functional activities performed by the wrist and hand generate forces. This includes a variety of daily activities, such as digging a hole with a trowel to plant flowers or twisting and tightening a water bottle lid. Sustained gripping or pinching, such as holding the steering wheel or writing, requires strength and stability in the wrist and hand. Other activities that involve higher loads at the wrist and hand are upper extremity weight bearing. As noted in the chapters on the shoulder and elbow, all the joints and muscles of the upper extremity are used when an individual ambulates with crutches, a walker, or a cane. The upper extremities must be used in propulsion of a wheelchair when the lower extremities are nonfunctional. In forceful, spontaneous hand activities, such as hitting a golf ball, hammering a nail, or using a jackhammer, the wrist is subject to very large loads. During moderate grasping activities involving only a 2-lb weight, the forces to the wrist are found to be up to 35 lbs (Oatis, 2004).

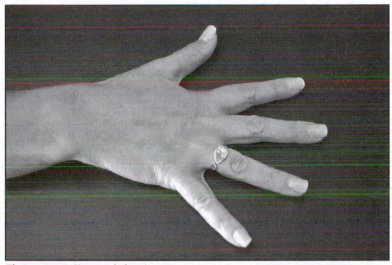

Figure 9-14. Finger abduction.

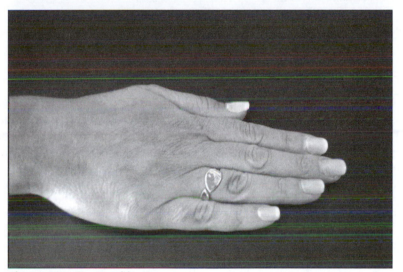

Figure 9-15. Finger adduction.

Laura, in the occupational profile, is unable to perform numerous occupational roles including gripping the steering wheel when driving. In addition to addressing her problems of stiffness, edema, and pain, wrist stability and strength will need to improve before she can drive to work. Table 9-1 identifies the functional roles of the joints, muscles, and nerves of the wrist and hand while gripping a steering wheel.

Of course, the activity of driving requires strength and coordination of all of the joints of the upper extremities. Safe driving also requires acute visual and hearing skills and the coordination of the lower extremities. Clients who may have driving deficits can be evaluated and taught compensatory techniques or can be instructed in the use of adaptive equipment by a trained OT practitioner. Please see Laura's functional outcome in Appendix C.

According to Rybski (2004), the wrist makes an active contribution to a task, a movement, or stabilization during hand function. The position of the wrist is important to the position of the fingers and thumb (Hertling & Kessler, 2006). The wrist serves a kinetic function in transmitting forces from the forearm to the hand and back to the forearm. Positional adjustments are required

Table 9-1	Gripping a Steering Wheel: Movements, Muscles, and Innervations of the Wrist and Hand		
	Muscles	Nerves	Nerve Roots
Wrist extension	ECRL	Radial	C6, C7, C8
	ECRB	Radial	C6, C7, C8
	ECU	Radial	C6, C7, C8
Wrist ulnar deviation	ECU	Radial	C6, C7, C8
Finger flexion of MCP, PIP, and DIP joints	FDS	Median	C7, C8, T1
	FDP	Median and Ulnar	C8, T1
	Lumbricals	Median and Ulnar	C7, C8
Thumb flexion of CMC, MCP, and IP joints	FPL	Median	C8, T1
	FPB	Median	C8, T1
Thumb CMC opposition	OP	Median	C6, C7

Adapted from Lippert, L. S. (2000). *Clinical kinesiology for physical therapist assistants* (3rd ed.). Philadelphia, PA: F. A. Davis.; American Medical Association. (2008). *Guides to the evaluation of permanent impairment* (6th ed.). Chicago, IL: Author.

by the wrist to increase fine motor control of the fingers. This in turn can allow fine degrees of prehension as well as a powerful grasp. There is an ideal position for the wrist and hand. This position is called the *functional position* and is most effective in terms of strength and precision during activities (Lippert, 2000). In the functional position, the wrist is slightly extended at 20 degrees, the fingers are slightly flexed at all their joints, with the degree of flexion increasing slightly from the index to the small finger, and the thumb is in opposition with the MCP joint moderately flexed and the IP joint slightly flexed (Hertling & Kessler, 2006). Figure 9-16 illustrates the functional position of the hand and wrist.

Because humans have the ability to oppose the thumb to the fingers, they exhibit a wide variety of prehension grasping patterns. These patterns are classified by the position of the fingers, the area of contact between the thumb and fingers, and the object grasped. Prehension can be either pinching or grasping. Pinch is primarily used for precision manipulation and involves the thumb and the pads of the index and long fingers. Grasp typically involves all of the hand, including the palm and the fingers (Oatis, 2004).

The grasp is sometimes called the power grip and is used when an object needs to be held forcefully while being moved by more proximal joints. The power grip involves an isometric contraction with very little movement occurring between the hand and the object. The most common power grips are the cylindrical, spherical, and hook. In the cylindrical grip, all of the fingers are flexed around the object in one direction, and the thumb is flexed in the opposite direction. Examples of the cylindrical grip include holding a golf club, steering wheel, or hammer. A spherical grip has all the fingers and thumb abducted around the object with the fingers more apart. Activities requiring a spherical grip include holding an orange, turning a doorknob, or opening a jar. The hook grip involves the fingers flexed around an object in a hook-like manner. The thumb is not necessarily involved. Examples of a hook grip are seen when holding onto a handle, such as in carrying a briefcase or bucket (Lippert, 2000). Figures 9-17 through 9-19 illustrate the three power grips of cylindrical, spherical, and hook.

A precision grip, commonly called a pinch, provides finer movements and accuracy. The object is usually small, and the palm does not tend to be involved. The intrinsic muscles of the hand are

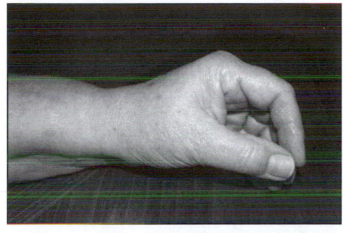

Figure 9-16. Functional position of the hand and wrist.

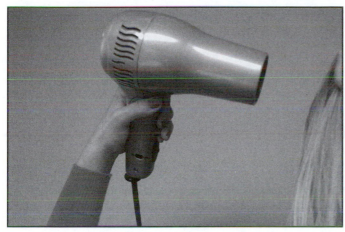

Figure 9-17. Cylindrical grip.

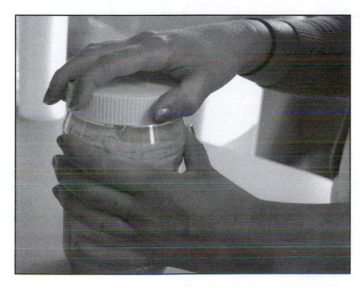

Figure 9-18. Spherical grip.

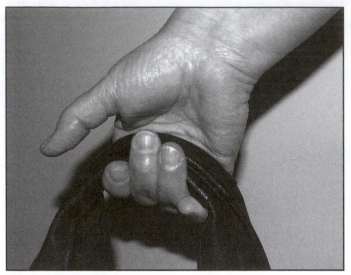

Figure 9-19. Hook grip.

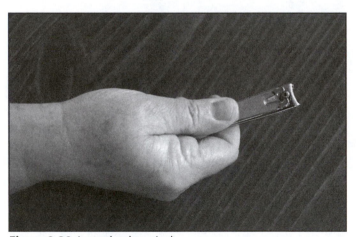

Figure 9-20. Lateral or key pinch.

used more with pinching. There are three commonly recognized pinches. The lateral or key pinch holds the object between the thumb and the radial side of the index finger. This is the strongest pinch used and is seen during activities such as turning a key to start a car or unlocking a door. The palmar or three-point pinch involves the thumb and two fingers, usually the index and long fingers. This pinch is used the most in functional activities. A good example of the palmar pinch is holding a pen during writing (Benbow, 2001). The tip or two-point pinch holds the object between the tips of the index finger and thumb. This pinch is used often when a very small object is picked up, such as a sewing needle or small coin. Figures 9-20 through 9-22 illustrate the three most common pinches: lateral, palmar, and tip.

Table 9-2 shows the frequency of functional patterns of prehension pinch.

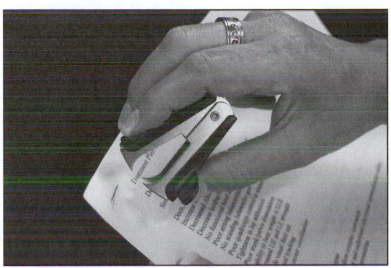

Figure 9-21. Palmar or three-point pinch.

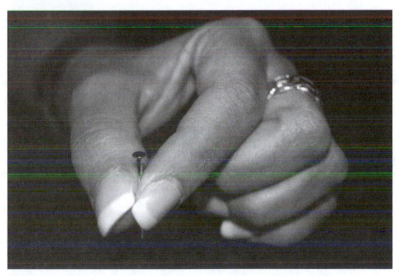

Figure 9-22. Tip or two-point pinch.

Table 9-2	**Frequency Patterns of Prehension Use**		
	Lateral Pinch	**Palmar Pinch**	**Tip Pinch**
Functional pick-up	33%	50%	17%
Hold during functional use	10%	88%	2%
Adapted from Rybski, M. (2004). *Kinesiology for occupational therapy.* Thorofare, NJ: SLACK Incorporated.			

Hand strength can be assessed by the OT practitioner using a dynamometer for grip strength and a pinch gauge for pinch strength. Comparisons to the uninvolved hand along with consideration of dominance and normative data are used during the assessment. Please refer to Appendix D for averages in pounds for varying age groups of both men and women. Figures 9-23 and 9-24 show the dynamometer and pinch gauge.

Figure 9-23. Dynamometer.

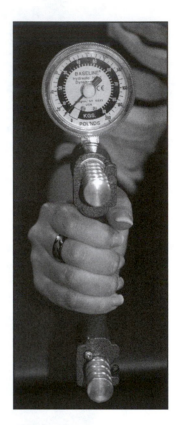

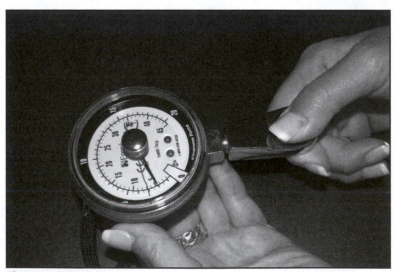

Figure 9-24. Pinch gauge.

Common Problems of the Wrist and Hand

Three problems commonly seen in OT will be defined and discussed in the following section of this chapter. These injuries and diseases specifically affecting the function of a client's wrist and/or hand can be seen in a variety of OT settings, including hospitals, skilled nursing facilities, outpatient clinics, and rehabilitation units.

Wrist and hand problems seen in OT can bridge the lifespan. The majority of clients with injuries and diseases defined below will be adults. As we age, the wrist and hand become more susceptible to injury. As an analogy of our hands compared to tires on a car, we replace the tires after about 50,000 miles or the car will have a blow-out or flat tire. Unfortunately, we cannot replace our hands when they get tired, injured, or worn out. An occupational therapy assistant (OTA) can significantly help clients rehabilitate their hands and wrists after injury or disease. The OTA can also help clients learn techniques to use their upper extremities more efficiently and independently as they age.

Think about Laura's functional limitations and her signs and symptoms. Try to identify her diagnosis while learning about these three injuries and diseases seen in OT. As in previous chapters, information about Laura's outcomes during and after OT intervention is located in Appendix C.

Distal Radius Fractures

Distal radius fractures most often occur when an individual falls on an outstretched hand with the wrist extended (Aaron & Stegink, 2000). This is commonly called FOOSH, which is the acronym for "**F**all **O**n an **O**ut**S**tretched **H**and." Distal radius fractures are the most common fracture of the upper extremity and are more common in postmenopausal women ages 51 to 75 years who may present with primary osteoporosis (Riley, 1998). Bone loss after menopause is more prevalent, making the distal radius more vulnerable to fracture if a woman falls on an outstretched hand.

There are several different types of fracture patterns present that can occur with a distal radius fracture. The most common fracture pattern is called a Colles' fracture, which was first identified by Abraham Colles in 1814 (Aaron & Stegink, 2000). A Colles' fracture is a distal radius fracture with dorsal displacement of the distal bone fragment (Weiss & Falkenstein, 2005). Colles' fractures will be the only fracture type discussed in regard to distal radius fractures in this chapter. Figure 9-25 provides an illustration of a Colles' fracture.

There are a variety of approaches to treating a Colles' fracture. It is most important that the fracture site is aligned anatomically to allow normal wrist and forearm movement to return. Closed reduction may require manipulation to align the fracture followed by casting (Cannon, 2003). If the fracture is unstable, fixation may be necessary for the best outcome. Numerous techniques can be used by the surgeon including percutaneous pin fixation, external fixation, and open reduction with internal fixation (ORIF). The technique used is contingent upon numerous variables, which may include the surgeon's preference and expertise, the client's age and medical condition, and the type of fracture displacement (Burke, Higgins, McClinton, Saunders, & Valdata, 2006). There is a recent trend to perform ORIF more often when appropriate after a Colles' fracture to begin gentle, controlled ROM earlier and avoid limiting conditions such as "fracture disease." Gold Box 9-1 provides a definition of fracture disease.

OT treatment techniques will vary according to the fixation techniques used by the physician. OT treatment goals for any distal radius fracture should be maximum pain-free forearm and wrist ROM and full ROM of the fingers, thumb, elbow, and shoulder with a return of upper extremity function (Hunter et al., 2002). It is beneficial to initiate OT while the wrist is still immobilized. The therapist can regain and maintain full shoulder, elbow, finger, and thumb ROM by the time the wrist is ready to be mobilized with early intervention. According to Hurou (1997), OT intervention assisted clients with distal radius fractures to resume functional activities by significantly increasing wrist and forearm AROM and grip and pinch strength. There is often edema in the thumb and fingers that is more difficult to resolve as it becomes chronic. Edema decreases mobility, reduces circulation, and leads to fibrosis if not resolved early (Hunter et al.,

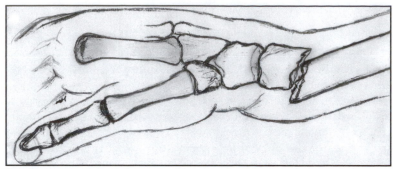

Figure 9-25. Colles' fracture. (Reprinted with permission of Angela Hartman.)

<u>**Gold Box 9-1**</u>

Fracture Disease

"**Fracture disease**" is a collection of symptoms caused by prolonged immobilization in a cast. It can lead to unresolved edema, pain, and stiffness even in the unaffected joints of the upper extremity. Muscle atrophy and osteoporosis can occur. Fracture disease can be avoided with early intervention of edema management and active range of motion of the fingers, elbow, and shoulder while the client is casted.

Weiss & Falkenstein (2005)

2002). Unfortunately, many clients are not instructed in edema control techniques immediately after casting or surgery. Clients should be individually instructed and provided handouts during OT. Figure 9-26 illustrates moderate edema in the left hand.

The best way to control edema is through the use of elevation. For elevation to be effective, the elbow should be positioned above the heart and the hand positioned above the elbow. Other edema control techniques include finger range-of-motion exercises, distal to proximal retrograde massage, lymphatic massage, compression garments such as gloves, and cardiovascular exercise. This is not an all-encompassing list, as there are many other approaches used to control edema. Gold Box 9-2 identifies an edema control technique handout used in an OT facility.

A client will be referred to OT after a Colles' fracture has healed and the doctor feels the client can begin treatment. The cast may be removed if surgery was not required, which usually occurs about approximately 6 weeks postinjury. If an ORIF was required for proper alignment, the client may be referred to OT from 2 to 6 weeks after surgery, depending on the referring physician.

Complications can occur after a distal radius fracture. The most common complications are carpal tunnel syndrome (CTS), malunion, complex regional pain syndrome (CRPS), and tendon rupture. In CTS, the median nerve, which supplies sensation to the thumb, index, and middle fingers, becomes compressed or irritated. CTS is sometimes seen after Colles' fracture due to edema and misalignment of the bone fragments. This can cause compression of the median nerve in the narrowed carpal tunnel.

Malunion can occur when the proper alignment of fracture slips, causing a deformity. This can occur more often with closed reduction and casting. As the swelling decreases, the cast sometimes loosens, allowing the aligned bone fragments to move. A client's function can be affected negatively due to pain or limited ROM if a malunion occurs. Surgery may be required to align the fracture (Weiss & Falkenstein, 2005).

CRPS, also known as **reflex sympathetic dystrophy (RSD)**, is a post-traumatic neuropathic syndrome characterized by pain and vasomotor and pseudomotor changes in the involved extremity (Stoykov, 2001). Signs and symptoms may include pain that is disproportionate to the initial

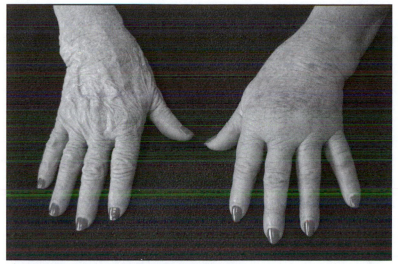

Figure 9-26. Moderate edema in the left hand.

Gold Box 9-2

Edema (Swelling) Control Techniques

The prevention of edema (swelling) is important in the rehabilitation of your hand/arm. These are techniques that can be used to decrease the edema in your hand/arm. Only perform the techniques that are circled and explained to you by your therapist.

1. **Elevation:** For elevation to be effective, the hand must be above the heart. Pillows may be used to elevate the arm and hand at night. During the day, keep your hand elevated as much as possible and not swinging at your side. This is especially important during the first 2 to 3 weeks after surgery or injury.

2. **Cold packs:** Use a gel wrap or frozen vegetables. Apply to affected area to decrease swelling and pain. Avoid placing directly on fingertips.
   Apply _____ times a day for _____ minutes.

3. **Movement:** Perform range-of-motion exercises as prescribed by your therapist. Movement especially of the fingers and hand will decrease swelling.

4. **Lymphatic massage:** Light massage proximal to the swollen region encourages the lymphatic system to "unclog," reducing the edema. Perform very gently three times daily for 1 minute to the area of your arm your therapist recommends.

5. **Use of an Isotoner (totes ISOTONER Corporation, Cincinnati, OH) glove:** Please wear as directed by your therapist. If it becomes too tight, please remove at once.

Tennessee Orthopaedic Clinic, P. C.

---

injury, excessive edema, discoloration, hypersensitivity, and increased stiffness (Burke et al., 2006). CRPS can be treated successfully if identified early.

Finally, a **tendon rupture** may occur as a result of a distal radius fracture. The tendon that ruptures most often after a distal radius fracture is the extensor pollicis longus (EPL). This is due to the position of the tendon located over the distal radius. The healing fracture site is sometimes rough, which can fray the EPL over time, eventually causing rupture. Gold Box 9-3 identifies this type of tendon rupture (Weiss & Falkenstein, 2005).

OT practitioners should be familiar with the signs and symptoms of the most commonly seen complications after a Colles' fracture. OTAs can then notify the physician and aid in early intervention, which can speed recovery and improve function.

Gold Box 9-3

Attrition Rupture

A tendon moving across a roughened bone may rupture. This type of rupture is called an **"attrition rupture"** and commonly involves the EPL tendon after a distal radius fracture.

Weiss & Falkenstein (2005)

Rheumatoid and Osteoarthritis of the Hand and Wrist

Rheumatoid arthritis (RA) is a systemic autoimmune disorder. The cause of RA is unknown, and it most commonly affects women between 20 and 50 years of age. RA most commonly affects the joints of the hands, wrists, elbows, shoulders, hips, and ankles. Signs and symptoms include fatigue, joint pain, inflammation, edema, warmth, and redness. The distinctive factors in RA are synovitis of the peripheral joints, causing progressive joint destruction, deformity, and disability. Synovitis is a thickening and inflammation of the synovial lining of the joints. Synovitis from RA can cause ligament and tendon destruction as well, leading to ligament laxity and possible tendon rupture. Hand involvement may include ulnar deviation of the MCP joints and swan neck or boutonniere deformities of the fingers and thumb. Clients with RA of the hand and wrist may be seen in OT for conservative management and postoperatively following joint replacement (Cannon, 2003).

OT goals for conservative treatment of hand and wrist RA may include preventing further deformity, providing instruction in joint protection, and energy conservation. OT practitioners may provide instruction in the use of assistive devices, instruct the client in pain control techniques, and provide instruction to maintain or increase strength (Hunter et al., 2002).

Clients may require static splinting of the hand and wrist for support, to decrease pain, and to avoid further deformities of the joints through positioning. A common deformity pattern seen in the wrist and hand of RA clients is the zigzag or Z pattern. This pattern is characterized by carpal supination with a secondary radial shift of the metacarpals followed by an ulnar deviation of the digits (Weiss & Falkenstein, 2005). Figure 9-27 illustrates the zigzag or Z deformity of the hand and wrist in RA. Figure 9-28 illustrates static splinting to prevent further deformity of the zigzag pattern.

RA clients may benefit from instruction in gentle ROM exercises to help maintain or increase flexibility. Because of the inflammatory nature of RA, gentle resistive exercises should be introduced gradually to maintain or increase grip strength. A soft ball or sponge squeezed in a bowl of warm water is a gentle way to add resistance. Clients also benefit from instruction in basic joint protection, proper lifting, and energy conservation techniques, which are included in basic protection principles. Table 9-3 gives an overview of protection principles.

Occupational therapists may also see RA clients in hand therapy postoperatively. The most common surgery performed on the hand of RA clients seen in OT is MCP joint implant arthroplasty. The indications for performing flexible MCP joint implant arthroplasty is severe RA of the MCP joints of the hands that result in deforming disability and pain, limiting function in daily activities (Cannon, 2003). The surgeon uses a flexible silicone spacer to replace the MCP joint. This allows for good alignment of the joint as well as proper tendon repositioning, enabling return of effective finger function (Burke et al., 2006).

Usually, the client will present with implants in four digits postoperatively. Therapy is indicated to maintain MCP joint alignment, reduce pain and edema, and enhance functional performance. Treatment consists of static and dynamic splinting and active and passive ROM exercises. At approximately 3 to 7 days after surgery, the therapist will fabricate a dynamic splint for continuous

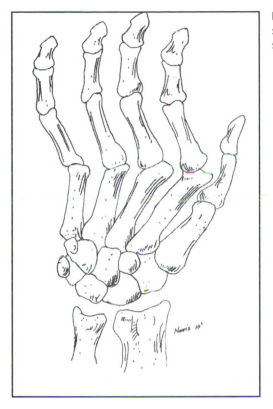

Figure 9-27. Zigzag deformity of the wrist and hand seen in rheumatoid arthritis. (Reprinted with permission of Kevin Norris.)

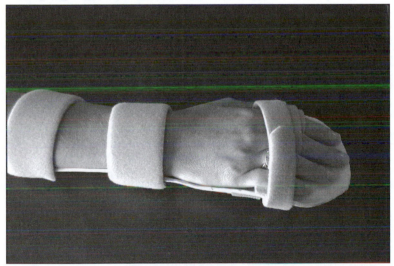

Figure 9-28. Resting splint with ulnar deviation correction to prevent further deformity.

daytime wear until 4 to 6 weeks. The splint will hold the wrist in 15 degrees of extension and MCP joints between 0 and 10 degrees of flexion with light rubber band traction at a 60-degree angle. The client should perform AROM within the splint every hour. A static resting splint is also fabricated with the wrist at 0 to 15 degrees of extension and the MCP joints at neutral and slight radial deviation. The IP joints are placed in neutral as well. If finger flexion is very limited, PROM to the digits can be initiated. Very light activities of daily living (ADL) tasks may be completed

Table 9-3	**Protection Principles**
Respect pain	Stop activities before the point of discomfort.
	Decrease activities that cause pain that lasts more than 2 hours.
	Avoid activities that put strain on painful joints.
Balance rest and activity	Rest before exhaustion and take frequent breaks.
	Avoid activities that cannot be stopped.
	Avoid staying in one position for a long time.
	Alternate heavy and light activities.
	Take more breaks when inflammation is active.
	Allow extra time for activities—avoid rushing.
	Plan your day ahead of time.
	Eliminate unnecessary activities.
Reduce the effort	Avoid excessive loads with carts, get help, and use appliances.
	Keep items near where they are used.
	Use prepared foods; freeze leftovers for later use.
	Avoid low chairs.
	Maintain proper body weight.
	Try to eliminate trips up and down stairs by completing work on each floor.
	Sit to work when possible.
Avoid positions of deformity	Avoid bent elbows, knees, hips, and back while sleeping.
	Practice good posture during the day.
	Use workstation evaluation for proper posture.
	See text for specific hand deformities.
Use the larger joints	Slide heavy objects on kitchen counters.
	Use palms, rather than fingers, to lift or push.
	Carry a backpack, instead of a handheld purse.
	Keep packages close to the body—use two hands.
	Push swinging doors open with side of body instead of the hands.
Use adaptive equipment	Use jar openers, button hooks, etc., that are specific to each patient's needs.
Distribute pressure	Use both hands, leverage, carts, etc.

Adapted from Hunter, J. M., Maklin, E. J., Callahan, H. D., Skirven, T. M., Schneider, L. H., & Osterman, A. E. (2002). *Rehabilitation of the hand and upper extremity* (5th ed.). St Louis, MO: Mosby.

without the splint, gradually starting about 6 weeks after surgery. The client may be allowed to fold clothes for 15 minutes then return to the splint, for example. At approximately 10 weeks after surgery, the client can stop wearing the dynamic splint and begin gentle strengthening exercises. The client should continue to avoid lateral pinching, which stresses the MCP joints in ulnar deviation. The MCP joints are most stable and functional at 60 to 70 degrees of flexion after this surgery (Cannon, 2003).

Osteoarthritis (OA), unlike RA, is caused by wear and tear of the joints. Degenerative changes from overuse or trauma cause destruction of joint surfaces. This results in pain and stiffness in the joints (Burke et al., 2006). OA is more prevalent in female clients older than 50. It is commonly seen in the PIP and DIP joints of the digits, CMC joint of the thumb, cervical and lumbar spine, shoulders, knees, and hips (Riley, 1998). Figure 9-29 illustrates OA joint deformities of the hand.

Conservative treatment for clients with OA in OT is quite similar to treatment for RA clients. Clients with OA who have pain and stiffness in their hands will benefit from protection principles that include assistive devices, gentle ROM, strengthening exercises, splinting, and the use of heat or other modalities. It is important to consider the client's needs when developing a home program for clients with RA or OA. A home program should also include treatment techniques that will be easy and cost-effective to increase compliance and carryover at home. Elderly clients with arthritis can use assistive devices at home to increase their independence in leisure, self-care, and home management activities (Mann, Hurren, & Tomita, 1995). According to Mann and colleagues (1995), clients with RA and OA used reachers, magnifying glasses, grab bars, jar openers, and other assistive devices in their homes and found them to be helpful in performing ADL and instrumental ADL (IADL). The clients were instructed in the use of the assistive devices by an OT practitioner (Mann et al., 1998). Because RA and OA are chronic and progressive diseases, clients seen in any setting will benefit from protection principles prior to discharge. Appendix A provides suggestions for online references that you can share with your clients when you practice OT in the future.

The CMC joint of the thumb is the most common site for surgical reconstruction of OA in the hand and upper extremity (Hunter et al., 2002). Indications for surgery include pain or deformity that interferes with daily function. Clients who present with severe symptomatic CMC OA usually complain of pain at the base of their thumb and weakness, especially with gripping and pinching. Clients often state they can no longer open their thumbs enough to pick up a bottle or glass for drinking. Clients may also report an inability to open jars, medication bottles, or pinch their thumbs to hold a book.

When surgery is indicated, soft tissue reconstruction is performed using a tendon as the soft tissue arthroplasty. Arthroplasty is joint replacement surgery. There are a variety of different styles of soft tissue arthroplasty depending on the surgeon and the anatomy and physiologic condition

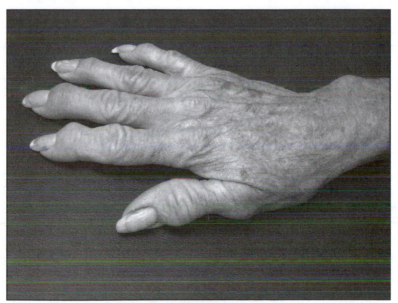

Figure 9-29. Osteoarthritis deformities of the hand.

of the client. Generally, CMC arthroplasty includes the removal of the diseased trapezium and the use of a tendon or portion of a tendon as the joint. According to Cannon (2003), the two tendons commonly harvested for this type of surgery are the flexor carpi radialis (FCR) or the abductor pollicis longus (APL). The goals of this highly successful surgery are to create a stable, pain-free joint with full function of the thumb. Gold Box 9-4 shows the basic guidelines for rehabilitation after CMC arthroplasty for OA of the CMC joint.

The information provided in this text is meant to be an introduction to some of the common problems the OTA may experience in arthritis hand and wrist treatment.

Gold Box 9-4

CMC Protocol

- A cast is applied for the initial 4 weeks to immobilize the wrist and thumb.
- After cast removal, a thumb spica splint is applied to be worn between exercise sessions and at night for protection.
- Edema, pain, and scar management techniques are used after cast removal.
- Active range of motion of the thumb and wrist is initiated at 4 weeks.
- Gentle passive range of motion is initiated at 6 weeks where joints are limited.
- Gentle gripping and pinching as well as use of the hand in light resistive ADLs is initiated at 6 to 8 weeks.
- The splint is discontinued at 6 to 8 weeks (and used as needed).
- Resistive use as tolerated is initiated at 10 to 12 weeks.
- Clients will continue to notice some discomfort, stiffness, and weakness for 6 to 12 months after this surgery.

Adapted from Cannon (2003); Weiss & Falkenstein (2005)

Repetitive Stress Injuries of the Wrist and Hand

Repetitive stress injuries (RSIs), also known as **cumulative trauma disorders** (CTDs), affect the wrist and hand more often than any other part of the body. RSI is an umbrella term that encompasses many specific conditions of the upper extremity, including lateral epicondylitis (tennis elbow), which was described in Chapter 8. Conditions limited to the wrist and hand will be discussed here, including CTS, trigger finger, de Quervain's disease, and tendonitis. OA of the CMC joint is considered an RSI as well but was covered in the previous section under arthritis.

Repetitive motion is required in many work and leisure activities. Jobs that require repetition include assemblers, mechanics, carpenters, computer programmers, and landscapers. Leisure activities such as gardening, quilting, reading, and cooking are repetitive. Factors that may increase the risk of RSI include repetitive activities, poor posture and body mechanics, an inherited predisposition to a health condition, and poor lifestyle choices (Weiss & Falkenstein, 2005). Clients cannot do anything about their inherent risk of arthritis, but they do have more control over their lifestyle choices. Making smart lifestyle changes can decrease the risk of developing or acquiring an RSI. Those changes should include no tobacco use, limiting caffeine and alcohol, and weight control, which includes a healthy diet and more aerobic exercise.

The use of communication devices such as handheld electronic devices (HEDs) is a described IADL in the *Occupational Therapy Practice Framework, 2nd Edition* (OTPF-2) and may increase the risk of an RSI. HEDs, including cell phones, BlackBerrys (Research in Motion, Waterloo, ON), computer note pads, and electronic readers require repetitive hand movements, according to the OTPF-2. The era we live in demands a fast-paced exchange of information in all areas of life, including work, leisure, and ADL. The ability to connect with coworkers, family, and friends around the world is not without its drawbacks. The use of HEDs and the repetitive hand movements required can place individuals at increased risk for developing RSIs (Amini, 2006). After briefly describing several RSIs of the wrist and hand frequently seen in OT, a discussion of preventative treatment will follow.

CTS is compression of the median nerve at the level of the wrist. It is believed to be caused by chronic tenosynovitis of the flexor tendons that run through the carpal tunnel. Chronic, progressive CTS can lead to sensory loss and motor weakness of the intrinsic muscles of the hand and consequently in a loss of hand function (Cannon, 2003). It is thought to be most common in women who perform repetitive tasks. Women have a smaller carpal tunnel and have more flexibility in their wrists than men, which increases the risk of developing CTS.

Numbness and tingling, more so at night, is the complaint that distinguishes CTS from other RSIs. Clients will complain of numbness and tingling in the median nerve distribution. Other signs and symptoms include pain, swelling, weakness in grip and pinch, and dropping objects (Novak & Mackinnon, 1997).

The good news regarding CTS is that surgical intervention can relieve the signs and symptoms. The surgeon completely releases the transverse carpal ligament, which forms the "ceiling" of the carpal tunnel. When this thickened ligament is divided, pressure on the median nerve is relieved, decreasing signs and symptoms of numbness and pain. Clients frequently recover strength and function of their hands after surgery. The client may benefit from several sessions of OT and a home exercise program. The client may complain of tenderness or "pillar pain" surrounding the small incision in the palm of the hand after surgery. There may also be weakness during gripping activities after carpal tunnel release surgery. These complaints usually resolve within 3 months after surgery.

Trigger finger is defined as pathological thickening of the sheath of the flexor tendon at or around the A1 pulley. If there is enough swelling in this area, the tendon can become locked in flexion, causing a snap with pain as the swollen tendon and sheath pulls under the pulley. A knot can be palpated at the distal palmar crease of the injured digit. The thumb is the most commonly affected digit, followed by the ring and long fingers (Weiss & Falkenstein, 2005). Clients with a history of RA or diabetes are more likely affected.

de Quervain's disease, another RSI, is tenosynovitis or inflammation of the tendon sheaths. de Quervain's disease was first named "washer woman's sprain" in 1893 and affects the APL, the EPL, and the extensor pollicis brevis (EPB) tendons. de Quervain's disease is typically caused from the combined repetitive movements of the thumb and wrist, combined with forearm rotation during resistive pinching activities. The client complains of pain along with localized tenderness and swelling over the anatomical "snuff box," which is a depression formed by the APL, EPL, and EPB, found just distal to the radial styloid. Gold Box 9-5 defines the origin of the **anatomical snuff box**.

Gold Box 9-5

Anatomical Snuff box

The **anatomical snuff box** is a small depression that is formed when the abductor pollicis brevis, the EPL, and the EPB tendons contract. The name anatomical snuff box originates from tobacco users' placing their snuff in this depression.

Floyd & Thompson (2001)

Tendonitis, as the name infers, is an irritation or inflammation of the tendons. Tendonitis is prevalent in the hand and wrist and can be a precursor to other RSIs. For example, tendonitis of the flexor tendons, which run through the carpal tunnel, can cause swelling in this small space, exerting pressure on the median nerve. This ultimately could lead to CTS. In tendonitis of the hand and wrist, microscopic tears of the tendons can occur, especially at the area where the tendon and muscle join, called the musculotendinous junction. This junction is a weaker part of the tendon-muscle complex and is more stressed during repetition and/or overuse of the hands and arms (Amini, 2006). The signs and symptoms of tendonitis are pain and swelling. The most common tendons affected are the flexor and extensor tendons of the wrist and the extensor tendons of the thumb.

Conservative treatment of RSI is always preferable to surgery, and this is where OT practitioners can make a difference through intervention. A comprehensive plan should include improving the symptoms of an existing RSI and preventing future trauma through education.

After the OT evaluation, OTAs may use physical agent modalities (PAMs) according to state licensure and the American Occupational Therapy Association (AOTA, 2008) guidelines in preparation for purposeful activity (Amini, 2006). PAMs, which include ultrasound or electrical stimulation, assist tissue healing, enhance movement, and decrease pain. PAMs also include the use of cold to reduce inflammation and pain during conservative treatment of RSIs. Splinting to rest the inflamed joints and tendon/nerve gliding exercises are also helpful in alleviating the symptoms of RSI and improving functional use of the client's upper extremities.

Client education is the key for prevention of RSIs in the future. OT practitioners possess the knowledge base to teach clients general protection principles as well as specific body mechanics and tool adaptations that can be used in home, work, and leisure activities. See Gold Box 9-6 for specific adaptations used in client education to prevent RSIs.

Gold Box 9-6

Prevention of Repetitive Stress Injuries

For healthy computer and handheld electronic device use:
- Maintain neutral wrists
- Take short, frequent rest breaks
- Stretch frequently to enhance blood flow
- Investigate the use of a cordless keyboard and mouse
- Use hands-free headsets with phone use
- Use a stylus (an inverted pencil) for tapping on miniature keyboards
- Be selective when responding to e-mails and text messages; use abbreviations

Additional prevention principles:
- Avoid a sustained grip or pinch in daily activities
- Avoid repetitive overuse of the wrist and hand in activity
- Avoid positioning the wrists in a flexed posture (fetal position) while sleeping
- Use ergonomic tools where possible (i.e., larger, cushioned handles and tool designs that avoid awkward wrist positions)
- Use vibratory diminishing devices or antivibratory gloves when using tools with high-frequency vibration

Adapted from Amini (2006); Cannon (2003); Keller, Corbett, & Nichols (1998); Weiss & Falkenstein (2005)

Table 9-4	Muscles of the Wrist
Action	**Muscles**
Wrist flexion	Flexor carpi ulnaris
	Flexor carpi radialis
Wrist extension	Extensor carpi radialis longus
	Extensor carpi radialis brevis
	Extensor carpi ulnaris
Wrist radial deviation	Flexor carpi radialis
	Extensor carpi radialis longus
Wrist ulnar deviation	Flexor carpi ulnaris
	Extensor carpi ulnaris

Adapted from Lippert, L. S. (2000). *Clinical kinesiology for physical therapist assistants* (3rd ed.). Philadelphia, PA: F. A. Davis.

BODY STRUCTURES OF THE WRIST AND HAND

The first part of this chapter introduced the amazing motions and functional input of the wrist and hand. This section will explore how all the body structures work together to produce the strong, yet intricate functions we possess through the use of our bodies, wrists, and hands. Muscles, nerves, tendons, and ligaments provide the body structures of our hands and arms and will be discussed as they relate to function.

Muscle Actions of the Wrist

The muscles that move the wrist but do not cross the hand to move the fingers and thumb will be presented first. The extrinsic muscles or the muscles that cross the wrist but have a more significant function at the thumb and fingers will be described in the next section. The six muscles that cause wrist motion are the flexor carpi ulnaris (FCU), FCR, palmaris longus (PL), extensor carpi radialis longus (ECRL), extensor carpi radialis brevis (ECRB), and the extensor carpi ulnaris (ECU). An overview of the wrist muscles can be found in Table 9-4.

The FCU is a prime mover in wrist flexion and ulnar deviation. Because of its origin at the medial epicondyle of the humerus, it is also a weak flexor of the elbow. Its distal attachment is the fifth metacarpal and the pisiform, making it the only wrist muscle with an attachment to a carpal bone (Lippert, 2000). The FCU is considered the strongest wrist flexor and is active in activities requiring a sustained power grip, such as using an ax or hammer (Rybski, 2004).

The FCR moves the wrist in flexion and radial deviation. It is not as strong as the FCU. Together with the FCU and PL, the FCR is powerful in stabilizing the wrist against resistance, especially with the forearm in supination (Floyd & Thompson, 2001).

The PL is the third wrist flexor and the weakest due to its small size and the fact that its distal attachment is the palmar fascia. The insertion on the palmar fascia does allow contribution by the PL to the production of a cupping motion of the hand (Rybski, 2004). This muscle is not present in approximately 15% to 20% of the population either unilaterally or bilaterally according to Lippert (2000).

Muscles providing extension primarily at the wrist are the ECRL, ECRB, and ECU. These muscles are the most powerful extensors. They also stabilize the wrist against resistance, particularly if the forearm is pronated. Performing the backhand in racquet sports, such as tennis, uses all of these muscles together (Floyd & Thompson, 2001).

The ECRL is a prime mover in wrist extension and radial deviation. It is a more effective wrist extensor when the elbow is also extended. The ECRB is a strong wrist extensor and works with the ECRL to extend the wrist. The ECRB also assists with wrist radial deviation. This is due to its distal attachment at the base of the third metacarpal. The attachment is close to the axis of motion for radial and ulnar deviation (Lippert, 2000).

The ECU moves the wrist in extension and ulnar deviation. According to Oatis (2004), the ECU is more effective in extending the wrist with the forearm in supination. The ECU is also a very weak elbow extensor due to the muscle's origin at the lateral epicondyle of the humerus (Floyd & Thompson, 2001).

It is important to note that of the six muscles primarily responsible for wrist movement, no single muscle moves the wrist in one plane. To produce pure wrist motions of flexion or extension and radial or ulnar deviation, pairs of muscles must contract together. For example, the FCR and the FCU are required to contract for pure wrist flexion (Oatis, 2004). Notice during a functional activity, such as using a hammer, that the wrist commonly moves in a diagonal pattern. This diagonal pattern moves from wrist extension with radial deviation to wrist flexion with ulnar deviation. These muscles appear specialized to support and move the wrist and hand in this functional, diagonal pattern.

Extrinsic Muscle Actions of the Hand

Muscles that originate in the forearm and cross the wrist to attach in the hand are called extrinsic muscles. These muscles have an assistive role in wrist function, but their primary role is the function of the fingers and thumb of the hand. The nine extrinsic muscles are the flexor digitorum superficialis (FDS), flexor digitorum profundus (FDP), flexor pollicis longus (FPL), APL, EPL, EPB, extensor digitorum communis (EDC), extensor digiti minimi (EDM), extensor indicis proprius (EIP), . An overview of these muscles and their motions can be found in Table 9-5.

The FDS muscle divides into four tendons on the palmar aspect of the wrist and hand to insert on each of the four fingers on the sides of the middle phalanx. The FDS is one of only two muscles that produce flexion of all four fingers. The FDS is vital in any type of gripping activity. It is the only muscle that can flex the PIP joints of the fingers without flexing the DIP joints. The FDS also assists in wrist flexion during finger flexion (Oatis, 2004).

The FDP is up to 50% stronger than the FDS but works with the FDS to flex all four fingers. The FDP is the only muscle that produces flexion of the DIP joints of all four fingers. It also flexes the PIP and MCP joints of the fingers and assists with wrist flexion. The FDP is the primary flexor of the fingers. The FDS is recruited to work with the FDP when additional strength is required, such as in forceful pinch and grasp (Rybski, 2004).

The FPL muscle is the prime mover of thumb flexion in all three joints, the CMC, MCP, and IP. Because of its palmar relationship to the wrist, it assists in wrist flexion. This muscle plays a vital role in pinching and gripping activities.

The APL muscle effectively abducts the thumb at the CMC joint. It forms the lateral border of the anatomical snuff box with the extensor pollicis brevis. The extensor pollicis longus forms the medial border of this landmark. Figure 9-30 illustrates the anatomical snuff box of the hand.

The EPL muscle extends the IP joint of the thumb. The EPL aids in extension of the thumb at the MCP and CMC joints. It also assists with wrist extension and radial deviation. The EPL winds around the dorsal tubercle of the distal radius, which allows it to act as a thumb adductor at the MCP and CMC joints of the thumb.

The EPB extends the thumb at the MCP joint, but because it shares a common tendon sheath with the APL, it has nearly the same actions. The EPB assists with CMC extension and wrist radial deviation. Movement of the thumb may alter its effect on wrist flexion and extension. It is one of the three snuff box muscles, forming the lateral border with the APL (Oatis, 2004).

Table 9-5	Extrinsic Muscles of the Hand and Their Movements
Muscle	**Action**
Flexor digitorum superficialis	• Finger flexion of the MCP and PIP joints • Wrist flexion
Flexor digitorum profundus	• Finger flexion of the MCP, PIP, and DIP joints • Wrist flexion
Flexor pollicis longus	• Thumb flexion of the CMC, MCP, and IP joints • Wrist flexion
Extensor digitorum communis	• Finger extension of the MCP joints • Wrist extension
Extensor digiti minimi	• Small finger extension of the MCP joints
Extensor indicis proprius	• Index finger extension of the MCP joints
Abductor pollicis longus	• Thumb abduction at the CMC joint
Extensor pollicis longus	• Thumb extension of the CMC, MCP, and IP joints • Thumb CMC adduction • Wrist extension
Extensor pollicis brevis	• Thumb extension of the MCP joint • Wrist extension

Adapted from Floyd, R. T., & Thompson, C. W. (2001). *Manual of structural kinesiology* (14th ed.). New York, NY: McGraw-Hill.

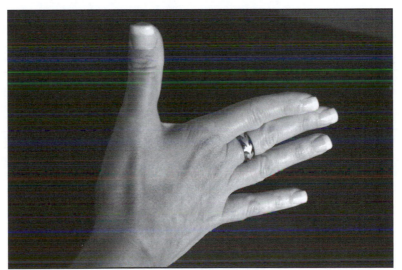

Figure 9-30. The anatomical snuff box of the hand.

The EDC muscle extends all the joints of the four fingers. It is the only common extensor muscle of the fingers. It originates at the lateral epicondyle of the humerus and passes under the extensor retinaculum at the wrist. It attaches on the distal phalanx of the fingers (Lippert, 2000). The EDC also assists with wrist extension. The extensor tendons of all four fingers are interconnected by fibrous bands at the level of the MCP joints called juncturae tendinae. These bands can impede individual finger extension; however, they provide stabilizing forces to the MCP joints while the fingers are flexed during forceful gripping (Oatis, 2004).

The EDM allows extension of the MCP joint of the small finger. The EDM is located on the ulnar side of the EDC and also acts to extend and abduct the PIP and DIP joints of the small finger due to its attachment in the extensor hood (Rybski, 2004).

The EIP allows independent extension of the MCP joint of the index finger and, due to a connection to the extensor hood, extends the PIP and DIP joints as well. The EIP is commonly titled the *pointing muscle* because it is responsible for extending the index finger, especially when the other fingers are flexed (Floyd & Thompson, 2001).

Intrinsic Muscle Actions of the Hand

The intrinsic muscles of the hand are called intrinsic because they originate and insert on the hand distal to the carpal bones. These muscles have a function on the thumb and fingers. They are also responsible for precise movements and fine motor control of the hand (Lippert, 2000). Although this text has separated the extrinsic and intrinsic muscle groups of the hand for learning purposes, it is important to understand how their function is interwoven. The hand functions by using a blended combination from the extrinsic and intrinsic groups of muscles (Oatis, 2004).

This section arranges the intrinsic muscles of the hand into four functional groups to help the student understand how the intrinsic muscles interact. The four functional groups include the thenar muscles, the hypothenar muscles, the interossei muscles, and the lumbricals. Table 9-6 presents an overview of the intrinsic muscles of the hand.

The four thenar muscles, or primary movers of the thumb, are the abductor pollicis brevis (APB), the flexor pollicis brevis (FPB), the opponens pollicis (OP), and the adductor pollicis (AP). These intrinsic muscles form the thenar eminence of the hand.

The APB acts to abduct the CMC joint of the thumb. Active abduction of the thumb is needed to position the thumb for grip or pinch. Due to the muscle being superficial, APB atrophy from median nerve palsy can lead to decreased strength in pinch and grip (Oatis, 2004).

The primary function of the FPB is to flex the MCP joint of the thumb. The FPB assists the FPL in CMC flexion only because it crosses the CMC joint. The FPB assists the APB in CMC joint abduction (Lippert, 2000).

The OP produces opposition of the CMC joint. Thumb opposition is the most important function of the hand, which probably explains why thumb movement is known to be up to 50% of hand function. The FPB and APB assist in this function because opposition is a combination of flexion, abduction, and rotation of the thumb. The OP is the second largest muscle of the thenar intrinsic group and reinforces the actions of the other thenar muscles. Weakness in the OP muscle affects positioning and stabilization of the CMC joint during pinching activities (Oatis, 2004).

The AP is the largest of the thenar muscles and adducts the CMC joint of the thumb. The AP is a deep muscle so it does not make up the bulk of the thenar eminence. It also flexes the thumb MCP joint. The AP adducts the thumb only to the palm, and then the EPL continues adduction through its full excursion (Oatis, 2004). This muscle supplies much of the force in pinch.

The **hypothenar** muscles are the intrinsic muscles of the hand that act on the small finger. They are the opponens digit minimi (ODM), abductor digit minimi (ADM), and flexor digit minimi brevis (FDMB). All the joints of the small finger are influenced by the above three muscles.

The ODM is the largest and strongest of the hypothenar muscles and opposes the small finger at the MCP joint. Opposition of the small finger contributes to the volar arch, which is formed while cupping the hand. The ADM abducts the small finger at the MCP joint and assists with MCP flexion as well. The FDMB flexes the small finger at the MCP joint. It is the smallest and weakest of the hypothenar muscles. Weakness of this muscle group could impair the intricate function of the small finger, especially in abduction. Individuals whose careers depend on finger movements,

Table 9-6	Intrinsic Muscles of the Hand and Their Movements	
Thenar Muscle Group	**Action**	
Abductor pollicis brevis	CMC abduction of the thumb	
Flexor pollicis brevis	CMC flexion and abduction	
	MCP flexion of the thumb	
Opponens pollicis	CMC opposition of the thumb	
Adductor pollicis	CMC adduction	
	MCP flexion of the thumb	
Hypothenar Muscle Group		
Opponens digiti minimi	MCP opposition of the small finger	
Abductor digiti minimi	MCP abduction of the small finger	
Flexor digiti minimi brevis	MCP flexion of the small finger	
Palmar Interossei	MCP adduction of the index, ring, and small finger	
Dorsal Interossei	MCP flexion and abduction	
	PIP/DIP extension of the index, long, and ring fingers	
	MCP adduction of the long finger	
Lumbricals	MCP flexion and PIP/DIP extension of the index, long, ring, and small fingers	

Adapted from Floyd, R. T., & Thompson, C. W. (2001). *Manual of structural kinesiology* (14th ed.). New York, NY: McGraw-Hill.

such as computer programmers or musicians, may be more negatively affected by hypothenar muscle weakness (Oatis, 2004).

The **palmar interossei** adduct the MCP joints of the index, ring, and small fingers to the long finger (Hunter et al., 2002). With the long finger as a central axis of the hand, the **dorsal interossei** muscles abduct the fingers. There are four palmar interossei muscles and four dorsal interossei muscles. If the client presents with weakness in the interossei muscles, he or she will not be able to completely spread the fingers or bring them tightly together. The client may also present with weakness in functional grip and pinch.

The **lumbrical** muscles are the last of the intrinsic muscles discussed. There are four lumbrical muscles located deep within the hand. The lumbrical muscles are unique because they have no bony attachments in the hand. They attach proximally to the tendons of the FDP and distally to the tendons of the EDC, which are antagonists (Oatis, 2004). The lumbricals flex the MCP joints and extend the PIP and DIP joints of all four fingers. This combined motion is called the "intrinsic plus" position (Lippert, 2000). If the intrinsic musculature is weakened due to an ulnar nerve injury, a "claw hand" deformity or "intrinsic minus" position can occur, negatively affecting hand function. The intrinsic plus position is the ultimate hand position for healing after injury because it maintains MCP joint flexion and a good hand posture for recovery of function. A good example of functional intrinsic plus hand posture is seen while an individual is holding a book by the binding. Figures 9-31 and 9-32 illustrate the functional intrinsic plus position and the claw hand deformity.

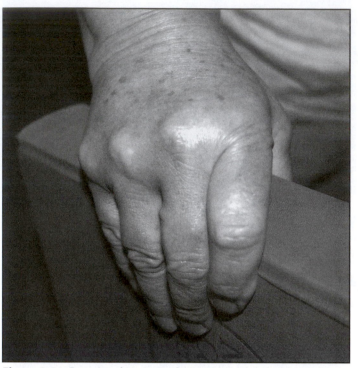

Figure 9-31. Functional intrinsic plus position while holding a book.

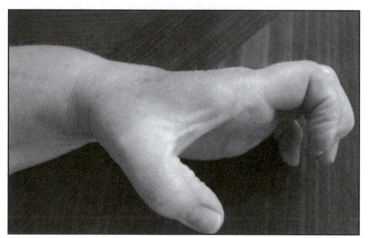

Figure 9-32. Claw hand deformity or intrinsic minus position.

Muscles, Nerves, and Spinal Cord Levels of the Wrist and Hand

Nerve roots C6, C7, C8, and T1 supply the joints and muscles of the wrist and hand. They form the peripheral nerves that innervate the wrist and hand, which are the radial, median, and ulnar nerves. Innervations of the wrist and hand are fairly direct with a few exceptions. Muscles on the posterior surface are mostly innervated by the radial nerve. Muscles on the thumb side are primarily supplied by the median nerve, except the AP, which is the only thumb muscle innervated by the ulnar nerve. Muscles on the ulnar side of the hand are supplied by the ulnar nerve. The FDP and the lumbrical muscles receive their innervations from both the ulnar and median nerves. This is not surprising because the lumbricals have a proximal attachment on the tendons of the FDP muscle (Lippert, 2000). Tables 9-7, 9-8, and 9-9 summarize the motions and innervations of the wrist and hand.

Sensation is extremely important to hand function. If an individual does not have intact sensation in his or her hand, he or she must compensate using vision, just as a person who is blind must use the sense of touch. Without intact sensory input, it would be impossible to tell what you are holding in your hand and how much force to use so as not to drop the item if you could not see. Sensory input can also help protect your hands from injury. Examples would be while using tools such as a knife or while working on or near a hot stove. Hand sensation is supplied by the median, radial, and ulnar nerves. Figure 9-33 illustrates the pattern of sensory distribution of the nerves of the hand.

The median nerve is known as the "nerve of function" to the hand. The median nerve gives sensation to the volar surface of the thumb, index, and long fingers and innervates the flexors of the thumb and fingers. It is easy to see that injury to the median nerve would become a functional challenge. Recall Laura in this chapter's occupational profile. She presented with deficits from her injury, but she also complained of numbness and tingling in the median nerve distribution of her injured hand. She presented with stiffness, pain, swelling, and weakness in her dominant wrist and hand. These signs and symptoms appeared to be limiting her function. Could the loss of sensation contribute to her ability to perform ADL and IADL?

Tendons and Ligaments of the Wrist and Hand

Tendons

The extrinsic tendons of the hand are more susceptible to inflammation due to their length from the musculotendinous junction to distal insertion and to the space limitations at the wrist. For example, the FDS, FDP, FCR, and FPL tendons all pass through the carpal tunnel. The tendons of the FDS and FDP share a common synovial sheath as well (Hertling & Kessler, 2006). The flexor

Table 9-7	**Motions and Innervations of the Wrist**								
		Nerve Root				Wrist Flexion 0 to 60 degrees	Wrist Extension 0 to 60 degrees	Radial Deviation 0 to 20 degrees	Ulnar Deviation 0 to 30 degrees
Muscle	Nerve	C6	C7	C8	T1				
Extensor carpi radialis longus	Radial	x	x				x	x	
Extensor carpi radialis brevis	Radial	x	x				x		
Extensor carpi ulnaris	Radial	x	x	x			x		x
Flexor carpi radialis	Median	x	x			x		x	
Palmaris longus	Median	x	x			x			
Flexor carpi ulnaris	Ulnar			x	x	x			x

Adapted from American Medical Association. (2008). *Guides to the evaluation of permanent impairment* (6th ed.). Chicago: Author.; Lippert, L. S. (2000). *Clinical kinesiology for physical therapist assistants* (3rd ed.). Philadelphia, PA: F. A. Davis.

Table 9-8 Motions and Innervations of the Thumb

Muscle	Nerve	Spinal Nerve Root				Thumb				
		C6	C7	C8	T1	Flexion* CMC (Palmar Abduction): 0 to 50 degrees MCP: 0 to 60 degrees IP: 0 to 80 degrees	Extension* CMC (Radial Abduction): 0 to 20 degrees MCP 60 to 0 degrees IP 80 to 0 degrees	Abduction: CMC 0 to 50 degrees	Adduction: CMC 50 to 0 degrees	Opposition CMC Measured in Centimeters Lacking
Extensor pollicis longus	Radial	x	x	x			x			
Extensor pollicis brevis	Radial	x	x				x			
Abductor pollicis longus	Radial	x	x					x		
Flexor pollicis longus	Median			x	x	x				
Flexor pollicis brevis	Median	x	x			x				
Abductor pollicis brevis	Median	x	x					x		
Opponens pollicis	Median	x	x							x
Adductor pollicis	Ulnar			x	x				x	

* Some muscles do not have actions at all joints listed in the category. For example, the FPB does not act at the IP joint as it inserts proximal to this joint.

Adapted from American Medical Association. (2008). *Guides to the evaluation of permanent impairment* (6th ed.). Chicago, IL: Author.; Lippert, L. S. (2000). *Clinical kinesiology for physical therapist assistants* (3rd ed.). Philadelphia, PA: F. A. Davis.

Table 9-9 Motions and Innervations of the Fingers

Muscle	Nerve	C6	C7	C8	T1	Flexion MCP: +20 to 90 degrees PIP: 0 to 100 degrees DIP: 0 to 70 degrees	Extension MCP: 90 to +20 degrees PIP: 100 to 0 degrees DIP: 70 to 0 degrees	Abduction MCP: 0 to 25 degrees	Adduction MCP: 25 to 0 degrees	Opposition Small finger Not Tested
Extensor digitorum communis	Radial	x	x	x			x			
Extensor indicis	Radial		x	x			x			
Extensor digiti minimi	Radial	x	x	x			x			
Flexor digitorum superficialis	Median		x	x	x	x				
Flexor digitorum profundus	Median and ulnar			x	x	x				
Lumbricals 1 and 2	Median	x	x			x (MCP)	x (DIP, PIP)			
Lumbricals 3 and 4	Ulnar			x	x	x (MCP)	x (DIP, PIP)			
Flexor digit minimi	Ulnar			x	x	x				
Abductor digiti minimi	Ulnar			x	x			x		
Opponens digit minimi	Ulnar			x	x					x
Dorsal interossei	Ulnar			x	x			x		
Palmar interossei	Ulnar			x	x				x	

Adapted from American Medical Association. (2008). *Guides to the evaluation of permanent impairment* (6th ed.). Chicago., IL Author.; Lippert, L. S. (2000). *Clinical kinesiology for physical therapist assistants* (3rd ed.). Philadelphia, PA: F. A. Davis.

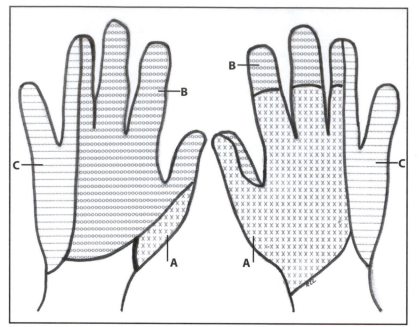

Figure 9-33. Pattern of sensory distribution of nerves in the hand. Key: (A) radial nerve = X; (B) median nerve = o; and (C) ulnar nerve = ~ (Reprinted with permission of Ruby Lowe.)

tendons of the fingers and thumb, as well as the palm of the hand, are protected their entire length by these sheaths that are lined with synovial fluid. This is to provide protection from impact, as well as repetitive movement, during the functional use of daily gripping and pinching.

The flexor tendons are held down at the fingers by annular, oblique, and cruciate fibers called pulleys, which prevent bowstringing of the tendons during composite finger flexion and gripping. The flexor tendons are cordlike in shape, which adds to their strength. In comparison, the extensor tendons are flatter and weaker and do not have synovial sheaths. The extensor tendons of the fingers and thumb do not have to work against resistance so they require less strength. Both the extensor and flexor tendons of the hands are prone to laceration because the tendons are superficial and are exposed to many dangers as the hands perform their duties. If an individual completely lacerates a tendon in his or her thumb or fingers, it will have to be surgically repaired to regain function. There will be a time of immobilization to allow healing, then rehabilitation to regain ROM and strength for return to functional use. To learn more about tendon repairs of the hand and OT treatment, see E-hand Web site in Appendix A.

Ligaments

The ligaments of the wrist can be divided into two large categories, extrinsic and intrinsic. Please refer to Table 9-10, which illustrates the ligaments of the wrist and their functions.

The extrinsic ligaments consist of the palmar radiocarpal ligament, the dorsal radiocarpal ligament, the ulnar collateral ligament, the radial collateral ligament, and the ulnocarpal complex. The palmar radiocarpal ligament is a tough, thick ligament that limits wrist extension. It attaches from the radius to the scaphoid, lunate, and triquetrum. Because most activities require wrist extension, this ligament is more likely to be sprained or stretched (Lippert, 2000). The dorsal radiocarpal ligament attaches to the same structures as the palmar radiocarpal ligament does but on the posterior surface. It limits the amount of flexion at the wrist. This ligament is not as strong as its counterpart.

Table 9-10	Ligaments of the Wrist and Their Function	
Extrinsic Ligaments	**Function**	
Palmar radiocarpal	Volarly stabilizes radius to carpal bones; limits excessive wrist extension	
Dorsal radiocarpal	Dorsally stabilizes radius to carpal bones; limits excessive wrist flexion	
Ulnar collateral	Provides lateral stability of ulnar side of wrist between ulna and carpals	
Radial collateral	Provides lateral stability of radial side of wrist between radius and carpals	
Ulnocarpal complex and articular disk (or triangular fibrocartilage complex)	Stabilizes and helps glide the ulnar side of wrist; stabilizes distal radioulnar joint	
Intrinsic Ligaments		
Palmar midcarpal	Forms and stabilizes the proximal and distal rows of carpal bones	
Dorsal midcarpal	Forms and stabilizes the proximal and distal rows of carpal bones	
Interosseous	Intervenes between each carpal bone contained within its proximal or distal row	
Accessory Ligament		
Transverse carpal	Stabilizes carpal arch and contents of the carpal tunnel	

Adapted from Hertling, D., & Kessler, R. (2006). *Management of common musculoskeletal disorders: Physical therapy principles and methods.* Philadelphia, PA: Lippincott, Williams & Wilkins.; Oatis, C. A. (2004). *Kinesiology: The mechanics and pathomechanics of human movement.* Philadelphia, PA: Lippincott, Williams & Wilkins.; Weiss, S., & Falkenstein, N. (2005). *Hand rehabilitation: A quick reference guide and review.* St. Louis, MO: Mosby Elsevier.

The radial and ulnar collateral ligaments provide lateral and medial support, respectively, to the wrist joint. The ulnocarpal complex is more likely to be referred to as the triangular fibrocartilage complex (TFCC) and includes the articular disk of the wrist. The TFCC is the major stabilizer of the distal radioulnar joint (DRUJ) and can tear after direct compressive force such as a fall on an outstretched hand. It is often seen in conjunction with a distal radius fracture. The client will complain of ulnar wrist pain with forearm rotation, ulnar deviation, and gripping (Weiss & Falkenstein, 2005). The articular disk is found at the distal end of the ulna where it articulates with the triquetrum and lunate. It functions as a shock absorber and spacer, filling the gap created between the ulna and the carpal bones. The gap occurs because the ulna does not extend as far distally as the radius (Lippert, 2000).

The intrinsic ligaments of the wrist include the palmar and dorsal midcarpal ligaments and the interosseous ligaments. The palmar and dorsal midcarpal ligaments form and stabilize the proximal and distal rows of the carpal bones. The interosseous ligaments stabilize the individual carpal bones to each other within their proximal or distal row. Like the extrinsic ligaments, the palmar midcarpal ligaments are stronger than the dorsal. The interosseous ligaments are considered the strongest in the wrist but are less rigid, which may allow larger loads of force to be sustained when falling on an outstretched arm. Despite the protective mechanical properties of the ligaments of the wrist, numerous sprains are reported (Oatis, 2004).

The transverse carpal ligament, or flexor retinaculum, supports the carpal arch, creating the carpal tunnel. It attaches medially on the pisiform and the hook of the hamate and laterally on the tubercles of the trapezium and scaphoid (Oatis, 2004).

The ligaments of the hand will be limited to discussion of the CMC and MCP joints of the thumb. A brief general description of the ligaments of the IP joints of the thumb and fingers and their main functions will follow. Finally, the fascia and arches of the hand will be described because these are important body structures with regard to function.

Providing support at the CMC joint of the thumb are the radial, dorsal, and volar oblique ligaments. These ligaments stabilize the CMC joint but also play a role in guiding the movement of the CMC joint. The pull of the oblique ligaments rotates the metacarpal during flexion/abduction and extension/adduction of the thumb (Oatis, 2004). The ligaments of the MCP joints of the thumb and fingers consist of collateral ligaments, which are thick bands running obliquely from the metacarpal to the proximal phalanges and the volar plate. The volar plate consists of fibrous connective tissue and fibrocartilage and limits hyperextension. The collateral ligaments protect the joints against radial and ulnar movement (Oatis, 2004). The ulnar collateral ligament of the thumb MCP joint is prone to strain or rupture when an individual falls on the hand, forcing the thumb into abduction. This injury is commonly called "skier's thumb" and can be treated with splinting of the MCP joint of the thumb. If the ligament is completely ruptured, it will require surgical repair and immobilization (Weiss & Falkenstein, 2005).

The ligaments of the IP joint of the thumb and the PIP and DIP joints of the fingers are quite similar. They consist of collateral ligaments and a volar plate. They also have a fan-shaped accessory ligament that attaches to the proximal portion of the volar plate. The collateral ligaments provide stabilization of the joints from the radioulnar direction throughout flexion and extension excursion. The accessory ligaments provide additional support to the joints, especially when the distal joints of the thumb and fingers are extended. The interphalangeal joints also receive stability from the surrounding tendons and their related connective tissue structures (Oatis, 2004).

In the hand, the connective tissue or fascia is quite different on the dorsum or the back of the hand than the palm. Dorsally, the fascia is loose, thin, and mobile, leaving it prone to avulsion injury and/or an accumulation of edema. The palmar fascia, often called the palmar aponeuroses, is deep, thick, and fibrous. The palmar aponeuroses fibers are oriented in many different directions including vertical, longitudinal, transverse, and oblique (Hunter et al., 2002). This thick and varied fascia stabilizes the skin to underlying structures and provides protection, more so during resistive grasping activities (Oatis, 2004).

When the hand is relaxed, the palm forms a cupped position. This posture is maintained by the skeleton and the ligaments. There are three arches that form this cupped shape. The first arch is the proximal transverse arch that is formed by the base of the metacarpals and the carpal bones and is maintained by the flexor retinaculum. The distal transverse arch is formed by the metacarpal heads. The longitudinal arch runs from the wrist to the length of the fingers (Lippert, 2000). Figure 9-34 illustrates the functional arches of the hand.

Summary

The two preceding chapters discussed the structure and function of the shoulder and elbow. The resulting functional relevance for both of these joint complexes, along with the wrist, is to position the hand. The mobility of the shoulder creates an immense space through which the hand can be moved. The elbow is much less mobile but stabilizes the hand along with the forearm and wrist for a variety of functional tasks. The hand carries out the performance of the upper extremity, including reaching nearly all parts of the body. Hand function shows variety and diversity, gentleness and strength, precision and emotion. This diversity requires structural complexity with a comparative ease of performance. If there is no pathology, there is complete synergy among the structures of the wrist and hand, which allows efficient completion of functional activities.

Figure 9-34. Functional arches of the hand and wrist. (A) The top, curved horizontal line is the longitudinal arch. (B) The proximal half circle is the proximal transverse arch. (C) The distal half circle is the distal transverse arch. (Reprinted with permission of Angela Hartman.)

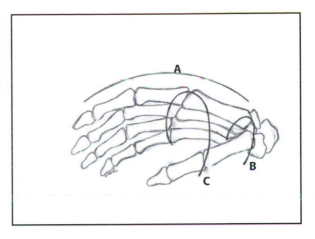

Through Laura, this chapter has explored how the wrist and hand move, grasp, and pinch. Knowledge of the normal wrist and hand and their supporting structures is necessary to understand the injuries and diseases that can affect them. Restoration of function is the objective of OT treatment. Effective wrist and hand function is a direct and critical link to independence.

APPLICATIONS

The following activities will help you apply knowledge of the wrist and hand in real-life applications. Activities can be completed individually or in a small group to enhance learning.

1. **Joints and Motions of the Wrist and Hand:** Complete the following activities to increase your familiarity with the functional aspects and movements of the wrist and hand.
    A. Locate and palpate the following landmarks on yourself or a partner:
        -   Radial styloid process
        -   Ulnar styloid process
        -   Hook of hamate
        -   Thenar eminence
        -   Hypothenar eminence
        -   Anatomical snuff box
    B. Identify all motions of the wrist and hand during the following functional activities:
        Button a shirt: _____
        Text using a cell phone: _____
        Remove a textbook from a backpack: _____
        Remove a glass from an overhead cupboard: _____
        Cut a piece of food using a knife and fork: _____
        Brush your teeth with a manual toothbrush: _____
    C. The PL is a small muscle that assists with wrist flexion. It is absent in approximately 15% to 20% of the population. The PL tendon is superficial and can be found in the volar distal forearm. Find and palpate the PL tendon in yourself and your partner. Is it present in you and your partner? What motions of the wrist and hand make the tendon more prominent?
    D. Demonstrate how the thumb and fingers work individually. First, produce the American Sign Language sign for "I love you" by following the steps below:
        a. Fully extend the index and small fingers
        b. Flex the long and ring fingers
        c. Radially abduct the thumb
        d. Move the wrist from radial to ulnar deviation

Did one hand seem easier than the other? Do you know why you cannot flex the DIP joints of the long and ring fingers?

Second, lace the fingers together, and supinate the forearms. Twiddle the thumbs in isolation from the fingers, rotate thumbs away from your body, and then rotate thumbs toward your body.

E.   Reliable and useful landmarks in the hand are skin creases. They are more prominent on the palmar surface and change during movement. The creases are valuable to the OT practitioner during observation, evaluation, and especially during splint fabrication. Observe and identify the following creases found in the palm of your hand:
- Thenar
- Distal palmar
- Proximal palmar
- Proximal phalangeal
- Distal phalangeal

F.   The arches of the hand are formed by bones and ligaments in the wrist and hand. Intrinsic muscles and the nerves that innervate them help to hold objects in the hand by means of cupping the palm. With the forearm supinated and the hand cupped, place small objects in your palm. Try vitamins, coins, dried beans, or marbles. Now, without closing your fingers around the objects, shake your arm and hand side to side. How many small objects can you and your partner hold in the "cup" of your hand without dropping them?

2.   **Strength and Dexterity of the Wrist and Hand:** Complete the following activities to familiarize yourself with functional stability, grip, and prehension of the wrist and hand.

A.   Perform push-ups using several different styles. Which style feels easier or more difficult? See how many you or your partner can perform of each style:
   a.   Palms flat on floor, forearms pronated
   b.   Weight bearing on fingertips
   c.   Hands in a fist, weight bearing on knuckles
   d.   Palms flat, forearms in mid-position

B.   Many clients you treat as an OTA will have lower extremity (LE) deficits that will require them to use an assistive device to ambulate. Demonstrate the use of the wrists and hands during the following:
- Ambulate using a standard or quad cane
- Ambulate using a standard walker with left LE weight bearing only
- Ambulate using crutches with no weight bearing through the LE bilaterally
- Propel yourself using a manual wheelchair

C.   Note how the ring and small fingers are inactive while the thumb, index, and middle fingers perform skilled activities during the following:
- Cut with scissors
- Write with a pen
- Snap your fingers
- Seal a sandwich bag

D.   Demonstrate the precision of the thumb and fingertips during the following:
- Thread a needle
- Hold a dime between the thumb, index, and middle fingers flipping it from heads to tails and back
- Continue to hold the dime as above, tails up, now rotate it to read the words

E.   As OT practitioners, you will educate clients in protection principles. Participate in the following, noting which task was easier on your hands:

    a.   Hold a bag of groceries with your fingers and your elbow extended next to your side; now place the handles over your forearm with your elbow bent to 90 degrees.

    b.   Carry a pillow by pinching it between your thumb and fingers, your elbow extended, arm to your side; now carry the pillow under your arm.

    c.   Carry a filled coffee mug in your hand using the handle; now, carry it with both hands, avoiding the handle.

    d.   Write using a ballpoint pen; now write using a gel pin with a built-in rubber grip.

    e.   Open a door with a round doorknob; now open a door with a lever-type handle.

3.   **Goniometric Measurements of the Wrist and Hand:** ROM norms can vary depending on the reference source. One norm is provided for each motion within this text to increase ease of applications. Additionally, while multiple muscles may influence a particular motion, only the main muscles responsible for a joint motion are included. References for the following information can be found in Gold Box 9-7. With your partner, practice using a goniometer to measure each motion available at the joints of the wrist and hand. You may record the available ROM in Table 9-11.

    A.   **Wrist Flexion ROM**

        a.   Goniometric landmark: Medial aspect of the ulnar styloid process

            Stable arm: Midline of ulna

            Moving arm: Midline of fifth metacarpal

        b.   Available ROM: 0 to 60 degrees

        c.   End feel: Firm

        d.   Muscles responsible: FCR, PL, FCU

        e.   Start and end position: Figure 9-35 displays the start position for wrist flexion and extension. The client is seated with the elbow resting on a table. The fingers are relaxed or extended. Bend the wrist down or into maximum flexion. Figure 9-36 displays the end position of ROM testing.

    B.   **Wrist Extension ROM**

        a.   Goniometric landmark: Medial aspect of the ulnar styloid process

            Stable arm: Midline of ulna

            Moving arm: Midline of fifth metacarpal

        b.   Available ROM: 0 to 60 degrees

        c.   End feel: Firm

        d.   Muscles responsible: ECRL, ECRB, ECU

Gold Box 9-7

Sections Referenced (a to e)	References for Range of Motion and Manual Muscle Testing
Goniometric landmark, end feel, and start and end position	Latella & Meriano (2003)
	Pendleton & Schultz-Krohn (2006)
Muscles responsible	Floyd, Floyd & Thompson (2001)
	Oatis (2004)
Available ROM	American Medical Association (2008)

Table 9-11	Range of Motion Application Table		
Joint	**Motions**	**Available ROM (degrees)**	**ROM of your partner**
Wrist	Flexion	0 to 60	
	Extension	0 to 60	
	Radial deviation	0 to 20	
	Ulnar deviation	0 to 30	
Finger MCP	Flexion	0 to 90	
	Extension	90 to 0	
	Hyperextension	0 to 20	
	Abduction	0 to 25	
	Adduction	25 to 0	
Finger PIP	Flexion	0 to 100	
	Extension	100 to 0	
Finger DIP	Flexion	0 to 70	
	Extension	70 to 0	
Thumb MCP	Flexion	0 to 60	
	Extension	60 to 0	
Thumb IP	Flexion	0 to 80	
	Extension	80 to 0	
Thumb CMC	Radial abduction (Extension)	0 to 20	
	Palmar abduction	0 to 50	
	Adduction	50 to 0	
	Opposition	Measured in centimeters lacking	

Adapted from American Medical Association. (2008). *Guides to the evaluation of permanent impairment* (6th ed.). Chicago, IL: Author.

  e. Start and End Position: Figure 9-35 displays the start position for wrist extension. The client is seated with the elbow resting on a table. Bend the wrist back or into maximum extension. Figure 9-37 displays the end position of ROM testing.

C. **Wrist Radial Deviation ROM**

  a. Goniometric landmark: Base of third metacarpal over the capitate

    Stable arm: Midline of forearm

    Moving arm: Midline of third metacarpal

  b. Available ROM: 0-20 degrees

  c. End feel: Firm

  d. Muscles responsible: ECRL, FCR

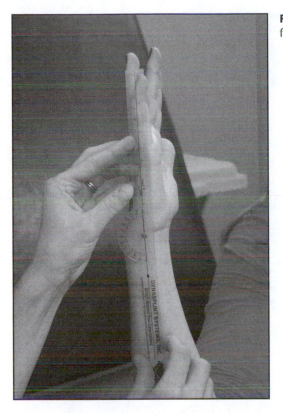

Figure 9-35. Start position for ROM testing of wrist flexion and extension.

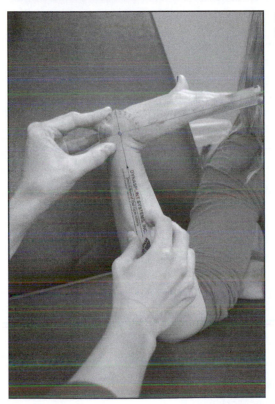

Figure 9-36. End position for ROM testing of wrist flexion.

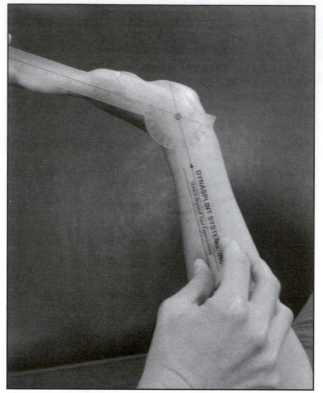

Figure 9-37. End position for ROM testing of wrist extension.

e.   Start and end position: Figure 9-38 displays the start position for radial and ulnar deviation. The client is seated with the arm pronated and resting on a table, wrist neutral and palm flat. Bend the wrist toward the thumb side or into maximum radial deviation. Figure 9-39 displays the end position of ROM testing.

D.   **Wrist Ulnar Deviation ROM**
    a.   Goniometric landmark: Base of third metacarpal over capitate
             Stable arm: Midline of forearm
             Moving arm: Midline of third metacarpal
    b.   Available ROM: 0 to 30 degrees
    c.   End feel: Firm
    d.   Muscles responsible: ECU, FCU
    e.   Start and end position: Refer to Figure 9-38 for the start position. Client is seated with arm pronated and resting on a table, wrist in neutral, and palm flat. Bend wrist toward the small finger side or into maximum ulnar deviation. Figure 9-40 displays the end position of ROM testing.

E.   **Finger MCP Flexion ROM**
    a.   Goniometric landmark: Dorsal surface of the MCP joint of the finger
             Stable arm: Midline of dorsal surface of finger metacarpal
             Moving arm: Midline of dorsal surface of proximal phalanx of finger
    b.   Available ROM: 0 to 90 degrees

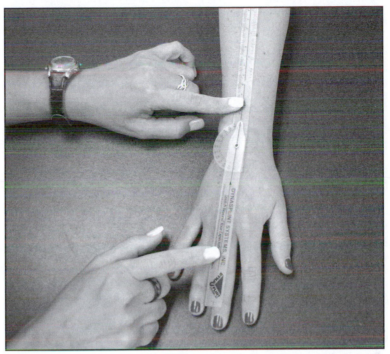

Figure 9-38. Start position for ROM testing of wrist radial and ulnar deviation.

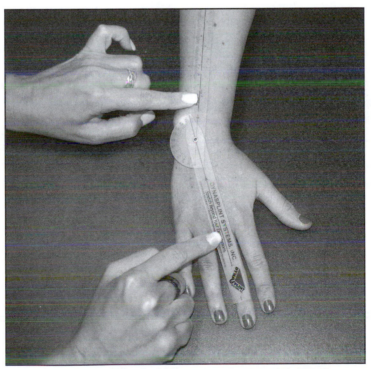

Figure 9-39. End position for ROM testing of wrist radial deviation.

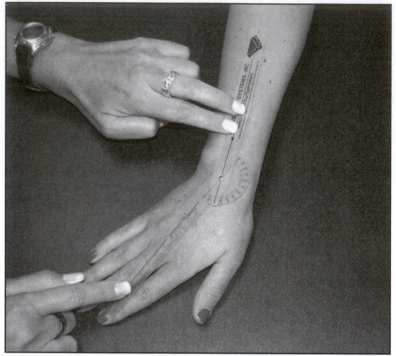

Figure 9-40. End position for ROM testing of wrist ulnar deviation.

    c.   End feel: Firm
    d.   Muscles responsible: FDS, FDP, lumbricals
    e.   Start and end position: Figure 9-41 displays the start position for finger MCP flexion. The client is seated with the arm resting on a table on the ulnar border with the wrist in neutral and the MCP joints straight. The client bends the MCP joint into maximum flexion. Figure 9-42 displays the end position of ROM testing.

        Note: Because MCP extension is simply a return from MCP flexion, the start position for MCP flexion will be the same as the end position for MCP extension. Similarly, the start position for MCP extension will be the same as the end position for MCP flexion. See Figures 9-41 and 9-42.

F.   **Finger MCP Extension ROM**
    a.   Goniometric landmark: Dorsal surface of the MCP joint of the finger
        Stable arm: Midline of dorsal surface of metacarpal of finger
        Moving arm: Midline of dorsal surface of proximal phalanx of finger
    b.   Available ROM: 90 to 0 degrees
    c.   End feel: Firm
    d.   Muscles responsible: EDC, extensor indicis, EDM, lumbricals
    e.   Start and end position: See Figure 9-42 for start position. The client is seated with the arm resting on a table on the ulnar border with the wrist in neutral and the MCP joints flexed. The client straightens or moves the MCPs into maximum extension as in Figure 9-41 or end position.

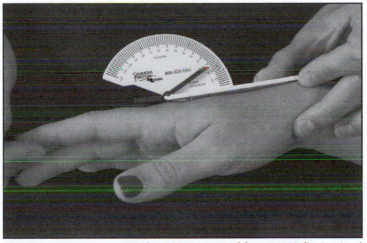

Figure 9-41. Start position for ROM testing of finger MCP flexion/end position for finger MCP extension.

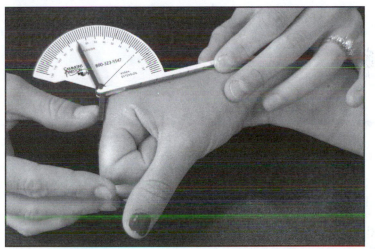

Figure 9-42. End position for ROM testing of finger MCP flexion/start position for finger MCP extension.

G. **Finger MCP Hyperextension ROM**

    a.   Goniometric landmark: Dorsal surface of the MCP joint of the finger

                Stable arm: Midline of dorsal surface of finger metacarpal

                Moving arm: Midline of dorsal surface of proximal phalanx of finger

    b.   Available ROM: 0 to 20 degrees

    c.   End feel: Firm

    d.   Muscles responsible: EDC, extensor indicis, EDM, lumbricals

    e.   Start and end position: Figure 9-43 displays the start position for finger MCP hyperextension. The client is seated with the arm resting on a table on the ulnar border with the wrist in neutral and MCP joints straight. The client extends or moves the MCP joints into maximum hyperextension. Figure 9-44 displays the end position of ROM testing.

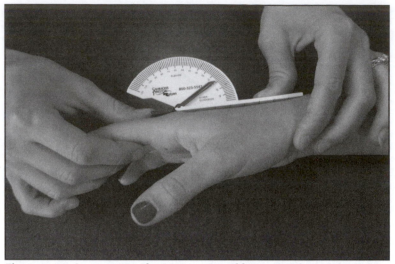

Figure 9-43. Start position for ROM testing of finger MCP hyperextension.

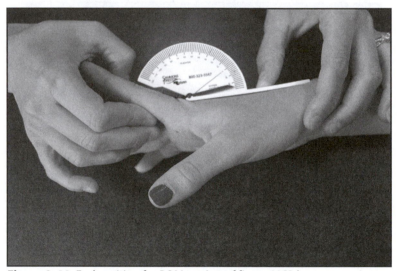

Figure 9-44. End position for ROM testing of finger MCP hyperextension.

H.   **Finger MCP Abduction ROM**
     a.   Goniometric landmark: Dorsal aspect of the MCP joint of the finger
              Stable arm: Dorsal and parallel to the corresponding metacarpal
              Moving arm: Dorsal and parallel to the proximal phalanx
     b.   Available ROM: 0 to 25 degrees
     c.   End feel: Firm
     d.   Muscles responsible: ADM, dorsal and palmar interossei
     e.   Start and end position: Figure 9-45 displays the start position for finger MCP abduction. The client is seated with the arm resting on a table with the forearm pronated, wrist neutral, palm flat, and the MCP joints adducted. The client moves the fingers into maximum MCP abduction. Figure 9-46 displays the end position of ROM testing.

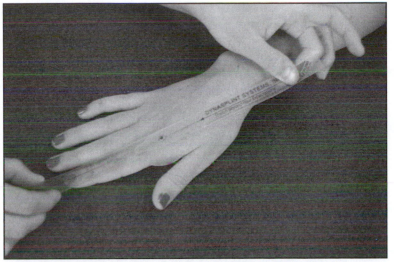

Figure 9-45. Start position for ROM testing of finger MCP abduction.

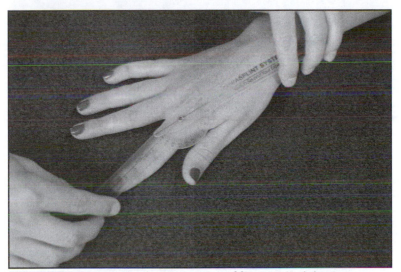

Figure 9-46. End position for ROM testing of finger MCP abduction.

I. **Finger PIP Joint Flexion ROM**
    a.   Goniometric landmark: Dorsal surface of the PIP joint of finger tested
                Stable Arm: Dorsal and midline of proximal phalanx of the finger
                Moving Arm: Dorsal and midline of the middle phalanx of the finger
    b.   Available ROM: 0 to 100 degrees
    c.   End Feel: Firm
    d.   Muscles Responsible: FDS, FDP, lumbricals
    e.   Start and end position: Figure 9-47 displays the start position for PIP flexion. The client is seated with the arm resting on a table on the ulnar border, with the forearm and wrist in neutral and the PIP joints straight. The client bends or moves the PIP joints into maximum flexion. Figure 9-48 displays the end position of ROM testing.

Note: Because PIP extension is simply a return from PIP flexion, the start position for PIP flexion will be the same as the end position for PIP extension. Similarly, the start position for PIP extension will be the same as the end position for PIP flexion (see Figures 9-47 and 9-48).

J. **Finger PIP Joint Extension ROM**

    a. Goniometric landmark: Dorsal surface of the PIP joint of finger tested

        Stable arm: Dorsal and midline of proximal phalanx of the finger

        Moving arm: Dorsal and midline of the middle phalanx of the finger

    b. Available ROM: 100 to 0 degrees

    c. End feel: Firm

    d. Muscles responsible: EDC, extensor indicis, EDM, lumbricals

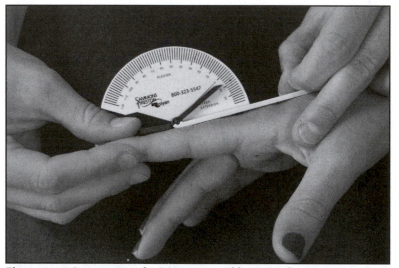

Figure 9-47. Start position for ROM testing of finger PIP flexion/end position for finger PIP extension.

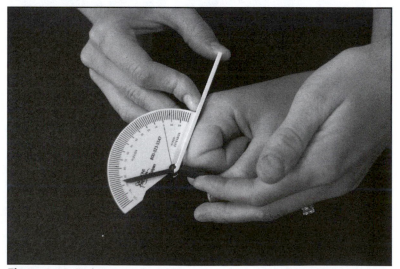

Figure 9-48. End position for ROM testing of finger PIP flexion/start position for finger PIP extension.

e. Start and end position: See Figure 9-48 for start position. The client is seated with the arm resting on a table on the ulnar border, with the forearm and wrist in neutral and the PIP joints flexed. The client straightens or moves the PIP joints into maximum extension as in Figure 9-47 or the end position.

K. Finger DIP Joint Flexion ROM

  a. Goniometric landmark: Dorsal surface of the DIP joint of finger tested

      Stable arm: Dorsal and midline of the middle phalanx of finger tested

      Moving arm: Dorsal and midline of distal phalanx of finger tested

  b. Available ROM: 0 to 70 degrees

  c. End feel: Firm

  d. Muscles responsible: FDP

  e. Start and end position: Figure 9-49 displays the start position for DIP flexion. The client is seated with the arm resting on a table on the ulnar border, with the forearm and wrist in neutral and DIP joints straight. The client bends or moves the DIP joints into maximum flexion. Figure 9-50 displays the end position of ROM testing.

    Note: Because DIP extension is simply a return from DIP flexion, the start position for DIP flexion will be the same as the end position for DIP extension. Similarly, the start position for DIP extension will be the same as the end position for DIP flexion (see Figures 9-49 and 9-50).

L. Finger DIP Joint Extension ROM

  a. Goniometric landmark: Dorsal surface of the DIP joint of finger tested

      Stable arm: Dorsal and midline of the middle phalanx of finger tested

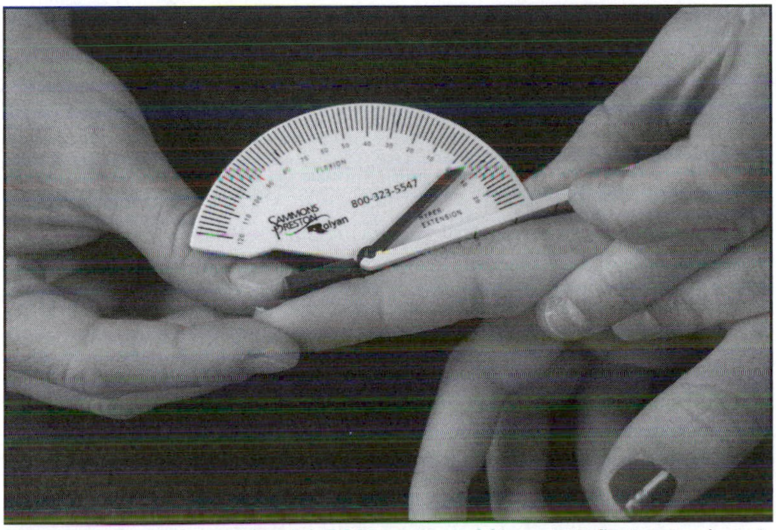

Figure 9-49. Start position for ROM testing of finger DIP flexion/end position for finger DIP extension.

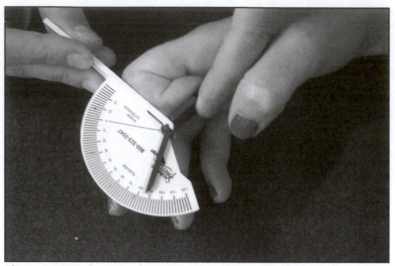

Figure 9-50. End position for ROM testing of finger DIP flexion/start position for finger DIP extension.

Moving arm: Dorsal and midline of distal phalanx of finger tested

b.   Available ROM: 70 to 0 degrees

c.   End feel: Firm

d.   Muscles responsible: EDC, extensor indicis, EDM

e.   Start and end position: See Figure 9-50 for start position. The client is seated with the arm resting on a table on the ulnar border, with the forearm and wrist in neutral, and the DIP joints flexed. The client straightens or moves the DIP joints into maximum extension or the end position as in Figure 9-49.

M.   **Thumb MCP Joint Flexion ROM**

a.   Goniometric landmark: Dorsal surface of the thumb MCP joint

Stable arm: Midline dorsal surface of the thumb MCP joint

Moving arm: Midline dorsal surface of the proximal phalanx

b.   Available ROM: 0 to 60 degrees

c.   End feel: Firm

d.   Muscles responsible: FPL, flexor pollicis brevis

e.   Start and end position: Figure 9-51 displays the start position for thumb MCP flexion. The client is seated with the arm resting on a table on the ulnar border, with the forearm and wrist in neutral and the thumb MCP joint straight. The client bends or moves the thumb into maximum flexion. Figure 9-52 displays the end position of ROM testing.

Note: Because thumb MCP extension is simply a return from MCP flexion, the start position for thumb MCP flexion will be the same as the end position for MCP extension. Similarly, the start position for thumb MCP extension will be the same as the end position for MCP flexion (see Figures 9-51 and 9-52).

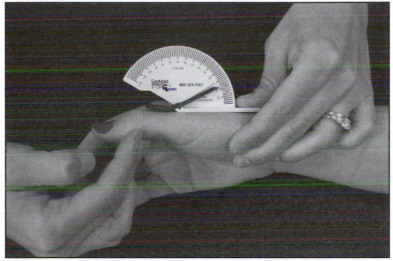

Figure 9-51. Start position for ROM testing of thumb MCP flexion/end position for thumb MCP extension.

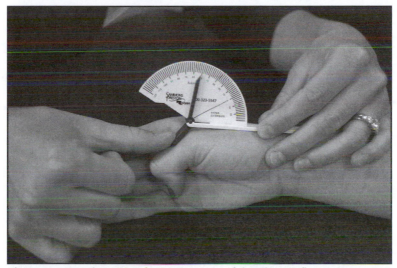

Figure 9-52. End position for ROM testing of thumb MCP flexion/start position for thumb MCP extension.

N.   **Thumb MCP Joint Extension ROM**

   a.   Goniometric landmark: Dorsal surface of the thumb MCP joint

         Stable arm: Midline dorsal surface of the thumb MCP joint

         Moving arm: Midline dorsal surface of the proximal phalanx

   b.   Available ROM: 60 to 0 degrees

   c.   End feel: Firm

   d.   Muscles responsible: Extensor pollicis longus, extensor pollicis brevis

   e.   Start and end position: See Figure 9-52 for start position. The client is seated with the arm resting on a table on the ulnar border, with the forearm and wrist in neutral and the thumb MCP joint flexed. The client straightens or moves the thumb into maximum extension as in Figure 9-51 or end position.

O. **Thumb IP Joint Flexion ROM**
   a. Goniometric landmark: Dorsal surface of the thumb IP joint

   Stable arm: Midline dorsal surface of the proximal phalanx

   Moving arm: Midline dorsal surface of the distal phalanx
   b. Available ROM: 0 to 80 degrees
   c. End feel: Firm
   d. Muscles responsible: FPL
   e. Start and end position: Figure 9-53 displays the start position for thumb IP joint flexion. The client is seated with the arm resting on a table on the ulnar border, with the forearm and wrist in neutral and the thumb IP joint straight. The client bends or moves the thumb into maximum flexion. Figure 9-54 displays end position for ROM testing.

   Note: Because thumb IP extension is simply a return from IP flexion, the start position for thumb IP flexion will be the same as the end position for IP extension. Similarly, the start position for thumb IP extension will be the same as the end position for IP flexion (see Figures 9-53 and 9-54).

P. **Thumb IP Joint Extension ROM**
   a. Goniometric landmark: Dorsal surface of the thumb IP joint

   Stable arm: Midline dorsal surface of the proximal phalanx

   Moving arm: Midline dorsal surface of the distal phalanx
   b. Available ROM: 80 to 0 degrees
   c. End feel: Firm
   d. Muscles responsible: EPL
   e. Start and end position: See Figure 9-54 for start position. The client is seated with the arm resting on a table on the ulnar border, with the forearm and wrist in neutral, and the thumb IP joint flexed. The client straightens or moves the IP joint of the thumb into maximum extension as in Figure 9-53 or the end position.

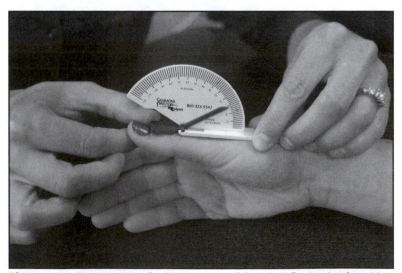

Figure 9-53. Start position for ROM testing of thumb IP flexion/end position for thumb IP extension.

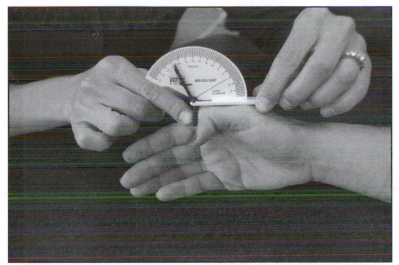

Figure 9-54. End position for ROM testing of thumb IP flexion/start position for thumb IP extension.

> **Note:** It is common to see hyperextension at the thumb IP joint; however, unless the injury involves the IP joint directly, it is not typically measured. Instructions for ROM testing of the IP joint hyperextension of the thumb are not provided in this chapter.

Q. **Thumb CMC Joint Radial Abduction (also called CMC extension) ROM**
    a.   Goniometric landmark: Over the CMC joint at the base of the thumb metacarpal
            Stable arm: Parallel to the second or index finger metacarpal
            Moving arm: Parallel to the first or thumb metacarpal
    b.   Available ROM: 0 to 20 degrees
    c.   End feel: Firm
    d.   Muscles responsible: EPL, EPB
    e.   Start and end position: See Figure 9-55 for start position. The client is seated with the arm resting on a table with the forearm pronated, palm flat, and the fingers and thumb adducted. The client moves the thumb into maximum CMC radial abduction or CMC extension. Figure 9-56 displays the end position of ROM testing.

R. **Thumb CMC Joint Palmar Abduction ROM**
    a.   Goniometric landmark: Over the CMC joint at the base of the thumb metacarpal
            Stable arm: Parallel to the second or index finger metacarpal
            Moving arm: Parallel to the first or thumb metacarpal
    b.   Available ROM: 0 to 50 degrees
    c.   End feel: Firm
    d.   Muscles responsible: APL, abductor pollicis brevis

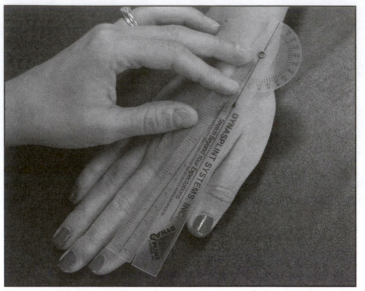

Figure 9-55. Start position for ROM testing of thumb CMC radial abduction (extension).

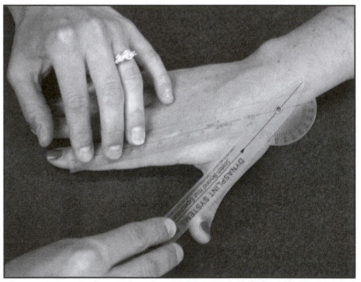

Figure 9-56. End position for ROM testing of thumb CMC radial abduction (extension).

    e.   Start and end position: See Figure 9-57 for start position. The client is seated with the arm resting on a table on the ulnar border, the forearm and wrist in neutral, and the fingers straight with the thumb adducted. The client moves the thumb into maximum CMC abduction. Figure 9-58 displays the end position of ROM testing.

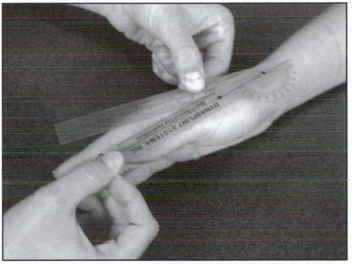

Figure 9-57. Start position for ROM testing of thumb CMC palmar abduction.

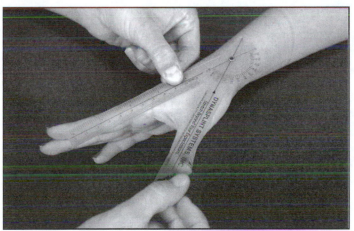

Figure 9-58. End position for ROM testing of thumb CMC palmar abduction.

S.   **Thumb CMC Adduction**
Deficits in thumb adduction may be recorded by measuring the distance between the index finger MCP joint and the thumb IP joint with a centimeter ruler as displayed in Figure 9-59. The muscle responsible is the AP.

T.   **Opposition**
Deficits in opposition may be recorded by measuring the distance between the centers of the pads of the thumb and the small finger using a centimeter ruler as displayed in Figure 9-60. The muscles responsible are the OP, ODM, and ADM.

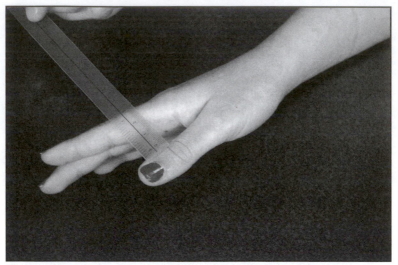

Figure 9-59. Position for measuring lack of thumb CMC adduction.

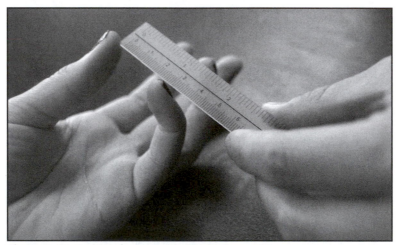

Figure 9-60. Position for measuring lack of opposition.

4. **Manual Muscle Testing (MMT) of the Wrist and Hand:** Complete gross MMT of the joints of the wrist and hand using Table 9-12.
    A. **Wrist Flexion and Extension**
        a. Muscle Palpation (if applicable)
        b. Testing Procedure: Figure 9-61 displays the start position for wrist joint flexion. The client is seated with arm resting on a table, forearm supinated, and wrist and fingers relaxed. The client moves his or her wrist into flexion. The therapist stabilizes the distal forearm to avoid

Table 9-12	Manual Muscle Testing Application Table		
Joint	Motions	Palpate Muscle Group/ Muscle	Gross MMT Score
Wrist	Flexion		
	Extension		
	Radial deviation		
	Ulnar deviation		
Finger MCP	Flexion		
	Abduction		
	Adduction		
Finger PIP	Flexion		
	Extension		
Finger DIP	Flexion		
	Extension		
Thumb MCP	Flexion		
	Extension		
Thumb IP	Flexion		
	Extension		
Thumb CMC	Radial abduction (Extension)		
	Palmar abduction		
	Opposition		

Adapted from American Medical Association. (2008). *Guides to the evaluation of permanent impairment* (6th ed.). Chicago, IL: Author.

compensation, and resistance is applied to the palm of the hand in the direction of wrist extension. Figure 9-62 displays the testing position. Figure 9-63 displays the start position for testing wrist joint extension. The client is seated with the arm resting on a table, forearm pronated, and wrist and fingers relaxed. The client moves his or her wrist into extension. The therapist stabilizes the distal forearm to avoid compensation. Resistance is applied to the dorsum of the hand in the direction of wrist flexion. Figure 9-64 displays the testing position.

B. **Wrist Radial and Ulnar Deviation**
    a. Muscle Palpation (if applicable)
    b. Testing Procedure: Figure 9-65 displays the start position for wrist radial and ulnar deviation. The client is seated with arm resting on a table, forearm pronated, wrist in neutral, and fingers and thumb relaxed. The therapist stabilizes the distal forearm to avoid compensation. To test radial deviation, the client moves his or her wrist into radial deviation. Resistance is applied at the second

Figure 9-61. Start position for MMT of wrist flexion.

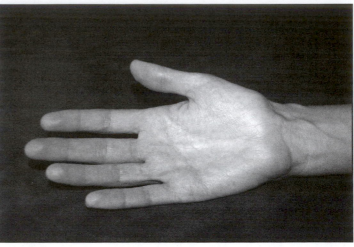

Figure 9-62. Testing position for MMT of wrist flexion.

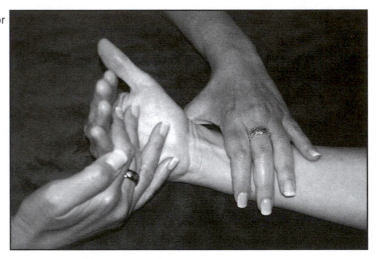

Figure 9-63. Start position for MMT of wrist extension.

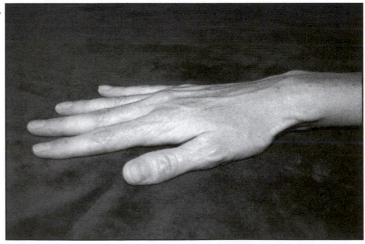

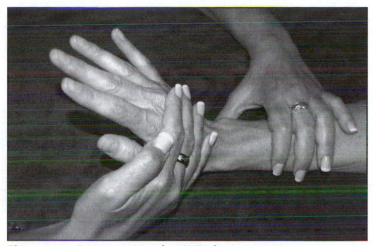

Figure 9-64. Testing position for MMT of wrist extension.

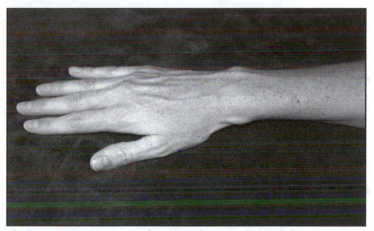

Figure 9-65. Start position for MMT of wrist radial and ulnar deviation.

metacarpal in the direction of ulnar deviation. Figure 9-66 displays the testing position.

To test ulnar deviation, the client moves his or her wrist into ulnar deviation. Resistance is applied at the fifth metacarpal in the direction of radial deviation. Figure 9-67 displays the testing position.

C. **Finger MCP Flexion**
   a. Muscle palpation (if applicable)
   b. Testing procedure: Figure 9-68 displays the start position. The client is seated with the arm resting on a table, forearm supinated, wrist in neutral, and fingers extended. The therapist stabilizes proximal to the MCP joints at the metacarpals to avoid compensation. The client moves his or her fingers in the direction of MCP flexion. Resistance is applied at the proximal phalanges in the direction of MCP extension. Figure 9-69 displays the testing position.

Figure 9-66. Testing position for MMT of wrist radial deviation.

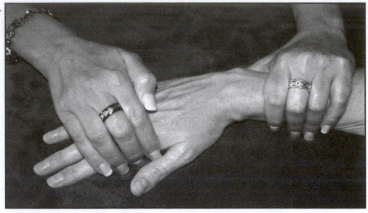

Figure 9-67. Testing position for MMT of wrist ulnar deviation.

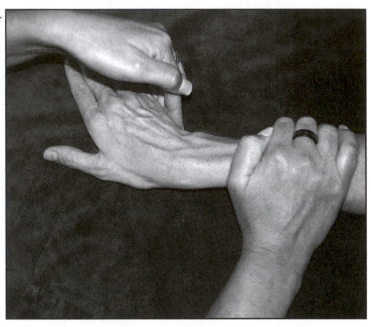

Figure 9-68. Start position for MMT of finger MCP flexion.

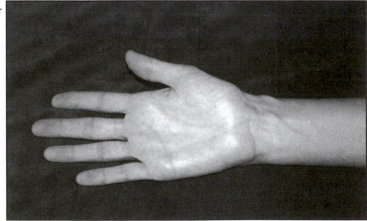

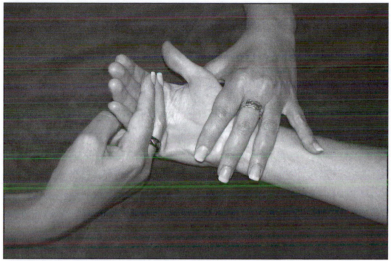

Figure 9-69. Testing position for MMT of finger MCP flexion.

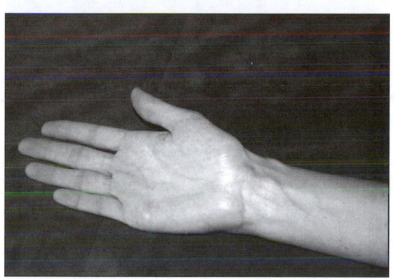

Figure 9-70. Start position for MMT of finger PIP/DIP flexion.

D.   **Finger PIP/DIP Flexion**
    a.   Muscle palpation (if applicable)
    b.   Testing procedure: Figure 9-70 displays the start position. The client is seated with the arm resting on a table, forearm supinated, wrist in neutral, and fingers extended. The therapist stabilizes at the MCP joints and metacarpals. The client moves fingers tested in the direction of PIP/DIP flexion while keeping MCP joints in extension. Resistance is applied at the middle and distal phalanges in the direction of PIP/DIP extension. Figure 9-71 displays the testing procedure.
E.   **Finger MCP/PIP/DIP Extension**
    a.   Muscle palpation (if applicable)
    b.   Testing procedure: Figure 9-72 displays the start position. The client is seated with the arm resting on a table, forearm pronated, wrist in

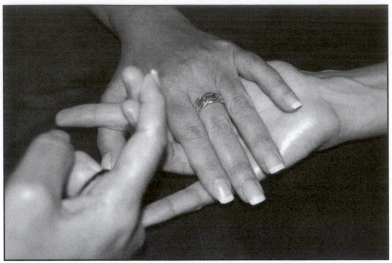

Figure 9-71. Testing position for MMT of finger PIP/DIP flexion.

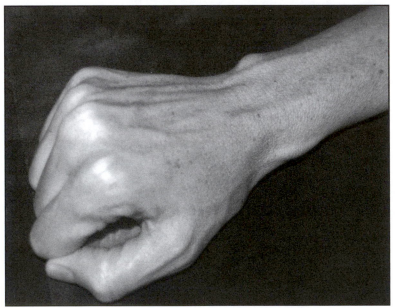

Figure 9-72. Start position for MMT of finger MCP/PIP/DIP extension.

neutral, and fingers flexed. The therapist stabilizes at the wrist and metacarpals to avoid compensation. The client moves the fingers tested in the direction of MCP/PIP/DIP extension. Resistance is applied to each finger individually on the dorsum of the proximal, middle, or distal phalanges in the direction of MCP/PIP/DIP flexion. Figure 9-73 displays the testing position.

F.   **Finger MCP Abduction and Adduction**
    a.   Muscle palpation (if applicable)
    b.   Testing procedure: Figure 9-74 displays the start position for finger MCP abduction. The client is seated with arm resting on a table,

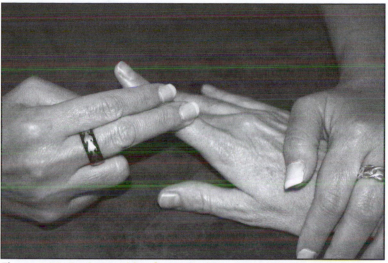

Figure 9-73. Testing position for MMT of finger MCP/PIP/DIP extension.

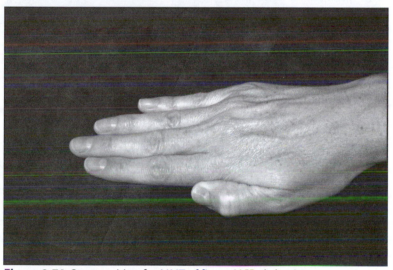

Figure 9-74. Start position for MMT of finger MCP abduction.

forearm pronated, wrist in neutral, fingers in extension, and MCP joints adducted. The client then moves the fingers in the direction of MCP abduction. The therapist stabilizes at the metacarpals to avoid compensation. Resistance is applied at the side of each individual finger in the direction of adduction. The long finger should be tested in both directions because it only abducts. Figure 9-75 displays the testing position.

Figure 9-76 displays the start position for testing finger MCP adduction. The client is seated with arm resting on a table, forearm pronated, wrist in neutral, fingers in extension, and MCP joints abducted. The client then moves his or her fingers into adduction. The therapist stabilizes at the metacarpals to avoid compensation. Resistance is applied at the side of the index, ring, and small fingers into abduction. Figure 9-77 displays the testing position.

Figure 9-75. Testing position for MMT of finger MCP abduction.

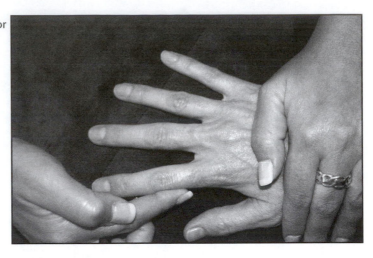

Figure 9-76. Start position for MMT of finger MCP adduction.

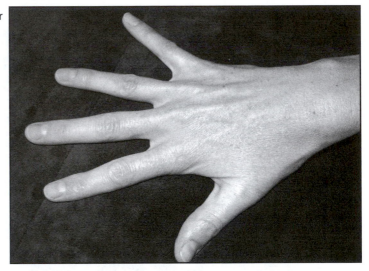

Figure 9-77. Testing position for MMT of finger MCP adduction.

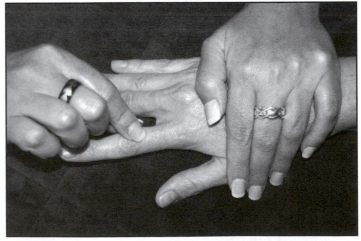

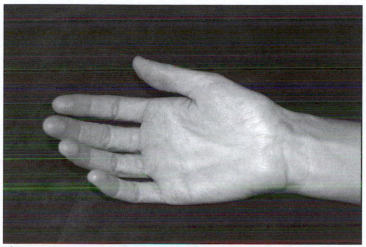

Figure 9-78. Start position for MMT of opposition.

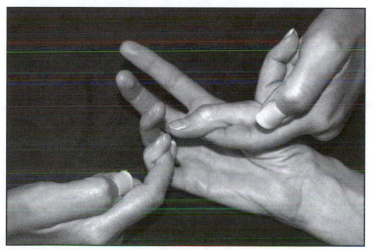

Figure 9-79. Testing position for MMT of opposition.

G. **Opposition of the Thumb to the Small Finger**
    a.   Muscle palpation (if applicable)
    b.   Testing procedure: Figure 9-78 displays the start position for opposition. The client is seated with arm resting on a table, forearm supinated, wrist in neutral, and fingers and thumb extended in a relaxed position. The client's wrist and forearm are stabilized against the table. The client moves in the direction of thumb opposition to the small finger. Resistance is applied at the thumb and small finger in the direction of extension. Figure 9-79 displays the testing procedure.

H. **Thumb MCP Flexion and Extension**
    a.   Muscle palpation (if applicable)
    b.   Testing procedure: Figure 9-80 displays the start position of thumb MCP flexion. The client is seated with arm resting on a table on ulnar border, forearm in mid-position, wrist in neutral, and fingers and

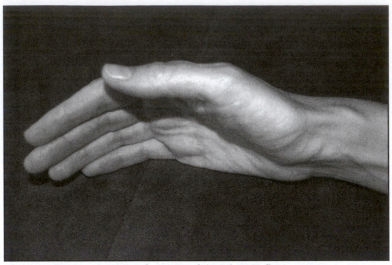

Figure 9-80. Start position for MMT of thumb MCP flexion.

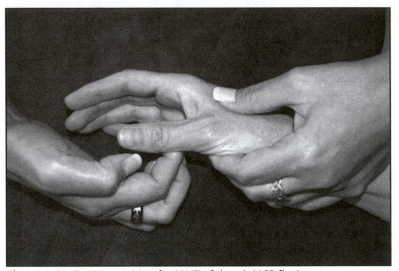

Figure 9-81. Testing position for MMT of thumb MCP flexion.

thumb extended in a relaxed position. The client's wrist and forearm are stabilized against the table. The client moves the thumb MCP in the direction of flexion. The therapist stabilizes the wrist and first metacarpal. Resistance is applied at the proximal phalanx in the direction of extension. Figure 9-81 displays the test position.

Figure 9-82 displays the start position for thumb MCP extension. The client is seated with the arm resting on a table on the ulnar border, forearm in mid-position, wrist in neutral, fingers extended, and thumb flexed into the palm at the MCP joint.

The client moves the thumb MCP in the direction of extension. The therapist stabilizes the wrist and first metacarpal. Resistance is applied at the proximal phalanx in the direction of flexion. Figure 9-83 displays the test position.

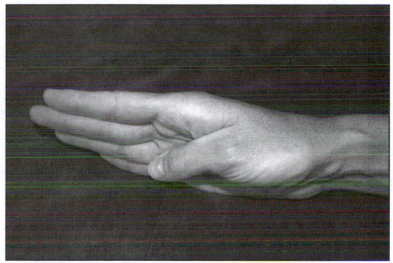

Figure 9-82. Start position for MMT of thumb MCP extension.

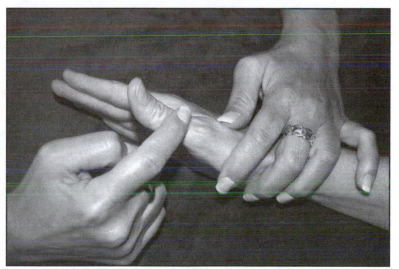

Figure 9-83. Testing position for MMT of thumb MCP extension.

I. **Thumb IP Flexion and Extension**
   a. Muscle palpation (if applicable)
   b. Testing procedure: Figure 9-84 displays the start position of thumb IP flexion. The client is seated with the arm resting on a table on the ulnar border, forearm in mid-position, wrist in neutral, fingers and thumb in a relaxed position. The client moves the thumb IP in the direction of flexion. The therapist stabilizes the thumb at the proximal phalanx, and resistance is applied at the distal phalanx in the direction of extension. Figure 9-85 displays the testing position.

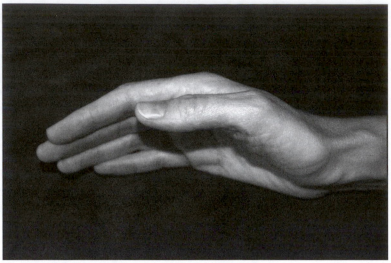

Figure 9-84. Start position for MMT of thumb IP flexion.

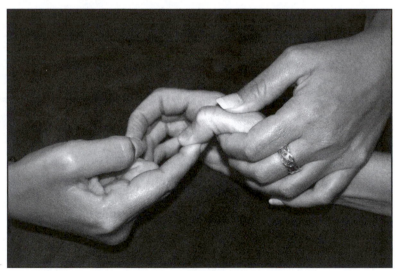

Figure 9-85. Testing position for MMT of thumb IP flexion.

Figure 9-86 displays the start position for thumb IP extension. The client is seated with the arm resting on a table on the ulnar border, forearm in mid-position, wrist in neutral, fingers extended, and thumb flexed into the palm at the IP joint. The client moves the thumb IP in the direction of extension. The therapist stabilizes the thumb at the proximal phalanx, and resistance is applied at the distal phalanx in the direction of flexion. Figure 9-87 displays the testing position.

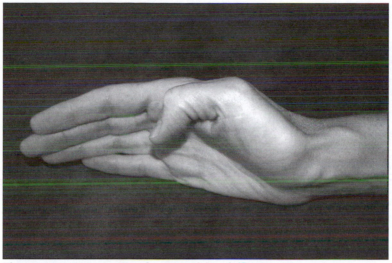

Figure 9-86. Start position for MMT of thumb IP extension.

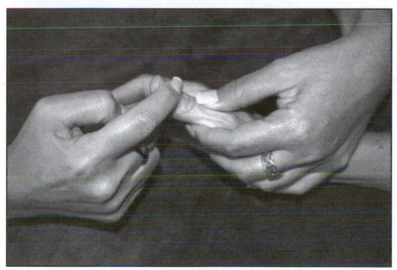

Figure 9-87. Testing position for MMT of thumb IP extension.

J. **Thumb CMC Palmar Abduction**
   a. Muscle palpation (if applicable)
   b. Testing procedure: Figure 9-88 displays the start position for thumb palmar abduction. The client is seated with the arm resting on a table with forearm supinated, wrist in neutral, and the thumb relaxed in adduction against the volar aspect of the index finger. The client moves the thumb up in the direction of palmar abduction. The therapist stabilizes the metacarpals and wrist to avoid compensation. Resistance is applied at the lateral aspect of the proximal phalanx in the direction of adduction. Figure 9-89 displays the test position.

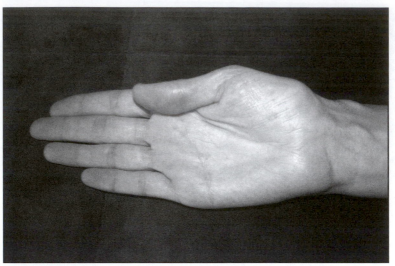

Figure 9-88. Start position for MMT of thumb CMC palmar abduction.

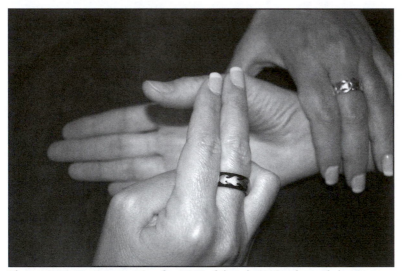

Figure 9-89. Testing position for MMT of thumb CMC palmar abduction.

K.   **Thumb CMC Radial Abduction (Extension)**
    a.   Muscle palpation (if applicable)
    b.   Testing procedure: Figure 9-90 displays the start position for thumb radial abduction. The client is seated with the arm resting on a table on the ulnar border, forearm in mid-position, wrist in neutral, fingers extended, and the thumb adducted and flexed slightly across the palm. The client moves the thumb up or away from the fingers in the direction of radial abduction. The therapist stabilizes the wrist and metacarpals. Resistance is applied at the lateral aspect of the proximal phalanx in the direction of adduction. Figure 9-91 displays the test position.

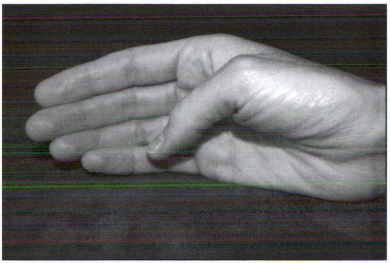

Figure 9-90. Start position for MMT of thumb CMC radial abduction.

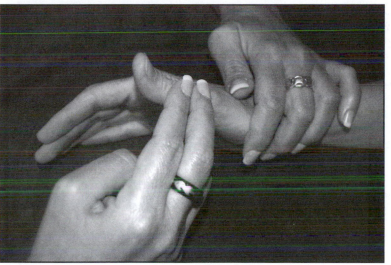

Figure 9-91. Testing position for MMT of thumb CMC radial abduction.

REFERENCES

Aaron, D. H., & Stegink, C. W. (2000). Hand rehabilitation: Matching patient priorities and performance with pathology and tissue healing. *Occupational Therapy Practice, 5*(8), 11–15.

American Medical Association. (2008). *Guides to the evaluation of permanent impairment* (6th ed.). Chicago: Author.

American Occupational Therapy Association. (2008). Occupational therapy practice framework: Domain and process (2nd ed.). *American Journal of Occupational Therapy, 62,* 625–683.

Amini, A. (2006). Repetitive stress injuries and the age of communication. *Occupational Therapy Practice, 11*(9), 10-15.

Benbow, M. (2001). *Hand skills and handwriting.* In S. A. Cermark & D. Larkin (Eds.). Developmental coordination disorders. Albany, NY: Singular Thomson Learning.

Burke, S. L., Higgins, J. P., McClinton, M. A., Saunders, R., & Valdata, L. (2006). *Hand and upper extremity rehabilitation: A practical guide* (3rd ed.). St. Louis, MO: Elsevier-Mosby.

Cannon, N. M. (2003). *Diagnosis and treatment manual for physicians and therapists: Upper extremity rehabilitation* (4th ed.). Indianapolis, IN: The Hand Rehabilitation Center of Indiana.

Floyd, R. T., & Thompson, C. W. (2001). *Manual of structural kinesiology* (14th ed.). New York, NY: McGraw-Hill.

Hertling, D., & Kessler, R. (2006). *Management of common musculoskeletal disorders: Physical therapy principles and methods.* Philadelphia, PA: Lippincott, Williams & Wilkins.

Hunter, J. M., Maklin, E. J., Callahan, H. D., Skirven, T. M., Schneider, L. H., & Osterman, A. E. (2002). *Rehabilitation of the hand and upper extremity* (5th ed.). St Louis, MO: Mosby.

Hurou, J. R. (1997). Fractures of the distal radius: What are the expectations of therapy? A two year retrospective study. *The Journal of Hand Therapy, 10*(4), 269–276.

Keller, K., Corbett, J., & Nichols, D. (1998). Repetitive strain injury in computer keyboard users: Pathomechanics and treatment principles in individual and group intervention. *Journal of Hand Therapy, 11*(1), 9–26.

Latella, D., & Meriano, C. (2003). *Occupational therapy manual for the evaluation of range of motion and muscle strength.* Clifton Park, NY: Delmar Carnage Learning.

Lippert, L. S. (2000). *Clinical kinesiology for physical therapist assistants* (3rd ed.). Philadelphia, PA: F. A. Davis.

Mann, W. C., Hurren, D., & Tomita, M. (1995). Assistive devices used by home-based elderly persons with arthritis. *American Journal of Occupational Therapy, 49*(8), 810–820.

Novak, C. B., & Mackinnon, S. E. (1997). Repetitive use and static postures: A source of nerve compression and pain. *Journal of Hand Therapy, 10*(2), 151–159.

Oatis, C. A. (2004). *Kinesiology: The mechanics and pathomechanics of human movement.* Philadelphia, PA: Lippincott, Williams & Wilkins.

Pendleton, H. M., & Schultz-Krohn, W. (2006). *Pedretti's occupational therapy practice skills for physical dysfunction* (6th ed.). St. Louis, MO: Mosby Elsevier.

Riley, M. A. (1998). The effects of medical conditions and aging on hand function. *Occupational Therapy Practice, 3*(6), 24–27.

Rybski, M. (2004). *Kinesiology for occupational therapy.* Thorofare, NJ: SLACK Incorporated.

Stoykov, M. E. (2001). OT treatment for complex regional pain syndrome. *Occupational Therapy Practice, 6*(15), 10–14.

Tennessee Orthopaedic Clinic, P. C. (2010). Edema (swelling) control techniques (Brochure). C. L. Roller: Author.

Weiss, S., & Falkenstein, N. (2005). *Hand rehabilitation: A quick reference guide and review.* St. Louis, MO: Elsevier Mosby.

Glossary

abnormal atypical movement: Movement characterized by the inability to produce the desired movement strategy necessary to complete an activity within generally accepted parameters.

abnormal end feel: The feel experienced when the typical quality of feel is different.

acceleration: "The rate in change of velocity with respect to time" (*Merriam-Webster's Online Dictionary*, n.d.).

accessory motion: Increase the pain-free movement available at a given joint. Accessory movements cannot be performed voluntarily. They occur between the articular surfaces of a joint in conjunction with voluntary movement. There are three types of accessory motions: roll, spin, and glide.

active assist range of motion (AAROM): Identifies that manual assistance is needed for the client to move the joint; however, the client also activates some joint motion.

active insufficiency: Occurs when a muscle cannot shorten or contract any further and fails to shorten to the extent required for simultaneous full range of motion at all joints crossed.

active range of motion (AROM): Describes the joint movements as the client alone moves a joint through the available ROM.

activity: A class of human actions that are goal directed (American Occupational Therapy Association [AOTA], 2008).

activity demands: The aspects of an activity that include the objects and their physical properties, space, social demands, sequencing or timing, required actions or skills, and required underlying body functions and body structures, needed to carry out the activity (AOTA, 2008).

activity limitation: Level of dysfunction identified by the ICF, including those that occur at the individual level.

adaptive motor behaviors: Certain ways the body acts in a situation (Horak, 1987). Appropriate and efficient movement strategies used by the body (Horak, 1987). The body's ability to apply normal movement strategies to achieve functional goals (Landel & Fisher, 1993).

afferent neurons: Sensory neurons are afferent, or ascending to the central nervous system, and send sensory information to the cortex for interpretation. Afferent neurons are located dorsally; also referred to as sensory neurons (Solomon, 2009).

agonist: A muscle that is the prime mover.

ampiarthrodial articulations: Sometimes called cartilaginous joints. Allow for limited movement as in the pubic symphysis.

Keough, J. L., Sain, S. J., Roller, C. L.
Kinesiology for the Occupational Therapy Assistant:
Essential Components of Function and Movement (pp. 321-330).
© 2012 SLACK Incorporated.

anatomical position: Reference position in which the subject is standing in an upright posture, eyes looking forward, feet parallel with toes pointed forward and the arms slightly abducted at the side of the body, and the palms facing forward (Solomon, 2009).

anatomical snuff box: A small depression formed where the thumb joins the wrist. The depression is formed when the abductor pollicus brevis, extensor pollicus longus, and extensor pollicus brevis tendons contract.

antagonists: Muscles that work against each other to equal or cancel out the movement and therefore gain stability.

anterior pelvic tilt: characterized as the pelvis *dipping forward*. The anterior superior iliac spine (ASIS) landmarks move forward of the pubic symphisis.

anticipatory postural movements: "Reflect movements of the trunk or posture in response to changes in task or environmental demands" (Shumway-Cook & Woollacott, 2001).

appendicular skeleton: Composed of the shoulder and pelvic girdles, the upper extremities, and the lower extremities.

areas of occupation: Various kinds of life activities in which people engage, to include activities of daily living (ADL), instrumental activities of daily living (IADL), rest and sleep, education, work, play, leisure, and social participation (AOTA, 2008).

articulations: More commonly known as joints, which connect bones.

atrophy: Wasting of tissue, in muscle especially due to lack of use.

attrition rupture: Tendon rupture caused by movement across a roughened bone.

autonomic: The autonomic division is part of the PNS and helps maintain an internal balance as it responds to internal stimuli, providing functions such as maintaining body temperature, regulating heart rate, and regulating blood pressure (Solomon, 2009).

axial skeleton: The skull and trunk comprise the axial skeleton.

axis: The center, or point, around which the object rotates.

ball and socket joint: Triaxial, able to move in all three planes including flexion and extension, abduction and adduction, horizontal abduction and horizontal adduction, internal and external rotation and circumduction; consists of spherical head on one bone that fits into cup- or saucer-like cavity on adjoining bone; an example is the hip joint (Luttgens & Wells, 1982).

beliefs: A person's basic truth that remains, regardless of what another person might say, think, or believe.

body functions: Focus on the physiological functions of body systems, such as sensory, neuro-muscular, psychological, respiratory, and cardiovascular.

body structures: Anatomy and specific body parts, such as organs, skin, muscles, bones, limbs, and other anatomical features.

brachial plexus: Relating to the arm, usually indicates nerve roots C5 through T1.

buoyancy: A phenomenon of water defined as an upward force equal to the weight of the dis placed liquid.

carrying angle: Of the elbow, is described as the angle formed by the long axis of the humerus and forearm.

center of gravity: Refers to the balance point of an object where all sides are equal (Lippert, 2006).

central nervous system (CNS): The CNS is commonly defined as the brain and spinal cord. The CNS ends at the point where nerve fibers exit the spinal cord. Motor neurons in the CNS are referred to as upper motor neurons.

client factors: Those factors residing within the client that may affect performance in areas of occupation. Client factors include values, beliefs, and spirituality; body functions; and body structures (AOTA, 2008).

closed kinematic chain: The distal segment past a joint is fixed or stabilized so movement in one joint will automatically necessitate movement at connecting proximal joints.

close-pack position of joint: Most stable position of joint. The two articulating bones in this position have the greatest amount of contact between surface areas—the ligaments and joint capsule are taut; often occurs one extreme of the range of motion; in the knee the close-pack position is flexion (Lippert, 2006).

complex regional pain syndrome (CRPS): A post-traumatic neuropathic syndrome characterized by pain and vasomotor and pseudomotor changes in the involved extremity. Also called *reflex sympathetic dystrophy (RSD)*.

compression: An external force causing two joint surfaces to be in closer contact with each other; the pushing together of the two bones in the joint. Also referred to as joint approximation.

concave: A concave curve refers to a curve that extends inward or anteriorly. The opening part of a curve.

concentric: An isotonic contraction is considered concentric when the muscle shortens and the joint angle is decreased.

condyloid joint: Allows for biaxial movement occurring in two planes including flexion and extension as well as abduction and adduction. When movements occur concurrently, the movement is termed circumduction. This joint is usually oval in shape with the end of one bone having a convex shape which fits into the concave surface on the articulating bone. An example is the metacarpophalangeal joints of the four lesser digits (Luttgens & Wells, 1982).

context: Consists of primarily internal conditions which may include cultural aspects such as customs, personal aspects such as demographics, temporal aspects and virtual aspects; interrelated conditions within and surrounding the client (AOTA, 2008).

contractility: A muscle's ability to shorten in length; however, not all contractions result in muscle shortening.

convex: A convex curve refers to a curve that extends outward or, in relation to the body, posteriorly; the closed part of a curve.

cranial nerve: Twelve pairs of nerves that transmit information directly to the brain.

cubital tunnel syndrome: Syndrome frequently involving pressure at the medial side of the elbow, which compresses the ulnar nerve.

cumulative trauma disorders: A group of signs and symptoms that, over time, affect the joints and soft tissues of the upper and lower extremities and back. Signs and sympoms may include pain, numbness, and tingling. Also known as repetitive stress injuries, repetitive motion injuries, or repetitive strain injuries,

decubitus: Short for decubitus ulcer; a lesion on the surface of the skin caused by superficial tissue loss often with inflammation present, may be caused by excessive pressure, shearing pressure or static postures over a period of time; commonly refered to as a bed sore (Steadman, 1982)

degree of freedom: The number of axes a joint can rotate around and the number of planes the joint can move in.

de Quervain's disease: Tenosynovitis that causes pain and swelling of the thumb and wrist over the *anatomical snuff box*.

dermatome: The area of skin that is innervated by cutancous (pertaining to the skin) branches form a single spinal nerve (Steadman, 1982).

diarthrodial articulations: Considered freely moving. Joint movement is limited primarily by muscles, tendons, and ligaments rather than by the joint structure itself. Diarthrodial joints are enclosed within a joint capsule that secretes synovial fluid to lubricate the joint; thus these joints are also referred to as synovial joints.

distraction: An external force causing slight separation between the two surfaces of a joint; slight pulling apart of a joint. Also referred to as traction or tension.

dorsal: Pertaining to the back of the body, synonymous with posterior (Steadman, 1982).

dorsal interossei: Muscles of the hand that abduct the metacarpophalangeal joints of the index, ring and small fingers away from the long finger.

double support: Position during walking when both feet are in contact with the ground.

drag: Resistance to forward motion.

eccentric: The muscle is actually lengthening under stress. Eccentric contractions work to decelerate the movement, as a brake would do for a car.

efferent neurons: Motor neurons are generally regarded as efferent, or exiting the CNS, which terminate on muscle fibers causing a contraction. Efferent neurons are located ventrally; interchangeable with the term motor neurons (Solomon, 2009).

elasticity: Describes the muscle's ability to return to its original length after it has been stretched.

elbow complex: Consists of the body structures that provide motion at the elbow and the forearm.

end feel: How the joint movement feels at the end of the ROM. See *abnormal end feel, firm end feel, hard end feel, soft end feel.*

environment: The external physical and social environment that surrounds the client and in which the client's daily life occupations occur (AOTA, 2008).

Erb's palsy: Disorder characterized by weakness or paralysis of the arm by affecting nerve roots C5, C6, and C7.

ergonomics: The study of the interaction between human capabilities and the demands of their occupational roles. Occupational therapy and ergonomics are both concerned with an individual's adaption to his or her physical environment (Hertfelder & Gwin, 1989).

excursion ratio: The difference between how long the muscle is when stretched as compared to its length when contracted. For most muscles, this ratio is 2:1, indicating that most muscles are capable of stretching twice as long as they can shorten (Gench, Hionson, & Harvey, 1999).

extensibility: Depicts a muscle's capacity to be stretched or lengthened.

extrinsic: Muscles that originate proximal to the wrist joint.

fasciculus: Fascicle, a bundle or band, usually of fibers muscle or nerve fibers (Steadman, 1982).

firm end feel: The end feel experienced when a normal joint or ligament is stretched.

flaccid paralysis: Loss of voluntary movement due to lack of muscle tone; tendon reflexes are also decreased or absent (*Merriam Webster Online Dictionary*)

force couple: Muscles that act as synergists to one another to provide a stronger action on the joint, resulting in stronger functional movement for the client. The resulting movement must be rotary in nature, and the line of force and the pull or angle of muscle fibers of all muscles involved must be in opposing directions.

friction: Force acting in the opposite direction to the desired movement and occurring at the area of contact between the two surfaces.

frozen shoulder: See *primary adhesive capsulitis.*

fundamental position: Reference position where the subject is standing in an upright posture, eyes looking forward, feet parallel with toes pointed forward, the arms slightly abducted at the side of the body, and the palms facing the side of the body (Solomon, 2009).

gait patterns: Walking patterns; body funtions commonly considered by occupational therapy (AOTA, 2008).

gait cycle: Describes the movement from the heel strike of one leg to the heel strike of the same leg on the ground.

gliding joint: Also referred to as irregular, arthrodial or plane joints; considered nonaxial as the only movement permitted is gliding in nature, as in one bone over another. An example is the carpal joints (Luttgens & Wells, 1982)

hard end feel: The feel experienced when two bones block motion.

hemiparesis: Paralysis affecting only one side of the body (Thomas, 1989).

hemiplegia: Paralysis of one side of the body after a cerebrovascular accident (CVA) or stroke.

hinge joint: Uniaxial, allowing movement in one plane to include flexion and extension; the end of one bone is spool-like, whereas the articulating bone is concave to fit around the spool. An example is the elbow joint (Luttgens & Wells, 1982).

humeral positioners: Muscles that position the humerus in space during or after actions of the scapular pivoters (Glinn, 2008).

humeral propellers: Muscles that propel or move the humerus (Glinn, 2008).

hypertonia: "Above or over tone," extreme tension of the muscles.

hypothenar: The muscular portion of the palm of the hand on the small finger side.

hypotonia: "Under tone," having a lesser degree of tension, diminished muscular tone.

impairment: Level of dysfunction identified by the ICF that occurs at the body part level.

inertia: "The state of a physical body in which it resists any force acting to move it from a position of rest or to change its uniform motion" (Steadman, 1982).

insertion: The end point of a muscle attachment. The insertion is usually distal, or further away from the trunk and midline of the body, and is considered the most movable part.

intrinsic: Muscles that originate distal to the wrist joint.

irritability: Describes the property of the muscle to receive and respond to a stimulus, whether the stimulus is chemical, electrical, or mechanical (Hall, 1999; Thompson & Floyd, 2004).

isometric: Muscle tension develops, but the muscle length does not change. This means that the joint angle or measurement does not change either.

isotonic: Isotonic contractions maintain the muscle at equal tension. This means that the length of the muscle changes, causing joint movement.

kinematic chain: Also referred to as kinetic chain; the linkage system of joints between bony segments in the body; in engineering terms a kinetic chain is a series of rigid links connected in a specific way to allow motion (Dail et. al., 2011). In human bodies, the rigid links are bones and the motion occurs at joints. See *closed kinematic chain*, *open kinematic chain*.

kinesiology: The study of the principles of mechanics and anatomy in relation to human movement (*Merriam-Webster Collegiate Dictionary*, 1991).

kyphosis: A spinal deformity and refers to an excessive curvature in the thoracic spine.

lift: Refers to a change in fluid pressure as a result of differences in air or liquid flow velocities around an object.

line of gravity: Line of gravity is the vertical line from the center of gravity to the earth, and base of support is the area contained within the area of the body parts in contact with the ground (Lippert, 2006).

locus of control: Refers to whom, or what, has impact over outcomes. Locus of control can be external to a person or internal in nature.

lordosis: An exacerbated curvature of the lumbar spine; also called swayback.

lumbosacral plexus: Relating to the lower back and lower extremity; usually refers to nerve roots L1 through L5 (lumbar portion) and L5 through S3 (sacral portion) (Thompson & Floyd, 2004).

lumbricals: Muscles of the hand that flex the metacarpophalangeal joints as they extend the PIP and DIP joints of all four fingers.

malunion: A deformity that can occur after a properly aligned fracture slips in the cast during healing.

manual muscle testing (MMT): A manual technique used for estimating the relative strength of specific muscles (Thomas, 1989).

motivation: An internal factor that might create good feelings about oneself for reaching a goal. External or social motivators might include a high grade, parental approval, or retention of scholarship monies. Motivation can be intrinsic, coming from internal sources, or extrinsic, reinforced by external factors.

motor behavior: Observable and measurable movement (Spaulding, 2005).

motor control: The outcome of motor learning involving the ability to produce purposeful movements of the extremities and postural adjustments in response to activity and environment demands (Pendleton & Schultz-Krohn, 2006).

motor development: Identifies the changes in movement behavior that occur as the client progresses through the lifespan from infancy until death (Whiting & Rugg, 2006).

motor learning: The acquisition and/or modification of learned movement patterns over time (Pendleton & Schultz-Krohn, 2006).

motor neurons: See *efferent neurons*.

motor skills: Voluntary movements used to complete a desired task or achieve a specific goal (Whiting & Rugg, 2006).

muscle fiber: Characteristic of direction of muscle fibers that includes pennate, unipennate, bipenate, flat, parallel, fusiform, strap, radiate, and sphincter.

negotiability: The ability of the person to interact with the environment and independently use common features, such as a toilet paper dispenser.

nerves: Transmit stimuli from the central nervous system to the periphery or vice versa; a microscopic bundle or one or more fascicles of either myelinated or unmeylinated fibers, can also be a mixture of both fiber types (Steadman, 1982).

neutral pelvic tilt: characterized as equal weight distribution across femurs in a sitting position.

normal atypical movement: Reflects the motor behavior response when typical movement strategies are temporarily or no longer feasible.

normal (enhanced) typical movement: Highly trained motor skills and motor control that allow for high efficiency, adaptability, and consistency in performance of a task in a variety of environments.

normal typical movement: Movement characterized by smooth, coordinated, efficient, automatic movements that reflect a variety of movement options, high complexity, decreased time, high velocity, and high acceleration.

occupation: What people do to occupy their time. Things that have individual and unique meaning for each person and may include anything from rest or sleep to work, incorporating everything that occurs throughout the day.

open kinematic chain: The distal segment past a joint is freely moving, and therefore one joint can move without impacting movement of the other proximal joints.

open-pack position of joint: Also referred to as loose-pack. Least amount of contact between the two articulating surfaces—ligaments and joint capsule are loose or lax. This position allows for normal accessory motions in the joint to occur, thus allowing for normal range of motion; considered to occur whenever the joint is not in a close-pack position (Lippert, 2006).

origin: Describes where a muscle begins or originates. This point is usually proximal or closer to the trunk or middle of the body and is often considered to be more stable.

osteoarthritis: A condition of the joints causing pain and stiffness. It is caused by degenerative changes of the joints over time.

palmar interossei: Muscles of the hand that adduct the metacarpophalangeal joints of the index, ring and small fingers to the long finger.

paralysis: Loss of voluntary movement; a complete or partial loss of function which may include movement and/or sensation; inability to move (*Merriam-Webster Online Dictionary*); see *flaccid paralysis*, *spastic paralysis*.

participation restriction: Level of dysfunction identified by the ICF that occurs at the societal level.

passive insufficiency: Occurs when a muscle cannot be stretched any further, yet it has not stretched the amount required for full range of motion at all joints crossed at the same time.

passive range of motion (PROM): Refers to joint movement created by manual assistance only creating joint movement.

performance skills: The abilities that clients demonstrate in the actions they perform (AOTA, 2008).

performance patterns: Patterns of behavior related to daily life activities that are habitual or routine. They can include habits, routines, rituals, and roles (AOTA, 2008).

peripheral nervous system (PNS): The motor neurons found in the PNS are called lower motor neurons (LMNs). Cell bodies of the LMN are located in the anterior horn of the spinal cord and sometimes are referred to as anterior horn cells.

pivot joint: Also termed screw, movement allowed is uniaxial, occurs in only one plane, and consists of rotation; joint is a peglike pivot where one bone can roll or rotate around another. An example is the atlantoaxial joint (Luttgens & Wells, 1982).

plexus: Bundle or interconnection of nerves. Includes the brachial plexus and lumbosacral plexus. Latin term for braid; network or interjoining of blood, nerve, or lymphatic vessels (Steadman, 1982); see *brachial plexus, lumbosacral plexus*.

posterior pelvic tilt: Characterized by the tailbone tucking beneath the body on the posterior superior iliac spine (PSIS) shifting backward. The ASIS landmarks move posteriorly to the public symphisis.

postural control: "The regulation of the body's position in space for the dual purpose of stability and orientation" (Shumway-Cook & Woollacott, 2001).

posture: "State of the body in relationship to gravity, the ground and to its body parts or extremities" (Martin, 1977).

praxis: The ability to plan and perform purposeful movement (AOTA, 2008).

primary adhesive capsulitis: Condition of the shoulder involving progressive stiffness and diffuse pain that limits function. Also called *frozen shoulder.*

proprioceptive: From the Latin terms to take, and from one's own; the ability to receive stimuli from within one's own body, such as from muscles, tendons and other internal tissues (Steadman, 1982).

qualitative: Includes information on movement that may come from observation or interview.

quantitative: Identifies numerical data under standardized situations to gather information.

range of motion (ROM): The arc of motion through which a joint moves.

reflex sympathetic dystrophy (RSD): See *complex regional pain syndrome (CRPS).*

repetitive stress injuries (RSIs): Known as repetitive motion injuries, repetitive strain injuries, or cumulative trauma disorders. A group of signs and symptoms that commonly affect the joints and the soft tissues of the arms, hands, knees, and back (Hertfelder & Gwin, 1989).

reversal of muscle function: This occurs when the muscle is used in such a way that the normally stable origin moves toward the insertion; in typical muscle function, the insertion moves toward the origin.

rheumatoid arthritis (RA): A systemic autoimmune disorder causing fatigue, joint pain, and inflammation that leads to deformity and joint destruction.

rotator cuff: Tendon connecting four muscles that cover the head of the humerus. The rotator cuff muscles together lift and rotate the humerus and maintain the humeral head in the glenoid fossa.

rotator cuff tendonitis: This most common cause of shoulder pain occurs when there is impingement of an inflamed rotator cuff tendon between the humeral head, the swollen bursa, and acromion process. Also called *shoulder impingement.*

saddle joint: Often considered a modified condyloid joint; the end surfaces of both bones are tipped up, somewhat like a western saddle for horses. This joint is also biaxial, allowing flexion and extension, abduction and adduction, and circumduction; the saddle joint has more mobility than a traditional condyloid joint. The only example in the human body is the carpometacarpal joint of the thumb (Luttgens & Wells, 1982).

scapular pivoters: Muscles that are involved with motion at the scapulothoracic joint (Glinn, 2008).

scapulohumeral rhythm: Describes the movement relationship between the scapula in the shoulder girdle and the glenohumeral joint.

scoliosis: A spinal deformity in the frontal plane characterized by a lateral curvature of the vertebra.

sensory neurons: See *afferent neurons.*

shear force: A force that attempts to move one object against another.

shoulder complex: Includes all of the body structures that provide motion at the glenohumeral joint and scapula.

shoulder dystocia: Condition that may occur more often in births involving larger than average babies in which one of the infant's shoulders becomes stuck under a portion of the mother's pelvic bone during childbirth.

shoulder impingement: See *rotator cuff tendonitis.*

shoulder protectors: Muscles that act as a force couple with the humeral positioners to keep the structures of the shoulder complex safe. These include the rotator cuff muscles (Glinn, 2008).

shoulder subluxation: Partial dislocation of the humerus at the GH joint that is seen in many individuals after a stroke (Ohio Health, 1995).

single support: Position during walking when one foot is in contact with the ground.

sitting balance: The ability to maintain a seated posture without falling; refers to the ability to reach.

soft end feel: The end feel experienced when two muscle groups are compressed.

somatic: The somatic division is part of the PNS and is primarily responsible for responding to the external environment, or things happening outside of the body.

spastic paralysis: Loss of voluntary movement due to increase in muscle tone including spasms; tendon reflexes are increased or hyperexcitable (*Merriam-Webster Online Dictionary*).

spinal nerves: Nerves that link the spinal cord with sensory receptors and with other parts of the body. The spinal nerves are all mixed nerves, transmitting sensory information to the spinal cord through afferent neurons and also relaying motor information from the spinal cord to the various parts of the body using efferent neurons.

spirituality: The search for meaning in all that one does, which includes values and beliefs.

stability: Refers to the ability to maintain the body in equilibrium.

stretch reflex: Slight stretching of a muscle lengthens fibers causing stimulation of sensory endings, which leads to contraction of the muscle. This is a protective reflex to avoid overstretching. One role of the muscle spindle is to detect stretch and respond to it via the stretch reflex; this phenomenon is in constant use and provides adjustment to muscle tone.

synarthrodial articulations: Joints that are immovable, such as the suture joints of the skull.

syndesmosis: Articulation in which the bones are united by ligaments (Thomas, 1989).

synergist: Muscles that work together to increase the strength of a desired movement as they work in unison.

synovial: Refers to *diarthrodial articulations.*

tendonitis: An irritation or inflammation of the tendons.

tendon rupture: A tendon weakened by disease or injury may rupture or separate. Also see *attrition rupture.*

thoracic kyphosis: Condition seen in older individuals that features forward head posture and rounded shoulders.

trigger finger: A thickening of the flexor tendon sheath at the A1 pulley in the palm of the hand can cause the finger to lock as a "trigger" while making a fist.

Valsalva maneuver: Attempt to forcibly exhale with the nose and mouth closed. This causes increased intrathoracic pressure, slowing of the pulse, decreased return of blood to the heart and increased venous pressure (Thomas, 1989).

values: Principles and standards that an individual considers to be essential to follow in order to lead a good life. A person might value honesty, integrity, hard work, or family relationships, to name a few.

ventral: Pertaining to the front of the body, synonymous with anterior (Steadman, 1982)

vestibular: Related to the vestibule of the ear; vestibule is a small space or region at the entrance of a canal; vestibular organ—the organ of equilibrium.

winging of the scapula: Seen when the inferior angle of the scapula protrudes or wings out due to serratus anterior muscle weakness.

REFERENCES

American Occupational Therapy Association. (2008). Occupational therapy practice framework: Domain and process (2nd ed.). *American Journal of Occupational Therapy, 62*, 625-683.

Gench, B. E., Hionson, M. M., & Harvey, P. T. (1999). *Anatomical kinesiology.* Dubuque, IA: Eddie Bowers Publishing, Inc.

Glinn, J. E., Jr. (2008). Shoulder biomechanics. *Physical Therapy's Clinical Educator,* 49-53.

Hall, S. (1999). *Basic biomechanics* (3rd ed.). Boston: WCB/McGraw-Hill.

Hertfelder, S., & Gwin, C. (1989). *Work in progress: Occupational therapy in work programs.* Rockville, MD: American Occupational Therapy Association.

Horak, R. (1987). Clinical management of postural control in adults. *Physical Therapy, 67*(12), 1881-1885.

Landel, R., & Fisher, B. (1993). Musculoskeletal considerations in the neurologically impaired patient. *Orthopaedic Physical Therapy Clinics of North America, 2*(1), 15-24.

Lippert, L. S. (2006). *Clinical kinesiology for physical therapy assistants* (3rd ed.). Philadelphia, PA: F. A. Davis Company.

Luttgens, K., & Wells, K. F. (1982). *Kinesiology: Scientific Basis of Human Motion* (7th ed.). New York, NY: Saunders College Publishing

Martin, J. P. (1977). A short essay on posture and movement. *Journal of Neurology Neurosurgery and Psychiatry, 40*, 25-29.

Merriam-Webster's Collegiate Dictionary (9th ed.). (1991). Springfield, MA: Merriam-Webster.

Merriam-Webster Online Dictionary. (n.d.) Retrieved from http://www.merriam-webster.com/dictionary.

Ohio Health. (1995). *Shoulder subluxation.* Retrieved December 7, 2009, from: www.ohiohealth.com.

Pendleton, H. M., & Schultz-Krohn, W. (2006). *Pedretti's occupational therapy: Practice skills for physical dysfunction* (6th ed.). St. Louis, MO: Mosby Elsevier.

Shumway-Cook, A., & Woollacott, M. H. (2001). *Motor control: Theory and practical applications* (2nd ed.). Philadelphia, PA: Lippincott Williams & Wilkins.

Solomon, E. P. (2009). Introduction to human anatomy and physiology. St. Louis, MO: Saunders Elsevier.

Spaulding, S. J. (2005). *Meaningful motion: Biomechanics for occupational therapists.* New York, NY: Elsevier Churchill Livingston.

Steadman, T. (1982). *Steadman's Medical Dictionary* (24th ed.). Baltimore, MD: Williams and Wilkins.

Thomas, C. L. (1989). *Taber's cyclopedia medical dictionary* (17th ed.). Philadelphia, PA: F. A. Davis Co.

Thompson, C. W., & Floyd, R. T. (2004). *Manual of structural kinesiology* (15th ed.). Boston, MA: McGraw Hill.

Whiting, W. C., & Rugg, S. (2006). *Dynatomy: Dynamic human anatomy.* Champaign, IL: Human Kinetics.

Web Address References

WEB RESOURCES

Accessibility

Americans With Disabilities Act Accessibility Guidelines (ADAAG): Checklist for Buildings and Facilities
http://www.access-board.gov/adaag/checklist/Restaurants.html

Americans With Disabilities Act: Checklist for Readily Achievable Barrier Removal
http://www.ada.gov/checkweb.htm
    Select PDF version for checklist. This checklist has been made available over the Internet with permission of Adaptive Environments. This checklist may be copied for your own use as many times as desired but may not be reproduced in whole or in part and sold for commercial purposes by any entity without written permission of Adaptive Environments, the author.

Checklist of Checkpoints for Web Content Accessibility Guidelines
http://www.w3.org/TR/WCAG10/full-checklist.html

Kentucky Cabinet for Workforce Development and Kentucky Department of Vocational Rehabilitation, 2001 Edition
http://ada.ky.gov/documents/Checklist_2000.pdf
    Based on the Americans with Disabilities Act guidelines.

WebAIM
http://www.webaim.org/standards/508/checklist
    Checklists for Web content accessibility.

Adaptive Equipment

Dynamic Living
www.dynamicliving.com
Plastic lever handles that fit over most doorknobs.

Keough J, Sain S, Roller C.
Kinesiology for the Occupational Therapy Assistant:
Essential Components of Function and Movement (pp. 331-334).

North Coast Medical
http://www.ncmedical.com
Variety of adaptive equipment.

Dynamic-Living
www.dynamic-living.com
Aids and gadgets to make living at home easier.

Life With Ease
www.lifewithease.com
Variety of adaptive equipment.

Hand Helpers
www.handhelpers.com
Adapted computer equipment.

Better Garden Tools
www.bettergardentools.com
Ergonomic ratchet garden tools.

Aids for Arthritis
www.aidsforarthritis.com
Aids for arthritis.

Cool Safety Products
www.coolsafetyproducts.com
Innovative safety and ergonomic products.

Active Forever
www.activeforever.com
Variety of medical supplies, adaptive and safety equipment, and braces.

Book Mate Store
www.bookmatestore.com
Hand-friendly book holders and stands.

Anatomy and Physiology Tutorials

Human Biodyssey: Exploring Anatomy and Physiology
http://www.gwc.maricopa.edu/home_pages/crimando/jcHumanBiodyssey.htm

University of Iowa Hospitals and Clinics: Health Content Library Index
http://www.vh.org
Virtual hospital, internal link to anatomy atlases.

Duke Orthopedics: Wheeless' Textbook of Orthopedics
http://www.wheelessonline.com
Extensive links, pictures, diagrams, explanations; very thorough; easy to search.

Foot and Ankle

Foot and Ankle Web Index
http://www.footandankle.com
Library in this site is helpful.

Hand

E-Hand
http://www.e-hand.com
Electronic textbook of hand surgery, diagrams, text, videos, other images; very thorough site.

Musculoskeletal

Arthroscopy
http://www.arthroscopy.com/sports.htm
Information on various musculoskeletal problems.

Shoulder Study Aids

Shoulderdoc
http://www.shoulderdoc.co.uk
Information, including online books, regarding every aspect of shoulder anatomy, physiology, function, illness, and treatment.

Study Aids

Study Stack
http://www.studystack.com
Find flashcards to study or create your own.

How to Study
http://www.howtostudy.org/resources.php
Ideas on how to study, organization, time management, note taking, concentration, and more.

Gliffy - Online Diagram Software and Flowchart Software
http://www.gliffy.com
Easily create flowcharts, diagrams, and more.

MyNoteIt
http://www.mynoteit.com
Take and store your notes online, edit and revise notes with peers, look-up and define words with your Workspace Utilities.

NoteCentric
http://www.notecentric.com
Store and share your classroom notes with this innovative site. It keeps your notes organized so you can reference them later, and you can easily access it through a Facebook account.

Quizlet
http://quizlet.com
Quizlet makes it easy to study things like vocabulary words with online study tools. You can make quizzes, use your friend's, or browse existing flashcards on the site.

Available Range of Motion Norms

AVAILABLE RANGE OF MOTION NORMS

Appendix B-1 presents range-of-motion norms for the upper extremity.
Appendix B-2 presents range-of-motion norms for the lower extremity.

Keough J, Sain S, Roller C.
Kinesiology for the Occupational Therapy Assistant:
Essential Components of Function and Movement (pp. 335-338).
© 2012 SLACK Incorporated.

Appendix B-1	Range-of-Motion Norms for the Upper Extremity	
Joint	**Joint Motion**	**Range of Motion (degrees)**
Glenohumeral joint	Flexion	0 to 180
	Extension (also referred to as Hyperextension)	0 to 50
	Abduction	0 to 180
	Adduction	180 to 0
	Internal rotation	0 to 90
	External rotation	0 to 90
	Horizontal abduction	0 to 45*
	Horizontal adduction	0 to 135*
Elbow joint	Flexion	0 to 140
	Extension	Extension is the return to 0
Forearm	Supination	0 to 80
	Pronation	0 to 80
Wrist joint	Flexion	0 to 60
	Extension (also referred to as hyperextension)	0 to 60
	Ulnar deviation	0 to 30
	Radial deviation	0 to 20
Finger digits #2 to 5 MCP joint	Flexion	0 to 90
	Extension	Extension is the return to 0
	Hyperextension	0 to 20
	Abduction	0 to 20*
	Adduction	Adduction is the return to 0 with fingers touching each other
PIP joint	Flexion	0 to 100
	Extension	Extension is the return to 0
DIP joint	Flexion	0 to 70
	Extension	Extension is the return to 0
	Hyperextension	0 to 30
Thumb MCP joint	Flexion	0 to 60
	Extension	Extension is the return to 0
IP joint	Flexion	0 to 80
	Extension	Extension is the return to 0
	Hyperextension	0 to 30

Adapted from American Medical Association. (2008). *Guides to the evaluation of permanent impairment* (6th ed.). Chicago, IL: Author.

*Identified from Latella, D., & Meriano, C. (2003). *Occupational therapy manual for the evaluation of range of motion and muscle strength*. Clifton Park, NY: Delmar Carnage Learning.

Appendix B-2	Range-of-Motion Norms for the Lower Extremity	
Joint	**Joint Motion**	**Range of Motion (degrees)**
Hip	Flexion	0 to 100
	Extension (also referred to as hyperextension)	0 to 30*
	Abduction	0 to 25
	Adduction	Adduction is the return to 0
	Internal rotation	0 to 20
	External rotation	0 to 30
Knee	Flexion	0 to 110
	Extension	Extension is the return to 0
Ankle	Plantar flexion	0 to 20
	Dorsiflexion	0 to 10
	Eversion	0 to 10
	Inversion	0 to 20
Lesser toes (#2 to 5) Metatarsophalangeal (MTP) joint	Flexion	0 to 40*
	Extension	Extension is the return to 0*
Lesser toes (#2 to 5) Metatarsophalangeal (MTP) joint	Adduction	Adduction is the return to 0
	Abduction	Compare to opposite side*
Lesser Toes (#2 to 5) PIP joint	Flexion	0 to 35
	Extension	Extension is the return to 0*
Lesser toes (#2 to 5) DIP joint	Flexion	0 to 60*
	Extension	Extension is the return to 0*
Great toe (#1) MTP joint	Flexion	0 to 45
	Extension	Extension is the return to 0*
Great toe (#1) IP joint	Flexion	0 to 20
	Extension	Extension is the return to 0*

Adapted from American Medical Association. (2008). *Guides to the evaluation of permanent impairment* (6th ed.). Chicago, IL: Author.

*Identified from Latella, D., & Meriano, C. (2003). *Occupational therapy manual for the evaluation of range of motion and muscle strength*. Clifton Park, NY: Delmar Carnage Learning.

Epilogue of Occupational Profiles

EPILOGUE CHAPTER 5—TERRENCE

Occupational Therapy Plan of Care

Terrence was seen in outpatient occupational therapy (OT) five times a week for the first 2 weeks and then three times a week for the following 4 weeks. Terrence remained at the assisted-living facility while he was receiving OT. Terrence's discharge from OT was determined by Terrence's input, progress in OT, third-party payer approval of OT services, and report from staff at the assisted-living facility.

Terrence remained at the facility upon discharge with no further OT recommended. OT recommended continued assistance as needed with activities of daily living (ADL) and simple instrumental activities of daily living (IADL) tasks to facilitate safe functional ability. It was recommended that Terrence did not need 24-hour supervision and assistance. A summary of his goals and functional outcome are provided below.

Occupational Therapy Outcomes

Short-Term Goals:

1. Client will demonstrate safe and independent use of power seat functions of tilt, recline, elevator, and leg elevation by 2 weeks. ***Goal met—Terrence demonstrated appropriate use of a powered mobility wheelchair by 2 weeks.***

2. Client will demonstrate safe and proficient use of power mobility device including on/off, steering, navigating doorways, and areas where furniture is in close proximity by 2 weeks. ***Goal met—Terrence demonstrated appropriate use of a powered mobility wheelchair by 2 weeks.***

3. Client will be safe and independent in sit-to-stand transfers using the seat elevator to assist by 2 weeks. ***Goal met—Terrence demonstrated independence with seat elevator in sit-to-stand by 2 weeks.***

4. Client will demonstrate improved endurance with use of power mobility device by 2 weeks. ***Goal met—Terrence reports improved engagement in daily tasks of interest by 2 weeks.***

Keough, J. L., Sain, S. J., Roller, C. L.
Kinesiology for the Occupational Therapy Assistant: Essential Components of Function and Movement (pp. 339-346).
© 2012 SLACK Incorporated.

Long-Term Goals:
1. Client will be independent in pressure relief with power wheelchair features after instruction by 4 weeks. *Goal met—Terrence was able to demonstrate pressure relief techniques with power wheelchair by 4 weeks.*
2. Client will be independent and safe in sit-to-stand transfers using appropriately placed grab bars in the bathroom by discharge. *Goal met—Terrence was independently able to use grab bars in bathroom for upper extremity support during stand, dynamic standing, and stand pivot transfers.*
3. Client will demonstrate improved respiration with appropriate use of tilt and recline position by 4 weeks. *Goal not met—while Terrence was able to demonstrate appropriate use of the tilt and recline position on the wheelchair, he continues to present with impaired respiration upon exertion similar to nonuse of the tilt and recline position.*
4. Client will demonstrate improved social interactions secondary to improved endurance and improved posture by 4 weeks. *Goal met—Terrence was able to resume his prior patterns of activities at the assisted-living facility and was able to return to his prior level of ability in daily tasks.*
5. Client will prevent the development of pressure ulcers and orthopedic deformities by discharge. *Goal met—no pressure ulcer or orthopedic deformity developed.*

Occupational Therapy Services Provided

OT services provided included ADL, simple IADL tasks, therapeutic activities, therapeutic exercise, safety, standing balance, functional transfers, activity tolerance, and graded functional tasks. OT services provided for wheelchair seating and positioning are described below.

The OT practitioner recommended a power mobility device for the client after taking linear and angular measurements, and determining the client's needs, goals, functional skills, and activities. Terrence sits with a flexible posterior pelvic tilt, slight obliquity to the right, and minimal rotation on the right. He exhibits mild thoracic kyphosis and mild cervical hyperextension. Having a flexible posterior pelvic tilt suggests that he is able to be supported into a neutral or anterior pelvic tilt. Once he is supported into a neutral pelvic tilt, the thoracic kyphosis is minimized and consequently realigns the cervical spine. Thus, from an anterior-to-posterior view, his weight can be more evenly distributed across his femurs. Remember, when one is in a posterior pelvic tilt, greater pressure is placed on the ischial tuberosities, thus increasing the risk of pressure ulcer development. Additionally, a posture of posterior pelvic tilt creates an overstretch to the latissimus dorsi, brings the arms into internal rotation, and limits the ability of the arms to reach above shoulder level.

The wheelchair has the following characteristics: mid-wheel drive, power mobility wheelchair with power tilt, recline, and elevating leg rest. It is necessary that his wheelchair and seating system allow him to be repositioned with power seat functions to prevent increased risk of orthopedic deformities and pressure ulcers. Improving his posture would allow greater access to his environment by improving his ability to reach. He will have less difficulty drinking from a glass, combing his hair, and reaching in front of his body to retrieve items.

Also recommended is a swing away joystick mounted on the right. The OT practitioner recommended an air-filled pressure-distributing seat cushion that fits into the seat and a supportive back rest with lateral support built into the back rest. Additionally, a pelvic positioning belt was recommended to maintain his posture in the chair, a lap tray for improved weight bearing for his upper extremities, and a head rest for use while in a tilted or reclined position.

EPILOGUE CHAPTER 6—SARAH

Occupational Therapy Plan of Care

Sarah was seen in OT seven times per week for the first 4 weeks and then five times per week for the following 2 weeks. Sarah returned home after 6 weeks in the long-term care facility. Sarah's discharge home was determined by information provided by the rehabilitation team, Sarah's progress in therapy, her desire to return home, and family support to enable the assistance needed to return home. A summary of her goals and functional outcome are provided below.

Sarah was discharged to home with orders for continued outpatient OT. It was recommended that Sarah not drive until further OT or until cleared from her physician. OT further recommend continued assistance as needed with simple IADL tasks to facilitate return to home. It was recommended that Sarah did not need 24-hour assistance. Sarah's family and friends coordinated assistance for simple IADL tasks and transportation needs. Sarah's family installed grab bars in the bathroom to increase independence and safety with ADL tasks.

Occupational Therapy Outcomes

Short-Term Goals:
1. Client will be educated in and demonstrate independence with a home exercise program for increased left upper extremity functional ability within 1 week. *Goal met—Sarah was trained in daily tasks she could perform to increase the use of her left upper extremity.*
2. Client will demonstrate supervision with stand pivot transfers using adaptive equipment appropriately by 2 weeks. *Goal met—Sarah demonstrated supervision with stand pivot transfers consistently by the end of 2 weeks.*
3. Client will demonstrate supervision with standing balance to sweep floors by 2 weeks. *Goal met—Sarah demonstrated static standing ability by 2 weeks.*
4. Client will demonstrate modified independence to supervision with all ADL tasks by 2 weeks. *Goal met—Sarah demonstrated independence with self-feeding, grooming, upper body dressing, and upper body bathing. Sarah demonstrates supervision with lower body dressing, lower body bathing, and self-toileting due to concern for safety with standing balance.*

Long-Term Goals:
1. Client will demonstrate modified independence with all functional stand pivot transfers by discharge. *Goal met—Sarah demonstrated modified independence with functional transfers due to the use of adaptive equipment (i.e., rolling walker and ankle-foot orthotic [AFO]).*
2. Client will demonstrate modified independence with self-care tasks using bilateral upper extremity by discharge. *Goal met—Sarah demonstrates the ability to complete ADL tasks using her bilateral upper extremity. Sarah independently completes her upper body ADL tasks but requires modified independence with lower body ADL tasks due to adaptive equipment and methods for success. Examples include using grab bars for upper extremity support during self-toileting when standing. She also uses a cane or rolling walker for upper extremity support during standing for lower extremity dressing.*
3. Client will demonstrate manual muscle testing (MMT) and grip pinch strength within functional limits in the left upper extremity by discharge. *Goal not met—Sarah demonstrated significantly improved UE ability; however, she demonstrated and reported continued problems using her left upper extremity as prior to onset. She stated at discharge, "I'm really disappointed that I can't move my left arm like I used to." Sarah was able to demonstrate at discharge left upper extremity active range of motion (AROM) at full available ROM with MMT left shoulder grossly 3+/5. Sarah continues to*

demonstrate left upper extremity impaired sequencing of muscle synergies and delayed initiation of muscle contractions. Sarah displays no continued increased tone in the left upper extremity.

4.   Client will demonstrate modified independence with simple home management tasks by discharge. *Goal met—Sarah demonstrated safety and the ability to make simple meals, wash and fold clothes, and sweep a floor. Sarah reported continued difficulty with vacuuming with supervision needed for dynamic standing balance safety. Sarah did not demonstrate adequate driving ability to return to self-driving.*

Occupational Therapy Services Provided

Sarah's OT included the use of ADL retraining, IADL retraining, therapeutic activities, therapeutic exercise, functional transfers, neuro re-education, caregiver and client education and training, and graded functional tasks. An occupational therapy assistant (OTA) provided treatment for client education on adaptive methods to complete self-care tasks and don and doff her AFO. Education also included a home exercise program to improve left upper extremity functional ability, safety, use of adaptive equipment, and functional transfer ability. Therapeutic exercise and therapeutic activities included AROM and passive ROM, exercises, and physical agent modalities (PAMs) of electrical stimulation to enhance movement, decrease pain, and improve functional use. Neuro re-education in the form of neurodevelopmental treatment was provided to also improve left upper extremity functional ability.

Occupation-based treatment approaches were also used. Sarah completed ADL tasks using her affected left upper extremity. Sarah also completed functional transfers as needed to complete functional tasks, such as transferring into the wheelchair and onto the commode. Sarah also performed simple IADL tasks to ensure ability upon return home. Overall, Sarah demonstrated good progress toward OT goals.

EPILOGUE CHAPTER 7—LINDA

Occupational Therapy Plan of Care

Linda was seen in occupational therapy three times per week the first 3 weeks, two times per week for the following 3 weeks, and then one time per week for an additional 3 weeks. Linda was discharged to a home exercise program after a total of 9 weeks or 18 visits. Her discharge from OT was determined with input from Linda, the doctor, and recommendations from the OT practitioner based on her progress in therapy. The Medicare outpatient cap on OT services also influenced Linda's time in therapy. A summary of her goals and functional outcomes are provided below.

Occupational Therapy Outcomes

Short-Term Goals:
1.   Client will be instructed in and comply with a home exercise program. *Goal met—Linda was instructed in a home exercise program within the first week of therapy consisting of daily tasks she could perform to increase use of her right upper extremity. She demonstrated compliance by performing her home exercise program during the therapy session.*

2.   Client will decrease pain from 3/10 to 0/10 at rest and will be able to sleep all night within 4 weeks by following ergonomic postural changes. *Goal met—Linda reported she had no pain in her right shoulder at rest after 4 weeks of therapy. Linda demonstrated the use of postural changes at night and reported improved sleeping habits within 4 weeks.*

3.   Client will decrease pain from 8/10 to 4/10 at worst during resistive functional activities within 4 weeks by using modified lifting techniques and adaptive equipment. *Goal*

met—Linda reported her pain had decreased with doffing her bra and changing her granddaughter's diapers to a 3/10 at worst after 4 weeks.

4. Client will increase AROM in all limited planes of right shoulder ROM by 10 degrees within 3 weeks. *Goal met—Linda presented with increased right upper extremity AROM within 3 weeks. Glenohumeral joint flexion was 100 degrees (an increase of 25 degrees); glenohumeral joint abduction was 75 degrees (an increase of 15 degrees); glenohumeral joint external rotation was 35 degrees (an increase of 10 degrees); and glenohumeral joint internal rotation was 45 degrees (an increase of 10 degrees).*

5. Client will increase right grip strength by 5 lbs within 4 weeks. *Goal met—Linda presented with an increase in her right grip to 50 lbs (an increase of 5 lbs) within 4 weeks.*

6. Client will be able to perform toileting tasks using right hand independently and with fewer complaints of pain within 4 weeks. *Goal met—Linda demonstrated the ability to perform toileting tasks using her right dominant upper extremity independently with only minimal reports of discomfort within 4 weeks.*

Long-Term Goals:

1. Client will demonstrate compliance and independence in home exercise program at discharge. *Goal met—Linda demonstrated independence and compliance in a home exercise program that was modified to accommodate her progress. She was discharged with a structured, progressive home exercise program.*

2. Client will be independent with use of right upper extremity in self-care and occupational roles with only minimal complaints of discomfort within 3 months. *Goal met—Linda demonstrated independent use of the right upper extremity in domains of occupation at discharge. She reported only minimal discomfort when reaching overhead or placing her granddaughter in the car seat.*

3. Client will demonstrate AROM and grip strength to within functional limits within 3 months. *Goal met—Linda demonstrated grip and AROM to within functional limits, even though she was slightly limited in all planes of right glenohumeral joint motion compared to her left shoulder.*

Occupational Therapy Services Provided

Linda's occupational therapy included the use of ADL and IADL retraining, client education and training, therapeutic activities, therapeutic exercises, and graded functional tasks. An OTA with training and experience in the upper extremity provided treatment for client education on adaptive methods to complete grooming, toileting, and donning/doffing her bra. Education consisted of a home exercise program and protection principles, which included sleeping postures and proper lifting and reaching techniques. The OTA also provided therapeutic exercise and therapeutic activities including AROM, active assist ROM, and PROM exercises. PAMs of electrical stimulation and ultrasound were implemented to decrease pain, stimulate tissue healing, and enhance movement for improved functional use. Graded functional tasks included upper body dressing, folding clothes, and reaching in a cabinet for example.

Linda demonstrated the use of occupation-based treatment approaches in therapy to ensure independent use of her right dominant upper extremity upon discharge. Linda was able to perform all domains of occupation independently, including caring for her grandchildren after occupational therapy discharge. Overall, Linda demonstrated excellent progress toward her OT goals.

EPILOGUE CHAPTER 8—DAVID

Occupational Therapy Plan of Care

David was seen in occupational therapy three times per week for the first 3 weeks and then two times per week for the following 3 weeks for a total of 15 treatment sessions over 6 weeks. The number of visits and date of discharge were determined by several factors, including the doctor's orders, therapist's recommendations, and David's progress in therapy. His work schedule and insurance coverage also influenced his number of therapy visits. A summary of David's goals and functional outcomes are provided below.

Occupational Therapy Outcomes

Short-Term Goals:
1. Client will be instructed in and comply with a home exercise program within 1 week. ***Goal met—David demonstrated compliance and independence in a home exercise program within 1 week.***
2. Client will present with decreased pain from 7/10 to 3/10 at worst during resistive functional tasks within 4 weeks by using modified lifting techniques, adapting tool handles, cold modalities, and performing stretches. ***Goal met—David demonstrated less pain in the right elbow during resistive functional tasks using adaptive tools, protection principles, modalities, and stretches within 4 weeks. Pain during resistive functional tasks was rated at a 3/10 at worst.***
3. Client will increase right grip strength by 5 lbs with less pain within 4 weeks. ***Goal met—David demonstrated an increase in right grip strength to 100 lbs in the standard position and 85 lbs in the stressed position within 4 weeks.***
4. Client will be able to drive his truck and brush his teeth with no complaints of pain in the right elbow within 3 weeks. ***Goal not met—David demonstrated the ability to brush his teeth without elbow pain but continued to report pain with driving tasks after 3 weeks.***

Long-Term Goals:
1. Client will demonstrate compliance and independence in a home exercise program at discharge. ***Goal met—David demonstrated compliance and independence in a structured and progressive home exercise program at discharge.***
2. Client will be independent in self-care and occupational roles using the right upper extremity with no complaints of pain and the use of ergonomic considerations within 12 weeks. ***Goal met—David was able to perform ADL and IADL tasks independently and with no reports of pain in his right elbow. David was able to drive, work with no restrictions, and practice baseball with his son using protection principles at discharge. He did choose to delay the remodeling project at home for 3 months to rest his injured right arm.***
3. Client will demonstrate MMT and grip pinch strength within functional limits in the right upper extremity within 12 weeks. ***Goal met—David presented with right wrist extensor strength grossly 5/5 with MMT. His right grip improved to 110 lbs in the standard position and 115 lbs in the stressed position. His right palmar pinch improved to 25 lbs.***
4. Client will demonstrate independence and pain-free use of his right upper extremity during the leisure activity of fishing at discharge. ***Goal met—David demonstrated the ability to participate in the leisure occupation of fishing independently with no pain at discharge.***
5. Client will be able to work with a 20-lb lifting restriction and fewer complaints of pain in the right elbow within 6 weeks. ***Goal met—David demonstrated the ability to perform carpenter duties at work requiring up to 20 lbs within 6 weeks.***

Occupational Therapy Services Provided

David's occupational therapy included client education and instruction in adaptive equipment, protection principles, and ergonomic considerations. His OT treatment included therapeutic activities, therapeutic exercises, and graded functional tasks including work conditioning. An OTA experienced and trained in upper extremity injuries provided treatment including tool adaption and proper body mechanics during lifting and tool use. The OTA educated David in a structured home exercise program including friction massage, tennis elbow stretching, the use of cold, and bracing to decrease pain and inflammation and to increase healing. Therapeutic exercises and activities included ROM, strengthening, and physical agent modalities of ultrasound and cold to decrease pain for improved functional use.

Occupation-based treatment included graded functional tasks during work conditioning of casting a fishing rod and using a hammer and power screwdriver, for example.

At the time of discharge, David was able to participate in his occupational roles of father, carpenter, and fisherman independently and without pain. Overall, David demonstrated excellent progress, meeting all of his OT goals at discharge.

EPILOGUE CHAPTER 9—LAURA

Occupational Therapy Plan of Care

Laura was seen in occupational therapy three times per week for the first 4 weeks. Due to complications from her injury, there was an interruption in Laura's therapy for 3 weeks. After 4 weeks in occupational therapy and continued complaints of weakness, stiffness, and numbness in the median nerve distribution of her left hand, she received a nerve conduction study, which revealed moderate carpal tunnel syndrome. Laura received surgical release of the carpal tunnel and resumed OT at 2 weeks after her surgery. She continued therapy three times per week for 3 weeks and then two times per week for the following 2 weeks. Laura completed a total of 25 therapy sessions, 12 before her carpal tunnel release and 13 after surgery. She was discharged at the 3-month mark from beginning occupational therapy or 5.5 months after her fall resulting in the left wrist Colles' fracture. Discharge was based on a team decision involving Laura, her doctor, and the OT practitioner. It was difficult for Laura to attend therapy the first 2 weeks because she was unable to drive and had to rely on family and friends for her transportation. A summary of Laura's goals and her functional outcomes are provided below.

Occupational Therapy Outcomes

Short-Term Goals:
1. Client will be instructed in and comply with a home exercise program within 1 week. *Goal met—Laura demonstrated compliance and independence in a home exercise program given to her by the OT within 1 week by performing in-home therapy sessions.*
2. Client will tolerate a formal evaluation of left grip and pinch strength when able and appropriate or within 4 weeks. *Goal met—Laura demonstrated the ability to tolerate an assessment of her left grip and pinch strength within 4 weeks.*
3. Client will demonstrate the ability to grade students' papers using the left, dominant hand and adaptive writing implements within 3 weeks. *Goal met—Laura demonstrated the ability to return to her occupational role of teacher after 3 weeks. She was able to drive to work with a left wrist brace in place, and she was able to grade papers using a gel pen with an enlarged rubber grip.*
4. Client will demonstrate self-feeding with the left hand and adaptive utensils within 2 weeks. *Goal met—Laura demonstrated the ability to feed herself using her left*

dominant hand after using adaptive foam or pipe insulation to enlarge the handles of her fork and spoon.

5. Client will demonstrate decreased edema by 30 mL using edema-control techniques of elevation, AROM, and wearing of an Isotoner glove within 3 weeks. *Goal met—Laura demonstrated a 50-mL reduction in edema in the left hand and wrist within 3 weeks, which allowed her to make a straight fist, experience less pain, and drive to her teaching position.*

6. Client will demonstrate an increase in AROM in all limited joints by 5 degrees each in 4 weeks. *Goal met—Laura demonstrated an increase of more than 5 degrees in all limited joints of her forearm, wrist, thumb, and fingers by the end of 4 weeks.*

Long-Term Goals:

1. Client will demonstrate compliance and independence in a home exercise program at discharge. *Goal met—Laura demonstrated compliance and independence in a modified and progressive home exercise program by discharge.*

2. Client will be independent in self-care and occupational roles using the left, dominant hand and adaptive equipment within 3 months. *Goal met—Laura demonstrated the ability to perform all occupational roles independently using her left dominant upper extremity and adaptive equipment at discharge. She was able to perform grooming and household activities as well as drive to work and perform the duties of a teacher including computer use and writing tasks at discharge.*

3. Client will demonstrate AROM to within functional limits in left forearm, wrist, and thumb and demonstrate a straight fist in left hand within 3 months. *Goal met—Laura was able to perform all functional roles independently, showing gains in AROM to within functional limits in the left upper extremity. However, she continued to show a limitation in AROM compared to her right upper extremity, especially in forearm supination, wrist extension, ulnar deviation, and thumb flexion at discharge.*

4. Client will demonstrate a decrease in edema by 50 mL in the left hand volumetrically in 3 months. *Goal met—Laura's whole-hand edema had decreased by 75 mL when measured volumetrically at discharge.*

5. Client will demonstrate functional ROM in left, dominant hand by knitting a scarf in 3 months. *Goal not met—Laura did demonstrate functional AROM in her left hand and wrist by discharge. She was enjoying knitting again but was unable to complete a scarf project within 3 months.*

Occupational Therapy Services Provided

Laura's occupational therapy included client education and instruction in adaptive equipment, therapeutic activities, therapeutic exercises, and graded functional tasks. An OTA trained and experienced in hand and wrist injuries provided treatment including instruction in edema control techniques, compensatory techniques, and a home exercise program. Treatment in OT also included the use of adaptive equipment, therapeutic exercises and activities, AROM and PROM, and PAMs of electrical stimulation to decrease edema, enhance movement, and decrease pain for improved functional use.

Occupation-based treatment approaches were used. Laura completed tasks in therapy such as feeding, writing, and peeling vegetables to prepare for independent participation with occupational roles at home and at work. Overall, Laura demonstrated excellent progress toward her OT goals.

Muscle Testing and Grip/Pinch Norms

NINE-HOLE PEG TEST NORM SCORES

Appendix D-1 presents Nine-Hole Peg Test Average Male Participant Scores.
Appendix D-2 presents Nine-Hole Peg Test Average Female Participant Scores.

BOX AND BLOCK TEST NORM SCORES

Appendix D-3 presents Box and Block Test Average Male Participant Scores.
Appendix D-4 presents Box and Block Test Average Female Participant Scores.

GRIP AND PINCH NORM SCORES

Appendix D-5 presents Grip Strength Average Performance of Normal Subjects (ages 6-19).
Appendix D-6 presents Average Grip Strength Performance.
Appendix D-7 presents Average Tip Pinch Strength Performance.
Appendix D-8 presents Average Key Pinch Strength Performance.
Appendix D-9 presents Average Palmar Pinch Strength Performance.

Keough J, Sain S, Roller C.
Kinesiology for the Occupational Therapy Assistant:
Essential Components of Function and Movement (pp. 347-356).
© 2012 SLACK Incorporated.

Appendix D-1	Nine-Hole Peg Test Average and Standard Deviation of Male Participants' Scores (N=314)			
Age	N	AVG-right (seconds)	AVG-left (seconds)	SD-right (seconds)	SD-left (seconds)
21 to 25	41	16.41	17.53	1.65	1.73
26 to 30	32	16.88	17.84	1.89	2.22
31 to 35	31	17.54	18.47	2.70	2.94
36 to 40	32	17.71	18.62	2.12	2.30
41 to 45	30	18.54	18.49	2.88	2.42
46 to 50	30	18.35	19.57	2.47	2.69
51 to 55	25	18.93	19.84	2.37	3.10
56 to 60	25	20.90	21.64	4.55	3.39
61 to 65	24	20.87	21.60	3.50	2.98
66 to 70	14	21.23	22.29	3.29	3.71
71+	25	25.79	25.95	5.60	4.54
All Male					
Subjects	314	18.99	19.79	3.91	3.66

Oxford, G. K., Vogel, K. A., Le, F., Mitchell, A., Muniz, S., & Vollmer, M. A. (2003) Brief report—Adult norms for a commercially available nine hole peg test for finger dexterity. *American Journal of Occupational Therapy, 57,* 570-573. Reproduced with permission of American Occupational Therapy Association in the format Textbook via Copyright Clearance Center.

Appendix D-2	Nine-Hole Peg Test Average and Standard Deviation of Female Participants' Scores (N=389)			
Age	N	AVG-right (seconds)	AVG-left (seconds)	SD right (seconds)	SD left (seconds)
21 to 25	43	16.04	17.21	1.82	1.55
26 to 30	33	15.90	16.97	1.91	1.77
31 to 35	32	16.69	17.47	1.70	2.13
36 to 40	35	16.74	18.16	1.95	2.08
41 to 45	37	16.54	17.64	2.14	2.06
46 to 50	45	17.36	17.96	2.01	2.30
51 to 55	42	17.38	18.92	1.88	2.29
56 to 60	31	17.86	19.48	2.39	3.26
61 to 65	29	18.99	20.33	2.18	2.76
66 to 70	31	19.90	21.44	3.15	3.97
71+	31	22.49	24.11	6.02	5.66
All Female					
Subjects	389	17.67	18.91	3.17	3.44

Oxford, G. K., Vogel, K. A., Le, F., Mitchell, A., Muniz, S., & Vollmer, M. A. (2003) Brief report—Adult norms for a commercially available nine hole peg test for finger dexterity. *American Journal of Occupational Therapy, 57,* 570-573. Reproduced with permission of American Occupational Therapy Association in the format Textbook via Copyright Clearance Center.

Appendix D-3		Average Performance of Normal Males on the Box and Block Test (Number of Cubes Transferred in 1 Minute)				
Age	Hand	Mean	SD	SE	Low	High
20 to 24	R	88.2	8.8	1.6	70	105
	L	86.4	8.5	1.6	70	102
25 to 29	R	85.0	7.5	1.4	71	95
	L	84.1	7.1	1.4	69	100
30 to 34	R	81.9	9.0	1.7	68	96
	L	81.3	8.1	1.6	69	99
35 to 39	R	81.9	9.5	1.9	64	104
	L	79.8	9.7	1.9	56	97
40 to 44	R	83.0	8.1	1.6	69	101
	L	80.0	8.8	1.7	59	93
45 to 49	R	76.9	9.2	1.7	61	93
	L	75.8	7.8	1.5	60	88
50 to 54	R	79.0	9.7	1.9	62	106
	L	77.0	9.2	1.8	60	97
55 to 59	R	75.2	11.9	2.6	45	97
	L	73.8	10.5	2.3	43	94
60 to 64	R	71.3	8.8	1.8	52	84
	L	70.5	8.1	1.6	47	82
65 to 69	R	68.4	7.1	1.4	55	80
	L	67.4	7.8	1.5	48	86
70 to 74	R	66.3	9.2	1.8	50	86
	L	64.3	9.8	1.9	45	84
75+	R	63.0	7.1	1.4	47	75
	L	61.3	8.4	1.7	46	74
All male subjects	R	76.9	11.6	0.66	45	106
	L	75.4	11.4	0.65	43	102

SD = Standard Deviation; SE = Standard Error

Mathiowetz, V., Volland, G., Kashman, N., & Weber, K. (1985). Adult norms for the box and block test of manual dexterity. *American Journal of Occupational Therapy, 39* (6), 386-391. Reproduced with permission of American Occupational Therapy Association in the format Textbook via Copyright Clearance Center.

Appendix D-4		Average Performance of Normal Females on the Box and Block Test (Number of Cubes Transferred in 1 Minute)				
Age	Hand	Mean	SD	SE	Low	High
20 to 24	R	88.0	8.3	1.6	67	103
	L	83.4	7.9	1.6	66	99
25 to 29	R	86.0	7.4	1.4	63	96
	L	80.9	6.4	1.2	63	93
30 to 34	R	85.2	7.4	1.5	75	101
	L	80.2	5.6	1.1	66	92
35 to 39	R	84.8	6.1	1.2	71	95
	L	83.5	6.1	1.2	72	97
40 to 44	R	81.1	8.2	1.5	60	97
	L	79.7	8.8	1.6	57	97
45 to 49	R	82.1	7.5	1.5	68	99
	L	78.3	7.6	1.5	59	91
50 to 54	R	77.7	10.7	2.1	57	98
	L	74.3	9.9	2.0	53	93
55 to 59	R	74.7	8.9	1.8	56	94
	L	73.6	7.8	1.6	54	85
60 to 64	R	76.1	6.9	1.4	63	95
	L	73.6	6.4	1.4	62	86
65 to 69	R	72.0	6.2	1.2	60	82
	L	71.3	7.7	1.4	61	89
70 to 74	R	68.6	7.0	1.3	53	80
	L	68.3	7.0	1.3	51	81
75+	R	65.0	7.1	1.4	52	79
	L	63.6	7.4	1.5	51	81
All female subjects	R	78.4	10.4	0.58	52	103
	L	75.8	9.5	0.53	51	99

SD = Standard Deviation; SE = Standard Error

Mathiowetz, V., Volland, G., Kashman, N., & Weber, K. (1985). Adult norms for the box and block test of manual dexterity. *American Journal of Occupational Therapy, 39* (6), 386-391. Reproduced with permission of American Occupational Therapy Association in the format Textbook via Copyright Clearance Center.

Appendix D-5	**Average Performance of Normal Subjects (Age 6-19) on Grip Strength (lb)**						
		Males			Females		
Age	Hand	Mean	SD	Range	Mean	SD	Range
6 to 7	R	32.5	4.8	21 to 42	28.6	4.4	20 to 39
	L	30.7	5.4	18 to 38	27.1	4.4	16 to 36
8 to 9	R	41.9	7.4	27 to 61	35.3	8.3	18 to 55
	L	39.0	9.3	19 to 63	33.0	6.9	16 to 49
10 to 11	R	53.9	9.7	35 to 79	49.7	8.1	37 to 82
	L	48.4	10.8	26 to 73	45.2	6.8	32 to 59
12 to 13	R	58.7	15.5	33 to 98	56.8	10.6	39 to 79
	L	55.4	16.9	22 to 107	50.9	11.9	25 to 76
14 to 15	R	77.3	15.4	49 to 108	58.1	12.3	30 to 93
	L	64.4	14.9	41 to 94	49.3	11.9	26 to 73
16 to 17	R	94-0	19.4	64 to 149	67.3	16.5	23 to 126
	L	78.5	19.1	41 to 123	56.9	14.0	23 to 87
18 to 19	R	108.0	24.6	64 to 172	71.6	12.3	46 to 90
	L	93.0	27.8	53 to 149	61.7	12.5	41 to 86

SD = Standard Deviation
Mathiowetz, V., Wiemer, D., & Federman, S. (1986). Grip and pinch strength: Norms for 6- to 19- year- olds. *American Journal of Occupational Therapy, 40*(10), 705-711. Reproduced with permission of American Occupational Therapy Association in the format Textbook via Copyright Clearance Center.

Appendix D-6	**Performance of All Subjects on Grip Strength (lbs)**									
		Men					Women			
Age	Hand	Mean	SD	SE	Low	mm	Mean	SD	SE	Low	High
20 to 24	R	121.0	20.6	3.8	91	167	70.4	14.5	2.8	46	95
	L	104.5	21.8	4.0	71	150	61.0	13.1	2.6	33	88
25 to 29	R	120.8	23.0	4.4	78	158	74.5	13.9	2.7	48	97
	L	110.5	16.2	3.1	77	139	63.5	12.2	2.4	48	97
30 to 34	R	121.8	22.4	4.3	70	170	78.7	19.2	3.8	46	137
	L	110.4	21.7	4.2	64	145	68.0	17.7	3.5	36	115
35 to 39	R	119.7	24.0	4.8	76	176	74.1	10.8	2.2	50	99
	L	112.9	21.7	4.4	73	157	66.3	11.7	2.3	49	91
40 to 44	R	116.8	20.7	4.1	84	165	70.4	13.5	2.4	38	103
	L	112.8	18.7	3.7	73	157	62.3	13.8	2.5	35	94
45 to 49	R	109.9	23.0	4.3	65	155	62.2	15.1	3.0	39	100
	L	100.8	22.8	4.3	58	160	56.0	12.7	2.5	37	83

(continued)

Appendix D-6		**Performance of All Subjects on Grip Strength (lbs) (continued)**									
		Men					Women				
Age	Hand	Mean	SD	SE	Low	mm	Mean	SD	SE	Low	High
50 to 54	R	121.0	20.6	3.8	91	167	70.4	14.5	2.8	46	95
	L	101.9	17.0	3.4	70	143	57.3	10.7	2.1	35	76
55 to 59	R	101.1	26.7	5.8	59	154	57.3	12.5	2.5	33	86
	L	83.2	23.4	5.1	43	128	47.3	11.9	2.4	31	76
60 to 64	R	89.7	20.4	4.2	51	137	55.1	10.1	2.0	37	77
	L	76.8	20.3	4.1	27	116	45.7	10.1	2.0	29	66
65 to 69	R	91.1	20.6	4.0	56	131	49.6	9.7	1.8	35	74
	L	76.8	19.8	3.8	43	117	41.0	8.2	1.5	29	63
70 to 74	R	75.3	21.5	4.2	32	108	49.6	11.7	2.2	33	78
	L	64.8	18.1	3.7	32	93	41.5	10.2	1.9	23	67
75+	R	65.7	21.0	4.2	40	135	42.6	11.0	2.2	25	65
	L	55.0	17.0	3.4	31	119	37.6	8.9	1.7	24	61
All Subjects	R	104.3	28.3	1.6	32	176	62.8	17.0	0.96	25	137
	L	93.1	27.6	1.6	27	160	53.9	15.7	.88	23	115

SD = Standard Deviation; SE = Standard Error

This table was published in *Archives of Physical Medicine & Rehabilitation*, *66*, Mathiowetz, V., Kashman, N., Volland, G., Weber, K., Dowe, M., & Rogers, S., "Grip and pinch strength: Normative data for adults." pp. 69-72, Copyright Elsevier (1985).

Appendix D-7		**Average Performance of All Subjects on Tip Pinch (lbs)**									
		Men					Women				
Age	Hand	Mean	SD	SE	Low	High	Mean	SD	SE	Low	High
20 to 24	R	18.0	3.0	0.57	11	23	11.1	2.1	0.42	8	16
	L	17.0	2.3	0.43	12	33	10.5	1.7	0.34	8	14
25 to 29	R	18.3	4.4	0.84	10	34	11.9	1.8	0.35	8	16
	L	17.5	5.2	0.99	12	36	11.3	1.8	0.35	9	18
30 to 34	R	17.6	6.7	0.71	12	25	12.6	3.0	0.58	8	20
	L	17.6	4.8	0.93	10	27	11.7	2.8	0.54	7	17
35 to 39	R	18.0	3.6	0.73	12	27	11.6	2.5	0.50	8	19
	L	17.7	3.8	0.76	10	24	11.9	2.4	0.47	8	16
40 to 44	R	17.8	4.0	0.78	11	25	11.5	2.7	0.49	5	15
	L	17.7	3.5	0.68	12	25	11.1	3.0	0.54	6	17
45 to 49	R	18.7	4.9	0.92	12	30	13.2	3.0	0.60	9	19
	L	17.6	4.1	0.77	12	28	12.1	2.7	0.55	7	18
50 to 54	R	18.3	4.0	0.80	11	24	12.5	2.2	0.44	9	18
	L	17.8	3.9	0.77	12	26	11.4	2.4	0.49	7	16

(continued)

Appendix D-7		Average Performance of All Subjects on Tip Pinch (lbs) (continued)									
		Men					Women				
Age	Hand	Mean	SD	SE	Low	High	Mean	SD	SE	Low	High
55 to 59	R	15.0	3.7	0.81	10	26	10.4	1.4	0.29	8	13
	L	16.6	3.3	0.73	11	24	11.7	1.7	0.34	9	16
60 to 64	R	15.8	3.9	0.80	9	22	10.1	2.1	0.43	7	17
	L	15.3	3.7	0.76	9	23	9.9	2.0	0.39	6	15
65 to 69	R	17.0	4.2	0.81	11	27	10.6	2.0	0.39	7	15
	L	15.4	2.9	0.55	10	21	10.5	2.4	0.45	7	17
70 to 74	R	13.8	2.6	0.52	11	21	10.1	2.6	0.48	7	15
	L	13.3	2.6	0.51	10	21	9.8	2.3	0.43	6	17
75+	R	14.0	3.4	0.68	7	21	9.6	2.8	0.54	4	16
	L	13.9	3.7	0.75	8	25	9.3	2.4	0.47	4	13
All Subjects	R	17.0	4.1	0.23	7	34	11.3	2.6	0.15	4	20
	L	16.4	4.0	.023	8	36	10.8	2.4	0.14	4	18

SD = Standard Deviation; SE = Standard Error

This table was published in *Archives of Physical Medicine & Rehabilitation*, 66, Mathiowetz, V., Kashman, N., Volland, G., Weber, K., Dowe, M., & Rogers, S., "Grip and pinch strength: Normative data for adults." pp. 69-72, Copyright Elsevier (1985).

Appendix D-8		Average Performance of All Subjects on Key Pinch (lbs)									
		Men					Women				
Age	Hand	Mean	SD	SE	Low	High	Mean	SD	SE	Low	High
20 to 24	R	26.0	3.5	0.65	21	34	17.6	2.0	0.39	14	23
	L	24.8	3.4	0.64	19	31	16.2	2.1	0.41	13	23
25 to 29	R	26.7	4.9	0.94	19	41	17.7	2.1	0.41	14	22
	L	25.0	4.4	0.85	19	39	16.6	2.1	0.41	13	22
30 to 34	R	26.4	4.8	0.93	20	36	18.7	3.0	0.60	13	25
	L	26.2	5.1	0.98	17	36	17.8	3.6	0.70	12	26
35 to 39	R	26.1	3.2	0.65	21	32	16.6	2.0	0.40	12	21
	L	25.6	3.9	0.77	18	32	16.0	2.7	0.53	12	22
40 to 44	R	25.6	2.6	0.50	21	31	16.7	3.1	0.56	10	24
	L	25.1	4.0	0.79	19	31	15.8	3.1	0.55	8	22
45 to 49	R	25.8	3.9	0.73	19	35	17.6	3.2	0.65	13	24
	L	24.8	4.4	0.84	18	42	16.6	2.9	0.58	12	24
50 to 54	R	26.7	4.4	0.88	20	34	16.7	2.5	0.50	12	22
	L	26.1	4.2	0.84	20	37	16.1	2.7	0.53	12	22
55 to 59	R	24.2	4.2	0.92	18	34	15.7	2.5	0.50	11	21
	L	23.0	4.7	1.02	13	31	14.7	2.2	0.44	12	19

(continued)

| Appendix D-8 | **Average Performance of All Subjects on Key Pinch (lbs) (continued)** | | | | | | | | | |

		Men					Women				
Age	Hand	Mean	SD	SE	Low	High	Mean	SD	SE	Low	High
60 to 64	R	23.2	5.4	1.13	14	37	15.5	2.7	0.55	10	20
	L	22.2	4.1	0.84	16	33	14.1	2.5	0.50	10	19
65 to 69	R	23.4	3.9	0.75	17	32	15.0	2.6	0.49	10	21
	L	22.0	3.6	0.70	17	28	14.3	2.8	0.53	10	20
70 to 74	R	19.3	2.4	0.47	16	25	14.5	2.9	0.54	8	22
	L	19.2	3.0	0.59	13	28	13.8	3.0	0.56	9	22
75+	R	20.5	4.6	0.91	9	31	12.6	2.3	0.45	8	17
	L	19.1	3.0	0.59	13	24	11.4	2.6	0.50	7	16
All Subjects	R	24.5	4.6	0.26	9	41	16.2	3.0	0.17	8	25
	L	23.6	4.6	.026	11	42	15.3	3.1	0.18	7	26

SD = Standard Deviation; SE = Standard Error

This table was published in *Archives of Physical Medicine & Rehabilitation, 66*, Mathiowetz, V., Kashman, N., Volland, G., Weber, K., Dowe, M., & Rogers, S., "Grip and pinch strength: Normative data for adults." pp. 69-72, Copyright Elsevier (1985).

| Appendix D-9 | **Average Performance of All Subjects on Palmar Pinch (lbs)** | | | | | | | | | |

		Men					Women				
Age	Hand	Mean	SD	SE	Low	High	Mean	SD	SE	Low	High
20 to 24	R	26.6	5.3	1.03	18	45	17.2	2.3	0.45	14	23
	L	25.7	5.8	1.08	15	42	16.3	2.8	0.56	11	24
25 to 29	R	26.0	4.3	0.84	19	35	17.7	3.2	0.62	13	29
	L	25.1	4.2	0.82	19	36	17.0	3.0	0.58	13	26
30 to 34	R	24.7	4.7	0.91	16	34	19.3	5.0	0.99	12	34
	L	25.4	5.7	1.10	15	37	18.1	4.8	0.94	12	32
35 to 39	R	26.2	4.1	0.83	19	36	17.5	4.2	0.85	13	29
	L	25.9	5.4	1.17	14	40	17.1	3.4	0.69	12	24
40 to 44	R	24.5	4.3	0.85	17	37	17.0	3.1	0.56	10	23
	L	24.8	4.9	0.96	15	37	16.6	3.5	0.63	10	25
45 to 49	R	24.0	3.3	0.63	19	33	17.9	3.0	0.60	12	27
	L	23.7	3.8	0.71	18	33	17.5	2.8	0.57	12	24
50 to 54	R	23.8	5.4	1.08	15	36	17.3	3.1	0.63	12	23
	L	24.0	5.8	1.16	16	36	16.4	2.9	0.59	12	22
55 to 59	R	23.7	4.8	1.06	16	34	16.0	3.1	0.63	11	26
	L	21.3	4.5	0.99	12	8	15.4	3.0	0.61	11	21

(continued)

Appendix D-9		Average Performance of All Subjects on Palmar Pinch (lbs) (continued)									
		Men					Women				
Age	Hand	Mean	SD	SE	Low	High	Mean	SD	SE	Low	High
60 to 64	R	21.8	3.3	0.67	16	28	14.8	3.1	0.61	10	20
	L	21.2	3.2	0.65	15	27	14.3	2.7	0.54	10	20
65 to 69	R	21.4	3.0	0.58	15	25	14.2	3.1	0.59	8	20
	L	21.2	4.1	0.80	14	30	13.7	3.4	0.64	8	22
70 to 74	R	18.1	3.4	0.67	14	27	14.4	2.6	0.48	9	19
	L	18.8	3.3	0.65	13	27	14.0	1.9	0.35	10	17
75+	R	18.7	4.2	0.84	9	26	12.0	2.6	0.51	8	17
	L	18.3	3.8	0.77	10	26	11.5	2.6	0.52	6	16
All Subjects	R	23.4	5.0	0.28	9	45	16.3	3.8	0.21	8	34
	L	23.0	5.3	0.30	10	42	15.7	3.6	0.20	6	32

SD = Standard Deviation; SE = Standard Error

This table was published in *Archives of Physical Medicine & Rehabilitation, 66*, Mathiowetz, V., Kashman, N., Volland, G., Weber, K., Dowe, M., & Rogers, S., "Grip and pinch strength: Normative data for adults." pp. 69-72, Copyright Elsevier (1985).

Financial Disclosures

Jeremy L. Keough, MSOT, OTR/L has no financial or proprietary interest in the materials presented herein.

Teresa Plummer, PhD, MSOT, OTR/L, ATP has no financial or proprietary interest in the materials presented herein.

Carolyn L. Roller, OTR/L has no financial or proprietary interest in the materials presented herein.

Susan J. Sain, MS, OTR/L, FAOTA has no financial or proprietary interest in the materials presented herein.

Index

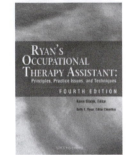
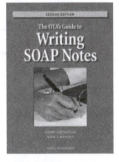
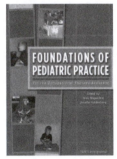
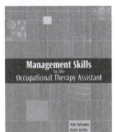
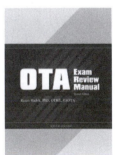

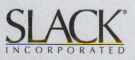